ADHD IN THE SCHOOLS

The Guilford School Practitioner Series

EDITORS

STEPHEN N. ELLIOTT, PhD
University of Wisconsin–Madison

JOSEPH C. WITT, PhD
Louisiana State University, Baton Rouge

Recent Volumes

ADHD in the Schools, Second Edition: Assessment and Intervention Strategies
George J. DuPaul and Gary Stoner

Helping Schoolchildren Cope with Anger: A Cognitive-Behavioral Intervention
Jim Larson and John E. Lochman

Child Abuse and Neglect: The School's Response
Connie Burrows Horton and Tracy K. Cruise

Traumatic Brain Injury in Children and Adolescents:
Assessment and Intervention
Margaret Semrud-Clikeman

Schools and Families: Creating Essential Connections for Learning
Sandra L. Christenson and Susan M. Sheridan

Homework Success for Children with ADHD:
A Family–School Intervention Program
Thomas J. Power, James L. Karustis, and Dina F. Habboushe

Conducting School-Based Assessments of Child and Adolescent Behavior
Edward S. Shapiro and Thomas R. Kratochwill, *Editors*

Designing Preschool Interventions: A Practitioner's Guide
David W. Barnett, Susan H. Bell, and Karen T. Carey

Effective School Interventions
Natalie Rathvon

DSM-IV Diagnosis in the Schools
Alvin E. House

Medications for School-Age Children: Effects on Learning and Behavior
Ronald T. Brown and Michael G. Sawyer

Advanced Applications of Curriculum-Based Measurement
Mark R. Shinn, *Editor*

Brief Intervention for School Problems: Collaborating for Practical Solutions
John J. Murphy and Barry L. Duncan

Academic Skills Problems: Direct Assessment and Intervention, Second Edition
Edward S. Shapiro

ADHD in the Schools

ASSESSMENT AND INTERVENTION STRATEGIES

Second Edition

♦ ♦ ♦

George J. DuPaul
Gary Stoner

♦

Foreword by Russell A. Barkley

THE GUILFORD PRESS
New York   London

Library of Congress Cataloging-in-Publication Data

DuPaul, George J.
  ADHD in the schools : assessment and intervention strategies / by George J. DuPaul, Gary Stoner.— 2nd ed.
      p. cm. — (The Guilford school practitioner series)
  Includes bibliographical references and index.
  ISBN 1-57230-862-1 (hardcover)
    1. Attention-deficit-disordered children—Education—United States.
  2. Attention-deficit hyperactivity disorder—Diagnosis. I. Title:
  Attention deficit hyperactivity disorder in the schools. II. Stoner,
  Gary D. III. Title. IV. Series.
  LC4713.4.D87 2003
  371.93—dc21   2002151253

About the Authors

◆

George J. DuPaul, PhD, is Professor and Coordinator of School Psychology at Lehigh University. His primary research interests are school-based treatment of disruptive behavior disorders as well as school-based interventions for children with chronic health conditions. He is the author of over 100 journal articles and book chapters regarding the assessment and treatment of attention-deficit/hyperactivity disorder. Dr. DuPaul's other books include *Promoting Children's Health: Integrating School, Family, and Community* (with Thomas J. Power, Edward S. Shapiro, and Anne E. Kazak) and *ADHD Rating Scale–IV: Checklists, Norms, and Clinical Interpretation* (with Thomas J. Power, Arthur D. Anastopoulos, and Robert Reid), both published by The Guilford Press. He also has served as Associate Editor for *School Psychology Review* and *School Psychology Quarterly*. He is a Fellow of Division 16 (School Psychology) and Division 53 (Clinical Child Psychology) of the American Psychological Association.

Gary Stoner, PhD, is Professor and Director of the School Psychology Program in the School of Education at the University of Massachusetts Amherst. He is known for his professional work in the areas of attention-deficit/hyperactivity disorder, interventions for achievement and behavior problems, and scientist-practitioner approaches to professional school psychology. Dr. Stoner is coeditor of the book *Interventions for Achievement and Behavior Problems, Second Edition* (2002, National Association of School Psychologists). His current professional interests are focused on the study and promotion of early school success with children at risk for learning and behavior problems.

106295

Foreword

♦

It is a special privilege and honor to be asked, once more, to prepare the Foreword for this unique addition to the vast literature on attention-deficit/hyperactivity disorder (ADHD) in children and adolescents. There was simply no other book akin to the first edition that filled the void of providing school personnel with the necessary scientifically based information on ADHD, and this remains true today. If the first edition was outstanding, the second one is even more so, encompassing the findings from hundreds of scientific studies published in the interim that have pertinence to the evaluation and management of children with ADHD in the educational setting.

What makes this book all the more important is the ever-growing body of evidence demonstrating that, more than any other domain of major life activities, the educational sphere is devastatingly affected by this relatively common childhood disorder. This fact is well established in this edition even more solidly than in the first. All education is founded on a single principle: deferred gratification. Individuals must be capable of putting off the seductions and reinforcers of the moment to attend to and acquire knowledge and skills, the payoff for which is long delayed into the future. Yet this is what ADHD so tragically disrupts: the capacity to value and be governed by the likely larger rewards of the future over the smaller, more assured consequences of the moment. Children must be able to work toward future goals, subject themselves to circumstances that are not immediately rewarding, restrain their impulses, and return again and again to education despite periodic distractions if they are to become fully effective adults who contribute to society. Children with ADHD struggle mightily in environments that demand restraint, goal-directed actions, single-mindedness of purpose, self-regulation, and, above all, delayed gratification. Success in such contexts demands far more effort on the part of ADHD than normal children because it taxes enormously their limited capacity for self-regulation toward time and the future. The educational fallout from these deficiencies is well established here. More importantly, so are the many strategies that can be used to preclude or minimize these risks and deficiencies. What is so special about those techniques so voluminously articulated here is that they are founded on science rather than educational fashion, folklore, or the mere "clinical wisdom" of senior educators unanchored to the empirical testing that adds veracity to that wisdom. This is the state of the science, not just the art, of the educational management of ADHD. The authors are to be congratulated for the substantial scholarship involved in bringing this edition to publication.

Also noteworthy here is the inclusion of detailed information on medical treatments for ADHD, and not just the psychosocial ones favored by educators, school psychologists, and social workers. Yes, the educational, behavioral, and other psychosocial treatment tactics are important for the management of children with ADHD. They are well covered here. As the information reviewed here attests, however, ADHD cannot be treated optimally without regard to combinations of treatments that often, though not always, include the need for various medications. It does not matter whether one "believes" in medication or not, as the question is so often phrased by the naive. Medication management is not a religious belief requiring a leap of faith to endorse it. Contrary to the political propaganda and scientifically illiterate blather one may discover in the popular media, some Congressional hearings, and zealotry-tainted websites against medication and even ADHD as a diagnosis, medication management of ADHD is a more well-established intervention in clinical science than is any other treatment strategy presented here. It deserves inclusion in any text aspiring to be a comprehensive handbook on educational intervention. I am pleased to see that the authors did not shy away from providing this requisite information on medical management so that school personnel can be well informed on the topic. Given that 70–80% of clinically diagnosed children having ADHD are likely to receive medication at some time in their childhood years, and that this is often initiated to address their educational problems and related behavioral difficulties, school staff must be fully cognizant of what is known about both ADHD and about treatments physicians are likely to use to address it. The advent of once-daily delivery systems for the major stimulants, such as Concerta, Metadate CD, Adderall XR, and Ritalin LA, not to mention the just recently FDA-approved once-daily nonstimulant, Strattera, has certainly reduced the involvement of school staff in the administration of medications. Nevertheless, school personnel are relied upon heavily, both directly and indirectly, in providing crucial information to physicians on the effectiveness of these medications in the school setting. Such personnel should not hesitate to advise their physician colleagues on the strengths, weaknesses, and problem areas of the student with ADHD and on the degree of success any medical approaches may be having in addressing them. Kudos to the authors for providing that medical information here in easily digestible form and for encouraging this team approach to the treatment of the total child.

Despite the various and serious educational problems posed by ADHD for the child in the school environment, there is a plethora of scientifically tested treatment approaches that can be used to address those problems. Indeed, there is no better time in history than now to have a child with ADHD in the classroom setting, for we know far more about the disorder and its management than ever before. Few are as well qualified as the authors to explicate these effective behavioral and educational treatment tactics. They have done so in a responsible and ethical manner, being clearly sensitive to the various moral and legal constraints that accompany efforts to control any child's behavior in institutional settings, such as the schools. They clearly appreciate that the child's parents are an essential part of the multiprofessional treatment team, perhaps the most important part. For it is the parents' support, both directly and indirectly, that can all too often determine the effectiveness of any efforts by the schools to address the problems of a particular child with ADHD in that setting.

I congratulate the authors here for another fine edition of this important text and trust that the reader will find it to be as informative and instructive as I have in approaching the evaluation and treatment of the child with ADHD in the school setting.

RUSSELL A. BARKLEY, PhD
Professor, College of Health Professions
Medical University of South Carolina

Preface

♦

Inattentive and disruptive students present significant challenges to educational professionals. In fact, many children and adolescents who exhibit behavior control difficulties in classroom settings are diagnosed as having an attention-deficit/hyperactivity disorder (ADHD). Students with ADHD are at high risk for chronic academic achievement difficulties, the development of antisocial behavior, and problems in relationships with peers, parents, and teachers. Traditionally, this disorder has been identified and treated by clinic-based professionals (e.g., pediatricians, clinical psychologists) on an outpatient basis. Given the fact that children and adolescents with ADHD experience some of their greatest difficulties in educational settings, increased attention has been paid to the needs of these students by school-based professionals. In addition, federal regulations governing special education eligibility have magnified the need for educators to receive training in assessing and treating students with ADHD in the schools. The purpose of this book is to assist school professionals in understanding and treating children and adolescents with ADHD.

Since the publication of the first edition of this book in 1994, there has been a virtual explosion of journal articles, book chapters, and textbooks devoted to the topic of ADHD. As has been the case for many years, most of the previous literature on this disorder has been written by and for clinic-based practitioners. We have attempted to address the problems associated with ADHD from a school-based perspective, while recognizing the need for a team effort among parents, community-based professionals, and educators. Specifically, we have focused on how to

(1) identify and assess students who might have ADHD; (2) develop and implement classroom-based intervention programs for these students; and (3) communicate with and assist physicians when stimulant medications are employed to treat this disorder.

In this second edition, we have updated information in these major areas to address the understanding and management of ADHD in a comprehensive fashion for school-based professionals. This book is intended to meet the needs of a variety of school-based practitioners, including school psychologists, guidance counselors, administrators, and both general and special education teachers. Given that students with ADHD are found in nearly every school setting and experience a wide breadth of difficulties, there should be something of interest to all professional groups in this text. In addition, graduate students who are receiving training in a variety of school-based professions should find this book helpful in understanding this complex disorder. The text has been written to facilitate its use by practitioners. We have included a number of figures and appendices containing forms (e.g., handouts, observation coding sheets) that should prove useful for educators. Readers are encouraged to copy and use these forms as they see fit.

Acknowledgments

♦

As was the case with the first edition, this book would not have reached fruition without the support and encouragement of a variety of people. We continue to owe a great deal to our former mentor and major professor, Dr. Mark Rapport of the University of Central Florida. His enthusiasm for the scientific study of ADHD, combined with his emphasis on conducting investigations that are clinically and practically relevant, provided us with an exemplar of the scientist-practitioner model in action. Further, the high scientific and academic standards that he set for us and other graduate students have led, at least indirectly, to the completion of this book. We also continue to be inspired by the work of Dr. Russell Barkley of the Medical University of South Carolina. One of the true "giants" in the field of ADHD research, his support and guidance were critical to the preparation of the first edition of this text. Next, we are grateful for the support and encouragement of our colleagues Drs. Arthur Anastopoulos, John Hintze, Asha Jitendra, Lee Kern, William Matthews, Thomas Power, Edward Shapiro, Terri Shelton, and Mark Shinn. Our students at Lehigh University and the University of Massachusetts, too numerous to name, also have been supportive and patient throughout the time that we were preparing this book. Our continued success is directly related to the innovative ideas and challenges presented by our students. Even greater levels of patience and support were evidenced by our families, specifically, our spouses, Judy Brown-DuPaul and Joyce Flanagan, respectively, as well as the DuPaul children, Jason and Glenn. Their willingness to tolerate "lost" evenings and weekends will not go unrewarded. In particular, we are grateful to Judy Brown-

DuPaul for offering valuable suggestions, included in Chapter 4, for preschool teachers working with young children at risk for ADHD. We remain indebted to the editorial staff at The Guilford Press, most especially Chris Jennison, for continuing to support our work with the ideal blend of patience and prodding. Finally, we would be remiss if we did not acknowledge the hundreds of students with ADHD, their families, and their teachers with whom we have worked over the past two decades. Much of this book represents what we have learned from them and we are most grateful for this learning experience.

Contents

◆

ADHD IN THE SCHOOLS

CHAPTER 1

♦ ♦ ♦

Overview of ADHD

♦

AMY, AGE 4

Amy is a 4-year-old girl who lives with her mother, stepfather, and younger brother (age 2). She attends preschool four mornings per week at a local church. Her mother reports Amy was "a terror" as an infant. She was colicky, frequently cried, and demanded to be held "constantly." At about 11 months old, when she began walking, Amy's activity level increased and she "was always into everything." In fact, on one occasion when Amy was 2 years old, she was brought into the emergency room following ingestion of some cleaning fluids that she had found under the kitchen sink. Amy has been asked to leave several daycare and nursery school settings because of her high activity level, short attention span, and physical aggression toward peers. Although she is beginning to learn letters and numbers, it is very difficult for her mother or teacher to get her to sit still for any reading or learning activities. Amy's preference is to engage in rough-and-tumble activities and she can become quite defiant when asked to sit and complete more structured or quiet activities (e.g., drawing or coloring).

GREG, AGE 7

Greg is a 7-year-old first grader in a general education classroom in a public elementary school. According to his parents, his physical and psychological development was "normal" until about age 3 when he first attended nursery school. His preschool and kindergarten teachers reported Greg to have a short attention span, to have difficulties staying seated during group activities, and to interrupt conversations frequently. These behaviors were evident increasingly at home as well. Currently, Greg is achieving at a level commensurate with his classmates in all academic areas. Unfortunately, he continues to evidence problems with inattention, impulsivity, and motor restlessness. These behaviors are displayed more frequently when Greg is supposed to be listening to the teacher or completing an independent task. His teacher is concerned that Greg may begin to exhibit academic problems if his attention and behavior do not improve.

TOMMY, AGE 9

Tommy is a fourth grader whose schooling occurs in a self-contained, special education classroom for children identified with "emotional disturbance" in a public elementary school. His mother reports that Tommy has been a "handful" since infancy. During his preschool years, he was very active (e.g., climbing on furniture, running around excessively, and infrequently sitting still) and noncompliant with maternal commands. He has had chronic difficulties relating to other children: he has been both verbally and physically aggressive with his peers. As a result, he has few friends his own age and tends to play with younger children. Tommy has been placed in a class for students in need of social/emotional support since second grade because of his frequent disruptive activities (e.g., calling out without permission, swearing at the teacher, refusing to complete seatwork) and related problematic academic achievement. During the past year, Tommy's antisocial activities have increased in severity: he has been caught shoplifting on several occasions and has been suspended from school for vandalizing the boy's bathroom. Even in his highly structured classroom, Tommy has a great deal of difficulty attending to independent work and following classroom rules.

HEATHER, AGE 13

Heather is a 13-year-old eighth grader who receives most of her instruction in general education classrooms. A psychoeducational evaluation conducted when she was 8 years old indicated a "specific learning disability" in math, for which she receives resource room instruction three class periods per week. In addition to problems with math skills, Heather has exhibited significant difficulties with inattention since at least age 5. Specifically, she appears to daydream excessively and to "space out" when asked to complete effortful tasks either at home or at school. Her parents and teachers report that she "forgets" task instructions frequently, particularly if multiple steps are involved. At one time, her inattention problems were assumed to be caused by her learning disability in math. This does not appear to be the case, however, because she is inattentive during most classes (i.e., not just during math instruction) and these behaviors predated her entry into elementary school. Heather is neither impulsive nor overactive. In fact, she is "slow to respond" at times and appears reticent in social situations.

ROBERTO, AGE 17

Roberto is a 17-year-old student who attends the 10th grade in a large urban high school. He was retained in grade twice during elementary school and has struggled academically throughout his academic career. Furthermore, he has been described by his teachers as impatient, disruptive, restless, and lacking in motivation. As a result of his academic and behavior difficulties, Roberto has been provided with a variety of special education services, including placement in a learning support classroom, individual counseling, and, briefly, placement in an alternative school environment. Furthermore, school professionals have attempted to involve Roberto's family with community-based counseling services and have recommended consultation with his physician regarding psychotropic medication; these recommendations have been followed inconsistently over the years. Despite these services, Roberto's difficulties have worsened and have been compounded in recent years by his involvement in a local gang. He has been arrested on two occasions for shoplifting and vandalism and also is truant from school quite often. He has asked his parents to allow him to drop out of high school so that he can obtain a full-time job.

Although the five children and adolescents described above are quite different, they share a common difficulty with attention, particularly to assigned schoolwork and household responsibilities. Furthermore, many children with attention problems, such as Amy, Greg, Tommy, and Roberto, display additional difficulties with impulsivity and overactivity. The current psychiatric term for children exhibiting extreme problems with inattention, impulsivity, and hyperactivity is *attention-deficit/ hyperactivity disorder*, or ADHD[1] (American Psychiatric Association, 2000). As can be discerned from the above case descriptions, the term ADHD is applied to a heterogeneous group of children and adolescents who are encountered in virtually every educational setting.

The purpose of this chapter is to provide a brief overview of ADHD. Specifically, we review information regarding the prevalence of

---

[1]Because multiple labels for attention-deficit/hyperactivity disorder have been used throughout the years and across disciplines, the term ADHD will be used in this text to promote simplicity. ADHD will be considered synonymous with other terms for the disorder, such as hyperactivity and ADD.

this disorder, the school-related problems of children with ADHD, associated adjustment difficulties, methods of subtyping children with this disorder, possible causes of ADHD, the impact of situational factors on symptom severity, and the probable long-term outcomes for this population. Furthermore, we review a theoretical framework for explaining the deficits underlying ADHD. This background material provides the context for later descriptions of school-based assessment and treatment strategies for ADHD. Readers who are interested in a more comprehensive discussion of the issues presented in this chapter should consult Barkley (1998), Goldstein and Goldstein (1998), or Teeter (1998).

PREVALENCE OF ADHD

Epidemiological (i.e., population survey) studies indicate that approximately 3–7% of children in the United States can be diagnosed with ADHD (Barkley, 1998; Pastor & Reuben, 2002). Because most general education classrooms include at least 20 students, it is estimated that one child in every classroom will have ADHD. As a result, children reported to evidence attention and behavior control problems are frequently referred to school psychologists and other education and mental health professionals. Boys with the disorder outnumber girls in both clinic-referred (approximately a 6:1 ratio) and community-based (approximately a 3:1 ratio) samples (Barkley, 1998; Pastor & Reuben, 2002). The higher clinic ratio for boys with this disorder may be a function in part of the greater prevalence of additional disruptive behaviors (e.g., noncompliance, conduct disturbance) among boys with ADHD (Gaub & Carlson, 1997). More than 50% of children diagnosed with ADHD receive psychotropic medication for this condition, while approximately 12% and 34% receive special education and mental health services, respectively (Pastor & Reuben, 2002). Thus, relative to other childhood conditions (e.g., autism and depression), ADHD is a "high-incidence" disorder that is particularly prominent among males. In a manner similar to these other disorders, it typically requires the services of multiple community and education professionals to achieve positive developmental outcomes.

SCHOOL-RELATED PROBLEMS
OF CHILDREN WITH ADHD

Core Behavior Difficulties

The core characteristics (i.e., inattention, impulsivity, and overactivity) of ADHD can lead to myriad difficulties for children in school settings.

Specifically, because these children often have problems sustaining attention to effortful tasks, their completion of independent seatwork is quite inconsistent. Their performance on classwork also may be compromised by a lack of attention to task instructions. Other academic problems associated with attention problems include poor test performance; deficient study skills; disorganized notebooks, desks, and written reports; and a lack of attention to teacher lectures and/or group discussion.

Children with ADHD often disrupt classroom activities, and thus disturb the learning of their classmates. For example, children with ADHD may exhibit impulsivity in a variety of ways, including frequent calling out without permission, talking with classmates at inappropriate times, and becoming angry when confronted with reprimands or frustrating tasks. Classwork and homework accuracy also may be affected deleteriously due to an impulsive, careless response style on these tasks.

In-class problems related to overactivity include children leaving their seats without permission, playing with inappropriate objects (e.g., materials in desk that are unrelated to the task at hand), repetitive tapping of hands and feet, and fidgeting in their chairs. Although the latter behaviors may appear relatively benign, when they occur frequently they can serve as a significant disruption to classroom instruction.

Difficulties Associated with ADHD

Students with ADHD are at risk for significant difficulties in a variety of functional areas. It appears as though problems with inattention, impulsivity, and overactivity serve as a "magnet" for other difficulties that are, in some cases, more severe than the core deficits of ADHD. Of these difficulties, the three most frequent correlates of ADHD are academic underachievement, high rates of noncompliance and aggression, and disturbances in peer relationships.

Teachers and parents frequently report that children with ADHD underachieve academically compared to their classmates (Barkley, 1998). As stated above, these children exhibit significantly lower rates of on-task behavior during instruction and independent work periods than those displayed by their peers (Abikoff, Gittelman-Klein, & Klein, 1977; Platzman et al., 1992). Consequently, children with ADHD have fewer opportunities to respond to academic material and complete less independent work than their classmates (Pfiffner & Barkley, 1998). Lower than expected rates of work completion may, in part, account for the association of ADHD with academic underachievement: up to 80% of children with this disorder have been found to exhibit academic performance problems (Cantwell & Baker, 1991). Furthermore, between 20 and 30% of children with ADHD are classified as "learning disabled" because of their deficits in the acquisition of specific academic skills (see Chapter 3 for details). Finally, the results of prospective follow-up studies of children with ADHD into adolescence and young adulthood indicate heightened risks for chronic academic failure as measured by higher rates of grade retention and dropping out of school relative to their peers (e.g., Barkley, Fischer, Edelbrock, & Smallish, 1990; Hansen, Weiss, & Last, 1999).

The strong correlation between hyperactivity and aggression is well documented in the research literature (Jensen, Martin, & Cantwell, 1997; Loney & Milich, 1982). Problems of aggression most frequently associated with ADHD include defiance or noncompliance with authority figure commands, poor temper control, and argumentativeness and verbal hostility, which presently comprise the psychiatric category of oppositional defiant disorder (American Psychiatric Association, 2000). Therefore, it is not surprising that oppositional defiant disorder is the most common codiagnosis with ADHD (i.e., associated or comorbid condition), as more than 40% of children with ADHD and 65% of teenagers with ADHD display significant oppositional defiant disorder-related behaviors (Jensen et al., 1997). More serious antisocial behaviors (e.g., stealing, physical aggression, and truancy) are exhibited by 25% or more of students with ADHD, particularly at the secondary school level (Barkley, Fischer, et al., 1990; Gittelman, Mannuzza, Shenker, & Bonagura, 1985). Children who display aggression and ADHD-related difficulties are at greater risk for interpersonal conflict at home, in school, and with peers than are children who display ADHD alone (Johnston & Mash, 2001). Not surprisingly, teachers report experiencing significant amounts of stress in interacting with students with ADHD, especially those who exhibit aggression along with ADHD symptoms (Greene, Beszterczey, Katzenstein, Park, & Goring, 2002). Finally, the combination of conduct problems and ADHD is strongly associated with the abuse of illicit drugs (Biederman et al., 1997; Gittelman et al., 1985).

It is very difficult for many children with ADHD to initiate and maintain friendships with their classmates (Stormont, 2001). Studies employing sociometric measures have found uniformly high rates of peer rejection for children displaying ADHD-related behaviors (e.g., Hinshaw, Zupan, Simmel, Nigg, & Melnick, 1997; Hodgens, Cole, & Boldizar, 2000). The rate of peer rejection is particularly high for children displaying both aggression and ADHD. Typically, peer rejection status is stable over time, reflecting the chronic nature of these children's interactional difficulties (Parker & Asher, 1987). Of additional concern, approximately 22% of boys and 15% of girls with ADHD can be characterized as having a "social disability" representing social functioning that is 1.65 standard deviations below age and gender means on standardized measures of social functioning (Greene et al., 1996, 2002). Preliminary evidence also indicates that children with ADHD tend to be on the periphery of classroom social networks and to "hang out" together, thereby increasing the probability of disruptive behavior (Kelly, 2001). Not surprisingly, therefore, children with this disorder perceive peers and classmates to provide less frequent social support than do their non-ADHD counterparts (Demaray & Elliott, 2001).

Presumably, the disturbed peer relations of children with ADHD are due to inattentive and impulsive behaviors disrupting their "social performance" (Stormont, 2001). The most common performance deficits associated with this disorder include inappropriate attempts to join ongoing peer group activities (e.g., barging in on games in progress), poor conversational behaviors (e.g., frequent interruptions, paying minimal attention to what others are saying), employing aggressive "solutions" to interpersonal problems, and being prone to losing temper control when conflict or frustrations are encountered in social situations (Guevremont, 1990). A related concern in the social arena is that boys with ADHD are involved in team or individual sports for shorter time periods than their typically developing counterparts and are more likely than control children to exhibit aggression, to display emotional reactivity, and to be disqualified during team athletic activities (Johnson & Rosén, 2000). Surprisingly, children with ADHD often are able to articulate the proper social behaviors to be exhibited in specific situations, although there may be a tendency for them to propose aggressive solutions to interpersonal problems (Stormont, 2001). At present, the most prudent conclusion is that ADHD-related symptoms lead to social *performance* difficulties for these children, rather than to social *skills* deficits per se (see Chapter 7 for details).

Children with ADHD require more frequent medical and mental health care than their non-ADHD counterparts. One recent study found that children with this disorder have more frequent primary care, pharmacy, and mental health service visits than do children without this disorder (Guevara, Lozano, Wickizer, Mell, & Gephart, 2001). As a result, health care costs for children with ADHD were more than double the costs for non-ADHD children. Costs for health care are even greater than for children with other chronic disorders, such as asthma (Chan, Zhan, & Homer, 2002). The "true" costs for treating ADHD may actually be underestimated given that these children receive services in school and mental health settings (Chan et al., 2002). Thus, school professionals need to be cognizant of the greater need for health care in this population and attempt to help families access needed services in the community.

SUBTYPES OF ADHD

The current definition of ADHD includes a list of 18 behavioral symptoms divided into two sets (inattention and hyperactivity–impulsivity) of nine symptoms each (American Psychiatric Association, 2000). There are three subtypes of ADHD: combined type (ADHD-CT), predominantly inattentive type (ADHD-IA), and predominantly hyperactive–impulsive type (ADHD-HI). Children with ADHD-CT exhibit at least six of the nine Inattention symptoms and at least six of the nine hyperactive–impulsive symptoms. ADHD-IA is indicated for children who exhibit at least six Inattention symptoms but less than six hyperactive–impulsive symptoms. Conversely, children with ADHD-HI exhibit at least six hyperactive–impulsive symptoms but less than six inattention symptoms.

Given that the symptomatic profile will vary across individuals, children classified with ADHD are a heterogeneous group. In fact, there are at least 7,056 possible combinations of 12 out of 18 symptoms that could result in a diagnosis of ADHD-CT. Broadening this inherent heterogeneity are the potential correlates of ADHD (i.e., academic underachievement, aggression, and peer relationship difficulties), as summarized above. Therefore, attempts have been made to identify more homogeneous subtypes of ADHD to facilitate searches for causal factors, to identify potential differences in long-term outcome, and, most importantly, to aid in treatment planning (for a review, see Jensen et al., 1997). A brief overview of each of the current subtypes is provided below, along with an exploration of the value of subtyping ADHD on the basis of the presence or absence of aggression or internalizing symptoms.[2]

ADHD Predominantly Inattentive Type

A previous American Psychiatric Association classification system (i.e., DSM-III; American Psychiatric Association, 1980) included two different subtypes of ADHD: attention deficit disorder with hyperactivity (ADD+H) and attention deficit disorder without hyperactivity (ADDnoH). The latter category included children who exhibited significant problems with inattention and impulsivity in the absence of frequent overactivity. When the DSM-III was revised in 1987, this subtype was removed from the classification schema because of its minimal empirical underpinnings at the time.

---

[2]The advantages and disadvantages of subtyping children with ADHD into those with versus without learning disabilities are discussed in Chapter 3.

Since the 1987 publication of the DSM-III-R (American Psychological Association, 1987), a variety of research studies have been conducted that support the existence of an ADDnoH subtype (for a review, see Carlson & Mann, 2000). On the basis of this empirical evidence, this subtype was reintroduced to the psychiatric nomenclature with the publication of the DSM-IV (American Psychiatric Association, 1994). Children with ADHD predominantly inattentive type (ADHD-IA) display significant problems with inattention in the absence of notable impulsivity and hyperactivity. There is initial evidence that children with ADHD-IA have greater problems with memory retrieval and perceptual–motor speed than their impulsive–hyperactive counterparts (Barkley, DuPaul, & McMurray, 1990). Furthermore, these children are described by parents and teachers as more "sluggish" cognitively, daydreamy, and socially withdrawn than children with ADHD-CT (Hodgens et al., 2000; McBurnett, Pfiffner, & Frick, 2001). These and other findings have led some investigators to postulate a greater incidence of learning disabilities among this subtype relative to other children with the full syndrome of ADHD. This hypothesis has not been borne out in any empirical studies, although at least one investigation (Barkley, DuPaul, & McMurray, 1990) found a greater percentage of students with ADHD-IA (i.e., 53%) placed in classrooms for students with learning disabilities relative to those with ADHD-CT (i.e., 34%).

In contrast to the ADHD-IA subtype, children with the full syndrome of ADHD exhibit higher rates of impulsivity, overactivity, aggression, noncompliance, and peer rejection (Carlson & Mann, 2000). Furthermore, children with ADHD-CT are more likely than their ADHD-IA counterparts to be diagnosed with other disruptive behavior disorders (e.g., oppositional defiant disorder and conduct disorder), to be placed in classrooms for students with emotional disturbances, to obtain a higher frequency of school suspensions, and to receive psychotherapeutic intervention (Barkley, DuPaul, & McMurray, 1990; Faraone, Biederman, Weber, & Russell, 1998; Willcutt, Pennington, Chhabildas, Friedman, & Alexander, 1999). Although comparative long-term outcome studies have not been conducted, it is assumed that children with the full syndrome of ADHD are at greater risk for antisocial disturbance and behavioral adjustment difficulties. Little is known about the chronicity and longitudinal outcome of ADHD-IA in childhood, although Willcutt and colleagues (in press; cited in Willcutt, Chhabildas, & Pennington, 2001) found that over 80% of children diagnosed with this subtype continued to display significant inattention symptoms over an 18-month period.

A handful of studies have examined the differential response to psychostimulant medication (i.e., Ritalin, or methylphenidate) in the two subtypes of ADHD. These studies generally indicate a positive response to medication among most members of both subtypes, with lower doses found to be sufficient for a greater percentage of children with ADHD-IA (e.g., Barkley, DuPaul, & McMurray, 1991). To date, no studies have compared response to nonpharmacological interventions between subtypes.

In clinical samples, a smaller percentage (i.e., approximately 1.3%) of children have ADHD-IA relative to those with the full syndrome (Szatmari, Offord, & Boyle, 1989), while there may be a higher percentage of children with the inattentive subtype (5%) among community samples (Wolraich, Hannah, Pinnock, Baumgaertel, & Brown, 1996). Furthermore, there is burgeoning evidence to indicate that such children should be identified separately from children with ADHD-CT. These subtypes clearly differ with respect to associated difficulties, and perhaps in the areas of treatment response and long-term outcome. Barkley (1998) has argued that children with ADHD-IA also may differ from hyperactive–impulsive children in the qualitative nature of their attention deficits. Specifically, children with ADHD-CT exhibit difficulties with sustained attention as a function of impaired delayed responding to the environment, while those with ADHD-IA are more likely to have problems with focused attention. Thus, different neural mechanisms may be involved, leading to discrepant behavioral response styles (Barkley, 1998). Furthermore, children with ADHD-IA who also display symptoms of sluggish cognitive tempo (e.g., confused, seems lost in a fog) exhibit outcomes such as social withdrawal and internalizing disorder symptoms that are not frequently found among children with ADHD-CT (Carlson & Mann, 2002). These important differences between subtypes have led researchers to suggest that ADHD-IA is a separate and distinct disorder from the combined type (Barkley, 1998: Milich, Balentine, & Lynam, 2001) and, at the very least, diagnostic criteria should include symptoms of sluggish cognitive tempo to allow more accurate identification of the inattentive subtype (Carlson & Mann, 2002).

ADHD Predominantly Hyperactive–Impulsive Type

The predominantly hyperactive–impulsive type of ADHD (ADHD-HI) was introduced in the DSM-IV (American Psychiatric Association, 1994). The field trials conducted prior to the publication of the DSM-IV indicated that a small percentage of children with this disorder evidenced significant hyperactive–impulsive behaviors in the absence of inattentive symptoms (Lahey et al., 1994). The vast majority of these children were of preschool and early elementary school age, leading to speculation that the ADHD-HI subtype may be a precursor of ADHD-CT. This speculation must be investigated through longitudinal studies of children with ADHD-HI. In fact, minimal research has been conducted regarding the epidemiology, clinical characteristics, school performance, and treatment outcomes of the ADHD-HI subtype. There is preliminary evidence that children with ADHD-HI are prone to the same comorbid disorders (i.e., oppositional defiant disorder and conduct disorder) as children with ADHD-CT (Willcutt et al., 1999). Therefore, given the dearth of research on this subtype, the most prudent conclusion is that ADHD-HI represents a less severe form or an early manifestation of the combined type of ADHD.

ADHD with versus without Aggression

As stated previously, the term "aggressive" has been used to describe children who display higher than average rates of noncompliance, argumentativeness, defiance, and poor temper control. Many children displaying such behaviors meet the criteria for the classification of oppositional defiant disorder. Although there is a great deal of overlap or comorbidity between ADHD and oppositional defiant disorder (Barkley, 1998; see "Difficulties Associated with ADHD" section, above), children with either disorder alone are distinct, especially with respect to long-term outcome, from those youngsters who are both hyperactive and aggressive (for a review, see Jensen et al., 1997).

Children with ADHD and aggression (i.e., oppositional defiant disorder or conduct disorder) exhibit greater frequencies of antisocial behaviors, such as lying, stealing, and fighting, than those who are hyperactive and not aggressive (Barkley, 1998). Furthermore, hyperactive–aggressive children are at higher risk for peer rejection than those displaying either ADHD or aggression in isolation. Greater levels of family dysfunction and parental psychopathology have been found among youngsters with both disorders as well (Jensen et al., 1997). Most importantly, children with both ADHD and aggression have the highest risk for problematic outcomes in adolescence and adulthood (e.g., greater prevalence of substance abuse) relative to any other subgroup of children with ADHD (Jensen et al., 1997).

Although these subtypes have not been found to exhibit different responses to psychostimulant medication (e.g., Barkley, McMurray, Edelbrock, & Robbins, 1989), there is considerable agreement among professionals that those children with ADHD *and* aggression will require more intensive and continuous professional service delivery to achieve favorable outcomes. The precursors to the combination of ADHD and aggression may hold some clues to the need for comprehensive multimodal treatment. A combination of within-child (i.e., irritable child temperament, shorter than average attention span, and high activity level) and environmental (i.e., coercive response style of family members, marital discord, and poor parental functioning) factors may lead to the coexistence of these disorders (Barkley, 1998). To the extent that these factors contribute to child maladjustment throughout development, the later the point of intervention, the greater the need for long-term, intensive, service delivery. The protracted and difficult nature of these behavior problems sometimes leads to children being placed in more restrictive placements outside of the public school and family environments.

ADHD with versus without Internalizing Disorder

Approximately 13–50% of children with ADHD exhibit symptoms of an anxiety or depressive disorder (Jensen et al., 1997). The presence of comorbid internalizing symptoms carries both positive and negative implications for children with ADHD. On the one hand, the association of internalizing symptoms with ADHD can serve as a protective factor wherein (1) hyperactive–impulsive behaviors are less severe than when internalizing symptoms are absent and (2) conduct disorder symptoms are less likely to be present (Pliszka, Carlson, & Swanson, 1999). Alternatively, the combination of ADHD and internalizing symptoms is associated with greater social impairment (as reported by teachers and parents) than ADHD alone (Karustis, Power, Rescorla, Eiraldi, & Gallagher, 2000). Furthermore, some studies have found a diminished effect of psychostimulant medication for children with ADHD and internalizing symptoms relative to children with ADHD without internalizing symptoms (e.g., DuPaul, Barkley, & McMurray, 1994). Thus, there may be important distinctions in clinical presentation, impairment, and treatment response between children with ADHD with and without internalizing symptoms, thereby supporting this as a viable subtyping scheme. This conclusion is tempered by the fact that what little research has been done in this area has (1) focused almost exclusively on anxiety rather than depressive disorders and (2) used a single-respondent (e.g., parent report) to assess internalizing symptomatology. Nevertheless, at the very least, practitioners need to assess both externalizing and internalizing symptoms when evaluating children suspected of ADHD because such symptoms are likely to influence both the trajectory of children's difficulties and their response to certain interventions.

POSSIBLE CAUSES OF ADHD

There is no apparent single "cause" of ADHD. Rather, ADHD symptomatology may result from a variety of causal mechanisms (Barkley,

1998). Most of the research examining the etiology of ADHD is correlational. Thus, caution is warranted in attributing causal status to identified variables. Nevertheless, empirical data have been gathered regarding the potential causal contributions of a number of factors to ADHD (see Barkley, 2002). Within-child variables, such as neurobiological factors and hereditary influences, have received the greatest attention in the literature (Barkley, 1998; Tannock, 1998). The contributions of these variables are summarized briefly below. Environmental influences (e.g., family stress, poor parental disciplinary practices) appear to modulate the severity of the disorder, but do not play a causal role per se (Barkley, 1998).

Neurobiological Variables

Historically, neurobiological factors have received the greatest attention as etiological factors. The earliest hypotheses postulated that children with ADHD had structural brain damage that contributed to attention and behavior control difficulties (Barkley, 1998). There appear to be minor structural differences between the brains of individuals with ADHD and those of normal controls. Specifically, studies using both structural (e.g., magnetic resonance imaging [MRI]) and functional (e.g., positon emission tomography [PET]) imaging techniques have indicated important differences and possible abnormalities in the fronto–striatal networks of the brain (for a review, see Tannock, 1998). Interestingly, one of the sections of the brain that has been studied in this regard is the prefrontal cortex, which purportedly is involved in the inhibition of behavior and mediating responses to environmental stimuli. In addition, the neurotransmitters, dopamine and norepinepherine, are presumed to be "less available" in certain regions of the brain (e.g., frontal cortex), thus contributing to ADHD symptomatology. This hypothesis has been based, in part, on the action of psychostimulants (e.g., Ritalin) in the brain wherein the availability of dopamine and norepinepherine is increased. Based on available evidence, it is presumed that these neurobiological differences are due to aberrations in normal brain development resulting from genetic, hormonal, and/or environmental factors (Tannock, 1998).

Hereditary Influences

There is consistent evidence that ADHD is a highly heritable disorder that runs in families (Faraone, 2000). Evidence supporting the primary role of genetic factors has been obtained in a number of ways. First, there is a higher rate of concurrent and past ADHD symptoms in immediate family members of children with ADHD relative to their non-

ADHD counterparts (e.g., Faraone et al., 1993). Furthermore, there is a higher incidence of ADHD among first-degree biological relatives relative to adoptive parents and siblings for children with ADHD that were adopted at an early age (e.g., Van der Oord, Boomsa, & Verhulst, 1994).

A second research strategy to investigate the heritability of ADHD symptoms has been to investigate symptom patterns in monozygotic (MZ) and dizygotic (DZ) twins. Specifically, the probability of one twin having ADHD given that the other twin has the disorder (referred to as a *concordance rate*) is significantly higher among MZ twin pairs than among DZ twin pairs (e.g., Levy, Hay, McStephen, Wood, & Waldman, 1997). Because MZ twins are genetically identical, while DZ twins share only 50% of their genes, it is presumed that higher concordance rates among MZ twins supports a substantial role for hereditary (rather than environmental) factors in the expression of ADHD symptoms. In fact, twin studies allow behavioral genetic researchers to estimate the variance of ADHD symptoms that are accounted for by genetic, shared environment, and nonshared environment factors. Most of the variance is accounted for by genetic factors, as indicated by heritability estimates ranging from .75 to .98 (for a review, see Tannock, 1998). A small but significant proportion of symptomatic variance is accounted for by nonshared environmental factors, while none of these studies support a significant role for shared environmental factors. Heritability estimates for ADHD are among the highest for any emotional or behavior disorder, exceeding estimates for schizophrenia and autism (Barkley, 1998).

Molecular genetic studies have provided initial support for the association of genes related to specific neurotransmitters and the phenotypic expression of ADHD symptoms (e.g., Comings et al., 2000). Although it is likely that multiple genes related to both the dopaminergic and the noradrenergic systems are involved (see Comings et al., 2000), two genes have received the greatest attention thus far. Specifically, important differences in the dopamine transporter gene (DAT; Dougherty et al., 1999) and the D4 dopamine receptor gene (DRD4; Swanson et al., 1998) have been found in ADHD relative to non-ADHD samples. These are interesting findings given that dopamine is an important neurotransmitter in those parts of the brain (e.g., frontal cortex) that have been implicated in ADHD and that stimulant medications temporarily increase the availability of dopamine in the synaptic cleft. Clearly, additional replication and extension studies are needed to identify genes that might play a role in ADHD symptomology.

Environmental Toxins

Over the years, a variety of environmental toxins have been hypothesized to account for ADHD symptoms. Some of the more popular theories have implicated nutritional factors, lead poisoning, and prenatal exposure to drugs or alcohol (Barkley, 1998). For example, Feingold (1975) argued that certain food additives (e.g., artificial food colorings, salicylates) led to childhood hyperactivity. Well-controlled studies that have examined this hypothesis, as well as similar assumptions about sugar, indicate that dietary factors play a minimal role in the genesis of ADHD (Barkley, 1998). More recently, investigators have found a significant relationship between maternal smoking (Milberger, Beiderman, Faraone, Chen, & Jones, 1996) or cigarette smoking (Mick, Biederman, Faraone, Sayer, & Kleinman, 2002) during pregnancy and later ADHD as well as low birth weight and later ADHD (Mick, Biederman, Prince, Fischer, & Faraone, 2002). Although the results of correlational studies implicate some environmental factors in ADHD, the exact role these factors play in actually "causing" this disorder is presumed to be minimal, at least for the majority of youngsters receiving this diagnosis.

Conclusions

The most prudent conclusion regarding the etiology of ADHD is that multiple neurobiological factors may predispose children to exhibiting higher rates of impulsivity and motor activity along with shorter than average attention spans compared to other children. The most promising evidence points to a hereditary influence that may alter brain (i.e., neurochemical) functioning, particularly in the frontal–striatal system. Furthermore, behavioral genetic studies have generally supported the notion of ADHD as a dimensional rather than a categorical disorder (Levy et al., 1997). Stated differently, everyone exhibits symptoms of this disorder on occasion. What sets children with ADHD apart from their nondiagnosed peers is that they may be genetically predisposed (through neurobiological differences) to exhibit these behaviors at a significantly higher rate than others of the same age and gender.

Several caveats should be kept in mind about etiological conclusions. First, research in this area has been fraught with methodological difficulties that reduce confidence in interpreting results (Tannock, 1998). Second, despite the fact that within-child variables appear to be the primary causal factors, this finding does not denigrate the role of the environment in the maintenance of ADHD symptoms. For instance, as discussed in Chapters 4 and 5, interventions that involve the manipulation of environmental conditions can be quite effective in enhancing the functioning of children with this disorder. Third, at present, there is no known connection between the "cause" of an individual's ADHD and treatment planning. As such, determination of etiology is minimally related to enhancing successful outcomes. Perhaps as the use of advanced assessment technologies, particularly in the realm of molecular genetics, becomes more widespread, clinically useful information about the etiology of ADHD will be forthcoming.

THE IMPACT OF SITUATIONAL
FACTORS ON ADHD SYMPTOM SEVERITY

Although biological variables are hypothesized to be the primary causes for ADHD, the role of environmental factors in setting the occasion for or reducing the probability of ADHD-related behaviors remains important for professional service delivery. Both antecedent and consequent stimuli are critical in determining the severity of attention problems, impulsivity, and behavior control. In fact, the development of classroom interventions for children with ADHD is enhanced by (1) determining the behavioral function of ADHD-related behaviors and (2) implementing strategies that are linked directly to behavior function (DuPaul & Ervin, 1996; see also Chapters 2 and 5). For example, if one determines that a child's inattentive disruptive behavior reliably results in access to teacher attention, then the classroom intervention should provide access to teacher attention contingent on nondisruptive behavior. The prevailing assumption is that although environmental factors affect the behavior of all children, the performance of children with attention and behavior control problems is much more sensitive to these events.

Important antecedent and/or setting events that affect the probability of ADHD-related behaviors occurring include the type of commands or instructions a child is given, the degree to which a child is supervised during independent work, the number of children present during instruction (Barkley, 1998), and the presentation of academic tasks that are perceived as difficult or aversive.

Teachers often state that children with attention and behavior control problems are able to complete work more accurately if they interact "one-to-one" with a "supervisor" (e.g., teacher, aide, peer). When asked to attend to seatwork or instruction in group settings, however, students with ADHD encounter frequent difficulties (Barkley, 1998). In a similar fashion, when independent work is closely supervised, children with ADHD are able to produce a greater quantity and a higher quality of output relative to minimal supervision situations. Children with ADHD also are more likely to complete tasks that are stimulating and interesting to them, as well as those that are within their range of skills (i.e., work that is at the instructional level). Furthermore, there is preliminary evidence that children with this disorder behave more appropriately when given a choice among several tasks rather than told to complete one specific assignment (Dunlap et al., 1994).

Children with ADHD are more likely to attend to commands that are given in a straightforward, declarative manner (e.g., "Get back to work") than those delivered as a question or as a request for a favor ("Will you please get back to work?") (Anastopoulos, Smith, & Wein, 1998). Furthermore, instructions are more likely to be followed when they are delivered once potential distractors (e.g., toys, television) have been removed and the student has made eye contact with the instructor. Finally, compliance with instructions is enhanced by continuing to supervise the child during the initial minute or so after giving the command (Barkley, 1997b). Thus, the antecedent conditions that will promote better behavior control and academic performance include provision of effective commands along with supervision of the child's work on a one-to-one basis.

A variety of factors affect the degree to which consequences control the behavior of children with ADHD. These include the latency between behavior and its consequences, the frequency of reinforcement, how salient or "motivating" the consequences are to the child, and the manner in which verbal reprimands are delivered (Pfiffner & Barkley, 1998).

Children with ADHD perform akin to their classmates under conditions of relatively immediate and frequent reinforcement (Pfiffner & Barkley, 1998). This is particularly the case when the type of reinforcement is highly salient and meaningful to the child. Unfortunately, reinforcement is delayed and infrequent in most general education classrooms. Furthermore, the typical reinforcers (e.g., grades, and teacher praise) provided in schools are usually on the low end of the saliency continuum.

Verbal reprimands are commonly used by teachers to reduce students' disruptive behaviors (White, 1975). Usually, reprimands are delivered in a loud voice in front of the class, while the teacher exhibits nonverbal cues (e.g., frown, ruddy complexion) that indicate anger with the perpetrating student(s). Alternatively, an impressive body of research indicates that reprimands are more likely to reduce behavior when delivered privately to the child, relatively immediately following a transgression, and with a minimum of discussion and affect (e.g., Pfiffner & O'Leary, 1987). The latter factors are particularly important when attempting to reduce the disruptive behavior of an inattentive student.

ADHD as a Disorder of Impaired Delayed Responding

The crucial role that the interaction of within-child biological factors and environmental events play in determining the severity of ADHD symptoms has led to recent changes in the conceptualization of the deficits underlying this disorder. In particular, the central feature of ADHD may be an impairment in delayed responding (i.e., behavioral inhibition) rather than a defict in attention, per se (Barkley, 1997a, 1998). Many important settings (e.g., classroom) and abilities (e.g., internalization of speech) require the capacity to delay responding to the environment. Thus, deficits in delayed responding lead to the exhibition of ADHD symptoms in multiple settings and deleteriously affect the development of rule-governed behavior.

Barkley (1997a) has articulated a theoretical model of ADHD as a disorder of behavioral inhibition wherein impaired delayed responding to the environment compromises the development of four critical executive functions. The latter include working memory, self-regulation of affect–motivation–arousal, internalization of speech, and behavioral analysis/synthesis. Impairments in the development of these executive functions in turn lead to myriad problems in cognitive, academic, and social functioning. This theoretical model makes intuitive sense and is consistent with the extant literature on this disorder (for a review, see Barkley, 1997a). Nevertheless, investigations using this theoretical model a priori to formulate hypotheses are just beginning to emerge in the literature. Thus, the full value of this theory for explaining ADHD and for formulating intervention strategies awaits further empirical scrutiny.

Despite the need for more research, the implications of this conceptualization of ADHD are clear. Interventions for this disorder must include changes in within-child variables (e.g., temporary change in brain functioning through stimulant medication) and/or changes in antecedent and consequent stimuli to increase the probability of delayed responding, thereby leading to attentive, productive behavior (Barkley, 1997a). Unfortunately, most classrooms are structured in a manner that provides delayed and infrequent reinforcement under the assumption that students become "internally motivated" to conform with rules and complete academic tasks. These are precisely the conditions most likely to lead to inattentive disruptive behaviors (i.e., impaired response inhibition) in children with ADHD. Thus, the challenge to education professionals is to incorporate environmental stimuli known to enhance student success into all classrooms where impulsive inattentive students are being taught (see Chapter 5).

LONG-TERM OUTCOME OF CHILDREN WITH ADHD

For many years it was assumed, particularly by members of the lay community, that children with ADHD would "outgrow" their behavior control difficulties upon reaching adolescence or early adulthood. Unfortunately, this assumption has not been borne out by longitudinal investigations of the disorder (see Weiss & Hechtman, 1993). As children with ADHD progress into their teenage years, the *absolute* frequency and intensity of their symptoms decline (Barkley, 1998). That is, they improve with respect to attention, impulsivity, and especially overactivity as compared to their own behavior during preschool and elementary school years. Of course, their peers are exhibiting similar improvements in behavior control, thereby contributing to an ongoing discrepancy between adolescents with ADHD and their classmates. In fact, 70–85% of children with ADHD will continue to exhibit significant deficits in inattention and impulsivity *relative* to their age-mates during their adolescence (Barkley, Fischer, et al., 1990; Biederman et al., 1996).

In addition to continued ADHD symptomatology, teenagers with ADHD display adjustment problems in a variety of areas of functioning. First, over 60% of adolescents with this disorder have been found to exhibit frequent defiance and noncompliance with authority figures and rules (Barkley, Fischer, et al., 1990; Biederman et al., 1997). Furthermore, more than 40% of teens with ADHD display significant antisocial behaviors such as physical fighting, stealing, and vandalism (Barkley, Fischer, et al., 1990; Gittelman et al., 1985). When compared to their non-ADHD classmates, adolescents with this disorder are at higher risk for grade retentions, school suspensions, dropping out of school, and substance abuse. The risk for drug use seems to be attributable to the presence of significant conduct problems in addition to ADHD-related behaviors (Biederman et al., 1997; Gittelman et al., 1985). Thus, for a large percentage of children with ADHD, it is unrealistic to assume that they will "outgrow" experiencing problems in daily living simply as a function of maturation.

Several prospective longitudinal investigations have followed children with ADHD into young adulthood (i.e., 18–25 years old). In general, these have found that over 50% of children with ADHD will continue to evidence symptoms of the disorder, especially with respect to inattention and impulsivity, into adulthood, especially when parent report rather than self-report data are used (Barkley, Fischer, Smallish, & Fletcher, 2002). Problems of academic achievement and antisocial behavior that were noted for adolescents with this disorder continue to be the highest risks for this group in adulthood. Almost a third of these adults will have dropped out of high school, with only 5% completing a university degree program as compared to over 40% of control group subjects (Barkley, Fischer, et al., 1990). Approximately 25% or more of these children will develop chronic patterns of antisocial behavior that persist into adulthood and that are associated with other adjustment problems (e.g., substance abuse, interpersonal difficulties, occupational instability). Older adolescents and young adults with ADHD are more likely than their non-ADHD counterparts to receive speeding tickets and to experience car accidents as the driver (Barkley, Guevremont, Anastopoulos, DuPaul, & Shelton, 1993; Barkley, Murphy, DuPaul, & Bush, 2002). On a positive note, approximately one-third of children followed into adulthood are seen as symptom-free and relatively well adjusted (Barkley, 1998). Yet this childhood disorder carries risks for long-term outcome that are quite high relative to the non-ADHD population.

Investigators have searched for childhood variables that can reliably predict the adolescent and adult outcomes of individuals with ADHD. Minimal specific predictors have been identified beyond those variables (e.g., intelligence test scores, socioeconomic status) that are predictive of outcome for the general population. Nevertheless, there are two classes of predictors that are noteworthy for practitioners to consider in their work. First, an early onset of antisocial behaviors, especially lying, stealing, and fighting, is predictive of later antisocial outcome and perhaps continued ADHD (Barkley, 1998; Biederman et al., 1996). *Early onset* is defined as prior to the ages of 8–10 years old. Second, being rejected by one's peers in childhood is predictive of continued interpersonal adjustment problems in later years (Barkley, 1998; Parker & Asher, 1987). Therefore, at the present time, the combination of the child's cognitive ability, the child's level of aggressiveness and peer rejection, family stability, psychosocial adversity, and childrearing practices represents the best predictive scheme (Barkley, 1998; Biederman et al., 1996).

Given the protracted nature of the disorder and the attendant long-term risks for a large percentage of children with ADHD, there is an emerging consensus that multiple treatment modalities are necessary throughout a child's school-age years (Barkley, 1998). Thus, rather than attempting to "cure" the disorder, school professionals and parents should help children "compensate" for their behavior control problems. Furthermore, it is assumed that ADHD is a disorder that lies at the interface of a child's biology (e.g., genetic differences in neurotransmitter functioning) and the environment (i.e., situational factors) wherein a child is predisposed to engage in higher frequencies of disinhibited and highly active behavior relative to peers, especially under certain environmental circumstances. Therefore, treatment may entail modifications to school and home environments as well as attempts to change within-child variables through the use of psychostimulant medication. With these perspectives in mind, our emphasis throughout this book is to promote methods to create and maintain "prosthetic environments" (Barkley, 1998) that allow children with ADHD to succeed academically, emotionally, and socially. To achieve these outcomes a concerted effort must be made by school professionals, parents, and other health practitioners over the course of multiple school years.

OVERVIEW OF SUBSEQUENT CHAPTERS

The purpose of this book is to provide school-based professionals with a guide to the assessment and treatment of students with ADHD. An attempt has been made to identify evaluation and intervention techniques that have a sound empirical basis and are practical for real-world application. In this second edition of our text, we have updated and expanded our coverage of assessment and intervention strategies that can be effectively used in school settings across the developmental spectrum.

A model for the school-based screening and assessment of ADHD is presented in Chapter 2. It is proposed that the evaluation of students who might exhibit ADHD-related behaviors involves the use of multiple assessment techniques across home and school settings. The purpose of assessment is not simply to arrive at a diagnosis, but, more importantly, to guide the development of an effective treatment plan. The use of functional behavioral assessment is particularly critical in making the connection between evaluation and treatment.

The relationship between ADHD and academic performance difficulties is examined in detail in Chapter 3. Although ADHD is not a learning disability per se, a significant minority of children with attention and behavior control problems display academic skills deficits. It is unclear whether ADHD "causes" academic skills deficiencies or vice versa. However, it is more likely that these disorders are simply correlated rather than one causing the other. Suggestions are offered for making special education eligibility decisions for students with ADHD.

ADHD is a disorder with an early onset, with symptoms typically exhibited prior to the age of 7. Thus, in Chapter 4, we outline methods for identifying young children who might be at risk for ADHD as well as strategies to minimize the severity of associated disruptive behaviors (e.g., aggression and defiance) and to promote early school success. Given that ADHD can be chronic and is associated with poor school outcomes, early identification and intervention may be critical in enhancing the long-term success of children with this disorder.

One of the most effective intervention approaches for ADHD is the manipulation of antecedent and consequent events in the classroom environment. In Chapter 5, behaviorally based methods that have been found to enhance behavior control, academic performance, and social behavior are described. We propose a data-based, problem-solving model for the development of academic and behavioral interventions that can be implemented with integrity, particularly in elementary school settings. The important connection between data derived from functional and curriculum-based assessments and intervention design is emphasized in the discussion of these techniques.

The most widely studied and cost-effective treatment for ADHD is the prescription of psychostimulant medications such as Ritalin (methylphenidate). These medications can lead to improvements in on-task behavior, impulsivity, social behavior, compliance, and academic productivity in as many as 70–80% of children with ADHD. Descriptions of the specific medications (including nonstimulants), behavioral effects, side effects, and dose–response factors are provided in Chapter 6. Furthermore, methods for school-based practitioners to aid physicians in evaluating medication response are delineated.

Multiple interventions across settings frequently are necessary to ameliorate ADHD symptomatology. Thus, medication and classroom-based behavioral interventions may be supplemented by social skills training, parent training, and/or behavioral family therapy. These treatments are described in Chapter 7. Furthermore, suggestions are provided on how to advise parents regarding "treatments" for ADHD that have minimal or lack empirical support (e.g., electroencephalogram [EEG] biofeedback training).

A team approach to treatment of ADHD is crucial to successful outcome. Communication among professionals and parents is discussed in detail in Chapter 8. All too often miscommunication between school and home or school-based professionals and community-based professionals (e.g., physicians) results in inefficient service delivery. Methods to foster appropriate communication among treatment team members are delineated in this chapter as well.

Potential future directions for school-based programming and research on ADHD are discussed in Chapter 9. Greater attention to direct instruction in study and organization skills and vocational counseling/programming is clearly needed for children with this disorder. The suggestions offered in this book are merely a starting point with an obvious need to develop school-based strategies that lead to more successful outcomes for students exhibiting ADHD-related difficulties.

CHAPTER 2

♦ ♦ ♦

Assessment of ADHD
in School Settings

♦

Multiple assessment techniques typically are employed across home and school settings in the comprehensive evaluation of children who may have ADHD (American Academy of Pediatrics, 2000; Barkley, 1998; National Institutes of Health, 1998). Although the diagnostic criteria for this disorder have been developed and published primarily by physicians (i.e., American Psychiatric Association, 2000), school professionals must be knowledgeable regarding appropriate evaluation procedures for a number of reasons. First, problems with attention and behavioral control are two of the most common reasons for referral to school and clinical child psychologists. Thus, school psychologists must be in a position to conduct an assessment of ADHD themselves, or, at least, to be cognizant of community-based professionals who could provide an appropriate evaluation. Second, school psychologists have direct access to sources of information and data (e.g., teachers, observations of child behavior in natural settings) crucial to the differential diagnosis of ADHD. Third, ADHD is prevalent among certain populations (e.g., children with learning disabilities) frequently served by school psychologists (Barkley, 1998). Finally, children with ADHD may be eligible for special education services under the "other health impairment" category of the 1997 federal Individuals with Disabilities Education Act (see Hakola, 1992). Thus, school psychologists will be called upon to help determine whether referred children are eligible for such services under this category.

The purpose of the present chapter is to describe a school-based assessment approach in the evaluation of ADHD that incorporates those techniques having the greatest empirical support in the literature.[1] Proper use of this evaluation methodology assumes that the professional conducting the assessment will have received appropriate training in the use of the DSM-IV (American Psychiatric Association, 1994) classification system as well as in clinical assessment techniques. First, the DSM-IV criteria for ADHD is reviewed in the context of a school-based assessment paradigm and its limitations for this purpose are delineated. Second, a behavioral assessment approach to the evaluation of ADHD is described, one that incorporates multiple sources of data collected across school and home settings. Finally, the specific steps of the assessment process are detailed in the context of an educational decision-making paradigm based on the model proposed by Salvia and Ysseldyke (1998). The stages of the ADHD evaluation described include screening, multimethod assessment, interpretation of obtained results to reach a diagnostic decision, development of a treatment plan based on assessment data, and ongoing evaluation of the success of the intervention program.

THE USE OF DIAGNOSTIC CRITERIA IN THE SCHOOL-BASED ASSESSMENT OF ADHD

Current Definition of ADHD

ADHD has been defined and conceptualized in a variety of ways over the past several decades, thus leading to confusion among professionals regarding proper diagnosis and evaluation procedures (Barkley, 1998). More recently, there is an emerging consensus that ADHD is characterized by the display of developmentally inappropriate frequencies of inattention and/or hyperactivity–impulsivity (American Psychiatric Association, 2000). These two dimensions of behaviors lead to impairment in functioning wherein the child with ADHD demonstrates difficulties with delaying responding to the environment, developing self-control, and maintaining consistent work performance over the course of time (American Psychiatric Association, 2000; Barkley, 1998).

The behaviors, or "symptoms," comprising ADHD according to DSM-IV criteria (American Psychiatric Association, 2000) are listed in

---

[1]For a demonstration of the use of our assessment model, readers should consult the video, *Assessing ADHD in the Schools* (DuPaul & Stoner, 1999a).

Table 2.1. To be considered symptoms of ADHD, the behaviors must have been initially exhibited early in childhood (i.e., prior to age 7) and must be chronically displayed across two or more settings (American Psychiatric Association, 2000). A child must be reported to exhibit at least six of the nine inattention symptoms and/or at least six of the nine hyperactive–impulsive behaviors. The ADHD diagnosis is usually determined by establishing the developmental deviance and pervasiveness of symptoms. At the same time, it is equally important to rule out alterna-

---

TABLE 2.1. DSM-IV Symptoms of Attention-Deficit/Hyperactivity Disorder

Inattention symptoms

(1) six (or more) of the following symptoms of **inattention** have persisted for at least 6 months to a degree that is maladaptive and inconsistent with developmental level:
   (a) often fails to give close attention to details or makes careless mistakes in schoolwork, work, or other activities
   (b) often has difficulty sustaining attention in tasks or play activities
   (c) often does not seem to listen when spoken to directly
   (d) often does not follow through on instructions and fails to finish schoolwork, chores, or duties in the workplace (not due to oppositional behavior or failure to understand instructions)
   (e) often has difficulty organizing tasks and activities
   (f) often avoids, dislikes, or is reluctant to engage in tasks that require sustained mental effort (such as schoolwork or homework)
   (g) often loses things necessary for tasks or activities (e.g., toys, school assignments, pencils, books, or tools)
   (h) is often easily distracted by extraneous stimuli
   (i) is often forgetful in daily activities

Hyperactivity–impulsivity symptoms

(2) six (or more) of the following symptoms of **hyperactivity–impulsivity** have persisted for at least 6 months to a degree that is maladaptive and inconsistent with developmental level:
   (a) often fidgets with hands or feet or squirms in seat
   (b) often leaves seat in classroom or in other situations in which remaining seated is expected
   (c) often runs about or climbs excessively in situations in which it is inappropriate (in adolescents or adults, may be limited to subjective feelings of restlessness)
   (d) often has difficulty playing or engaging in leisure activities quietly
   (e) is often "on the go" or often acts as if "driven by a motor"
   (f) often talks excessively
   (g) often blurts out answers to questions before the questions have been completed
   (h) often has difficulty awaiting turn
   (i) often interrupts or intrudes on others (e.g., butts into conversations or games)

Note. From American Psychiatric Association (1994). Copyright 1994 by the American Psychiatric Association. Reprinted by permission.

tive causes for the child's inattention, impulsivity, and motor restlessness. These may include poor academic instruction and management practices; gross neurological, sensory, motor, or language impairment; mental retardation; or severe emotional disturbance (Barkley, 1998).

There are three subtypes of ADHD. The combined type describes children who exhibit at least six inattention and at least six hyperactive–impulsive symptoms. This is the "classic" variant of ADHD that has been studied widely in the literature and is the most problematic subtype. ADHD predominantly inattentive type (previous terms have included "undifferentiated attention deficit disorder" and "attention deficit disorder without hyperactivity") is diagnosed in those children exhibiting at least six of the nine inattention symptoms and *no more than* five of the hyperactive–impulsive behaviors. Finally, ADHD predominantly hyperactive–impulsive type is diagnosed for those children who display at least six of the nine hyperactive–impulsive symptoms but less than six inattention symptoms. Very little is known about this subtype other than that it may be more prevalent among young children who appear to be at risk for later development of the combined type (Lahey et al., 1994). Furthermore, young children under age 6 may not have had sufficient opportunity to display inattentive symptoms, and therefore may fall into the hyperactive–impulsive group.

Advantages of the DSM Approach

Although the diagnostic criteria for ADHD have been developed in the context of a medical model for child behavior problems, there are several reasons why these criteria are useful in educational settings. First, the symptom list describes a set of problem behaviors that reliably covary in some children. The diagnosis (i.e., constellation of covarying behaviors) can be used to predict the relative success of possible interventions, to predict the risk for concurrent or future behavioral difficulties, and to suggest possible controlling variables (Barlow, 1981). Second, the use of DSM criteria structures the assessment in a standardized fashion, thus potentially increasing interprofessional agreement regarding diagnostic status. Third, such criteria guide the selection of competing hypotheses (i.e., other disorders or problems) that could potentially account for apparent symptoms of ADHD. Conclusions based on differential diagnosis may increase the chances of planning a successful intervention program in the classroom. For instance, if a child's attention problems were related to an anxiety disorder as opposed to ADHD, initial treatment strategies would be quite different.

Fourth, another advantage of the use of DSM criteria in the assessment protocol is that discussions of these symptom lists may indicate which problem behaviors should serve as targets for intervention. For example, those symptoms that are most frequently endorsed or are deemed most important by parents and teachers might become the initial focus of treatment. Fifth, incorporating agreed-upon diagnostic criteria into the evaluation (i.e., using a common language) will ultimately enhance communication with other mental health (e.g., clinical child psychologists) or medical professionals regarding the child's psychological status, thus fostering a team approach to treatment.

Limitations of the DSM Approach

Although DSM criteria are important components of the evaluation process, several limitations of this approach must be considered. First, the criteria for ADHD were developed in the context of a medical model, thus implying that the location of the "problem" is within the child. The characterization of the child as having a disorder could diminish attempts to assess environmental variables that may play a role in causing or maintaining the problem behaviors. Second, the use of a psychiatric classification system promotes a search for pathology that could, under certain conditions, result in overidentification of children with behavior disorders (i.e., identification of "false positives"). These circumstances suggest the need for a multimethod assessment approach wherein objective measures (e.g., behavioral observations) supplement the use of more subjective assessment techniques, such as a diagnostic interview (Achenbach & McConaughy, 1996). Third, the use of a psychiatric classification system and the resulting receipt of a diagnostic label may compromise a child's self-esteem if others come to view him or her as "disordered." Although frequently a topic of professional discussion, the possible iatrogenic effects of being diagnosed with ADHD have not been empirically investigated to date. A fourth important limitation of the DSM approach is that the psychometric properties (e.g., reliability, validity) of the various diagnostic criteria are not well established (Gresham & Gansle, 1992).

A number of skills are necessary to ensure the proper use of the DSM classification paradigm (adapted from Barlow, 1981). First, the school psychologist should have enough familiarity with child psychopathology to know which problem behaviors typically covary (e.g., inattention, impulsivity, and overactivity). Second, a working knowledge of current DSM criteria for most childhood disorders, not just ADHD, is necessary. This requires not only familiarity with symptom lists, but also criteria with respect to age of onset and minimum duration of problem behaviors. Finally, the psychologist must have had training in the use of a comprehensive assessment protocol to determine which symptoms are present in a specific student's repertoire.

ADHD is best viewed as a result of a "poor fit" between the biological endowment and characteristics of the child and the environment, such as the structure and prevailing contingencies in the classroom. In this context, diagnostic criteria provide suggestions about problem behavior covariation, controlling variables, and effective interventions based on what is known about ADHD in general (Barlow, 1981). Therefore, discussions of DSM criteria are supplemented with multiple assessment methods conducted across settings to determine the specific problem behaviors, controlling variables, and possible intervention strategies that are applicable for an individual student. The diagnosis of ADHD is but one step in the process of designing and evaluating interventions to promote greater classroom success.

OVERVIEW OF ASSESSMENT METHODS

Typically, a behavioral assessment approach is employed in the evaluation of ADHD wherein multiple methods of data collection are utilized across informants and settings (see Anastopoulos & Shelton, 2001; Barkley, 1998). In particular, emphasis is placed upon obtaining reliable information regarding a child's behavior from parents and teachers as well as from firsthand observations of student performance. Therefore, the major components of the evaluation include interviews with the child's parent(s) and teacher(s), questionnaires completed by parents and teachers, and observations of child behavior across multiple settings and under varied task conditions. Although many of these same procedures are used when evaluating adolescents, some modifications (e.g., inclusion of self-report measures) are necessary to maintain the reliability and validity of the assessment data (see "Developmental Considerations" section, below).

Each evaluation technique will be discussed in detail in the context of the stages of the assessment process in the next section. Interviews with the parent(s), teacher(s), and child are conducted to determine the presence or absence of various DSM symptoms as well as to identify historical and/or current factors possibly serving to maintain identified problem behaviors. Behavior rating scales completed by the student's parent(s) and teacher(s) provide data that establish the severity of ADHD-related behaviors relative to a normative sample. To supplement parent and teacher report, several direct measures of student behavior are used. The child's behavior is observed across settings (e.g., classroom and playground) on several occasions to establish the frequency and/or duration of various target behaviors. Behavioral frequencies are usually compared to those displayed by several of the student's classmates to determine the deviance of the referred child's behavior. Finally, the products of the child's behavior (e.g., academic productivity and accuracy, quality of desk organization) can be collected and/or examined. Although each of these techniques is limited in some manner, when used in a multimodal assessment package a system of "checks and balances" develops such that the drawbacks of any single measure are balanced by data obtained through other means (Anastopoulos & Shelton, 2001; Barkley, 1998).

Several assessment techniques typically employed by school psychologists have limited utility in the diagnostic evaluation of ADHD. Typically, the results of cognitive, neuropsychological, and educational tests are not helpful in determining whether a child has ADHD or not. To date, no individually administered test or group of tests has demonstrated an acceptable degree of ecological validity to be helpful in the diagnostic process (Barkley, 1991). For example, the test most frequently employed by school psychologists (i.e., Wechsler Intelligence Scale for Children–III [WISC-III]) has not been found to reliably discriminate children with ADHD from normal children or students with learning disabilities (Barkley, DuPaul, & McMurray, 1990). More importantly, scores on the Freedom from Distractiblity factor (i.e., Arithmetic, Digit Span, and Coding subtests) of the WISC-III are not reliable diagnostic indicators of ADHD (Anastopoulos, Spisto, & Maher, 1994). Poor performance on this factor may be due to a variety of possible causes, including performance anxiety. Furthermore, children with ADHD often display appropriate levels of attention and behavioral control under task conditions that are highly structured and involve one-to-one interaction with a novel adult, as is typically found in most testing situations (Barkley, 1998). Thus, although individually administered tests may be helpful in determining the child's intellectual and educational status, they are not necessary components of the diagnostic evaluation of ADHD.

Standardized measures of sustained attention and impulse control have been incorporated routinely into the diagnostic evaluation of ADHD (Anastopoulos & Shelton, 2001; Barkley, 1998). Purportedly, these tests provide objective data that are less influenced by factors (e.g., parental psychopathology) that may bias parent and teacher reports (Gordon, 1986). One of the more popular standardized measures is the Continuous Performance Test (CPT; Rosvold, Mirsky, Sarason, Bransome, & Beck, 1956) and its variants, including the Gordon Vigilance Task (Gordon, 1983) and the Conners Continuous Performance Test (Conners, 1995).

Although scores on CPTs appear to discriminate between children with ADHD and their normal counterparts at a *group* level, the utility of these measures in assessing *individual* children is limited by several factors. First, several investigations have failed to obtain significant correlations between criterion measures (e.g., teacher ratings) and scores on various CPTs (Halperin, Sharma, Greenblatt, & Schwartz, 1991; Lovejoy & Rasmussen, 1990). Second, when the effects of age, sex, and receptive vocabulary skills are partialled-out, scores on these measures have failed to discriminate among children with ADHD, children with conduct disorder, children with anxiety disorder, and their normal peers (Werry, Elkind, & Reeves, 1987). Even when significant correlations are obtained between CPT scores and criterion measures, these typically are of low magnitude (i.e., between absolute values of .21 to .50), suggesting that the results of clinic-based tasks account for minimal variance of criterion indices (Barkley, 1991). Furthermore, CPT scores, either alone or in combination, have been found to result in classification decisions that are frequently discrepant with a diagnosis of ADHD based on parent interview and behavior rating scale data (DuPaul, Anastopoulos, Shelton, Guevremont, & Metevia, 1992). Finally, even when clinically significant scores are obtained on CPTs, the degree to which these scores are specific to ADHD and aid in differential diagnosis is questionable (e.g., McGee, Clark, & Symons, 2000). Therefore, the most prudent conclusion, at present, is that the use of laboratory-based instruments in the evaluation of ADHD is limited by rather suspect ecological validity (Anastopoulos & Shelton, 2001; Rapport, Chung, Shore, Denney, & Isaacs, 2000).

Measures that typically are used by school psychologists to assess a student's emotional functioning are not useful in evaluating whether a child has ADHD. Projective techniques, such as the Thematic Apperception Test (Murray, 1943) or the Kinetic Family Drawing (Hammer, 1975), are based on a theoretical assumption that problem behaviors are caused by underlying emotional difficulties. This assumption has no empirical support, at least in relation to the behaviors comprising ADHD. Furthermore, projective tests have been criticized for their questionable levels of reliability and validity (Gregory, 1996)

Self-report questionnaires completed by children and adolescents have become increasingly popular in recent years (e.g., Conners et al., 1997). A number of psychometrically sound self-report checklists are available, including the Youth Self-Report (Achenbach, 1991a), the Youth Inventory–4 (Gadow et al., 2002), and the Conners–Wells Adolescent Self-Report of Symptoms (Conners et al., 1997). Although there have been long-standing concerns that children with disruptive behavior disorders are typically poor reporters of their own behavior (Landau,

Milich, & Widiger, 1991), growing evidence suggests adolescents with behavior disorders may be able to provide information that may aid in both diagnostic (Conners et al., 1997) and treatment (Smith, Pelham, Gnagy, Molina, & Evans, 2000) decisions. Also, self-report data are important to collect when evaluating adolescents who may be diagnosed with ADHD to allow assessment of covert areas of functioning (e.g., depressive symptoms) and to engender student cooperation with the evaluation and treatment process (see "Developmental Considerations" section, below).

STAGES OF ASSESSMENT OF ADHD

Following a teacher referral for attention and behavior control difficulties, the school-based evaluation of ADHD is conducted in five stages (DuPaul, 1992; see Figure 2.1). These stages are based on the educational decision-making model proposed by Salvia and Ysseldyke (1998). First, teacher ratings are obtained and a brief interview is conducted with the teacher to screen for the severity and frequency of possible ADHD symptoms. Second, if the findings of this screening are significant, then multiple assessment methods are used across sources and settings to document the child's functioning across a number of areas. Third, the evaluation results are interpreted such that classification and diagnostic decisions can be made. Fourth, a treatment plan is developed based on the obtained assessment data. Fifth, the child's school behavior and academic performance are assessed on an ongoing basis to determine the success of and the need for changes in the intervention program.

These stages of assessment are discussed in detail below. Initially, for each phase of the assessment, a series of questions to be addressed are identified, based in part on guidelines for behavioral assessment provided by Barrios and Hartmann (1986). Next, the process of assessment during each stage of the evaluation is delineated. Finally, the manner in which specific techniques are used to answer the assessment questions at each phase of the evaluation is reviewed.

Stage I: Screening

Questions to Be Addressed

The screening process is designed to answer the following questions:

1. Does this student have a problem related to possible ADHD?
2. Is further assessment of ADHD required?

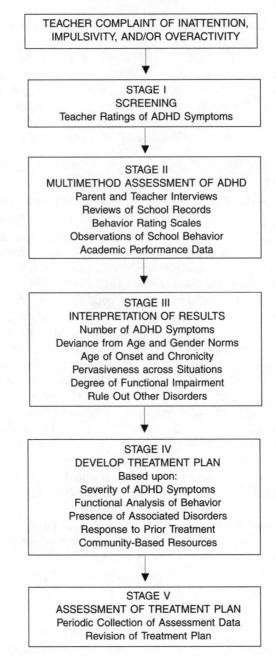

FIGURE 2.1. Five stages of the school-based assessment of attention-deficit/ hyperactivity disorder.

Screening Process

Screening for possible ADHD should be conducted whenever a teacher seeks assistance due to a student's difficulties paying attention during instruction, inconsistent completion of independent tasks, inability to remain seated at appropriate times, or display of impulsive disruptive behavior. A brief interview with the teacher is conducted to specify the behavioral concerns and to identify environmental factors that may be eliciting and/or maintaining the child's problem behaviors. Teacher ratings of the frequency of ADHD symptoms are then obtained.

Screening Techniques

The initial interview with the teacher should address the frequency, intensity, and/or duration of specific problem behaviors. The role of various environmental factors (e.g., task parameters, method of instruction, behaviors of classmates) also should be explored to establish antecedent and consequent events for the problem behaviors. To establish whether the problem behaviors may be related to ADHD, both the presence or absence of the 18 DSM-IV symptoms of this disorder should be determined, as should the chronicity of the apparent ADHD-related behaviors. If six or more inattention symptoms and/or six or more hyperactive–impulsive symptoms are reported to occur frequently, then further assessment of ADHD is warranted. Even if fewer than six symptoms in each dimension are reported, further assessment of ADHD may be warranted, especially for students at the secondary level.

The most efficient screening method is for the teacher to complete the ADHD Rating Scale–IV (DuPaul, Power, Anastopoulos, & Reid, 1998) regarding the child's typical behavior over the course of the school year. The teacher indicates on a 4-point Likert scale the frequency of the 18 behavioral symptoms of ADHD directly adapted from the DSM-IV (American Psychiatric Association, 1994). As with the teacher interview, if six or more of the items in either the inattention or hyperactivity–impulsivity domains are rated as occurring "pretty much" or "very much" of the time, then further assessment of possible ADHD is warranted. If a lesser number of items is endorsed in this frequency range, this does not rule out further assessment of ADHD but does necessitate strong consideration of other explanations (e.g., learning disabilities) for teacher concerns.

Stage II: Multimethod Assessment of ADHD

Questions to Be Addressed

Data from multiple assessment techniques are gathered to answer the following questions:

1. What is the extent and nature of the ADHD-related problems?
2. What environmental factors maintain these problems?
3. What are the frequency, duration, and/or intensity of the problem behaviors?
4. In what settings do the ADHD-related behaviors occur and for how long have these been exhibited?

Assessment Process

If the initial screening results are indicative of possible ADHD, then a more comprehensive evaluation of the child's overall functioning is warranted. Initially, the child's parent(s) and teacher(s) are interviewed to specify problem behaviors, to identify possible antecedent and consequent events for these behaviors, and to explore the causal role of various historical variables. A review of archival data (e.g., school records) is completed to provide additional historical data. Thus, the initial phase of the evaluation process is designed to identify specific problem behaviors, environmental factors, and historical variables that require further assessment.

The student's parent(s) and teacher(s) complete several questionnaires to provide more specific data regarding the frequency and/or severity of problem behaviors. These ratings help to establish the developmental deviance of ADHD-related behaviors relative to normative data, as well as to identify whether such behaviors are evident across settings and caretakers. The specific questionnaires utilized will vary as a function of the target behaviors to be assessed and the age of the child, as discussed below.

The final phase of the formal evaluation of ADHD is comprised of direct observations of child behavior across settings and the collection of academic performance data. These techniques can provide crucial information regarding the frequency and duration of target behaviors, whether specific antecedent and consequent events serve to elicit or maintain the problem behaviors, and the degree to which the ADHD-related behaviors compromise the child's social and academic functioning. From an intervention design perspective, the most critical activity is to gather data in the context of a functional behavioral assessment (DuPaul & Ervin, 1996).

Assessment Techniques

Teacher Interview. The teacher should be asked to describe the student's difficulties in specific behavioral terms in the context of a problem identification interview as described by Bergan and Kratochwill (1990).

Furthermore, the current DSM diagnostic criteria for a variety of child behavior disorders should be reviewed with the teacher. In addition to ADHD, the presence or absence of behaviors associated with oppositional defiant disorder, conduct disorder, generalized anxiety disorder, separation anxiety disorder, and depression should be ascertained. It is important to review this set of problems for two reasons. First, apparent symptoms of ADHD may actually be manifestations of another disorder. For instance, a child who is depressed may exhibit problems with concentration. Thus, the diagnosis of ADHD is arrived at by ruling out competing hypotheses (i.e., disorders) for the problem behaviors. A second reason to review these diagnostic criteria is that many children with ADHD also exhibit symptoms of other disorders. The most frequent associated diagnosis is oppositional defiant disorder; approximately 40–65% of children with ADHD exhibit symptoms of this disorder (Barkley, 1998). Furthermore, the combination of ADHD and other behavior or emotional disorders implicates the need for multiple interventions, as discussed below.

While ascertaining the presence or absence of each of the behavioral symptoms, the teacher also is asked to provide specific examples of those behaviors indicated to be present as well as to estimate their frequency. The typical antecedent (e.g., type of instruction) and consequent (e.g., teacher response to child misbehavior) events surrounding each problematic behavior should also be identified because these may be serving to maintain and/or exacerbate behavioral difficulties. Current management techniques and their relative degree of success then should be discussed.

It is imperative that information regarding the quality of the child's academic performance and social status be gathered. Some children with ADHD may exhibit significant academic skills deficits beyond task completion difficulties. Of course, an academic skills assessment (e.g., curriculum-based measurement) would be warranted in such situations. Teacher observations regarding the child's social interaction style and acceptance by peers are helpful in determining whether further assessment (e.g., sociometrics) in this area is necessary. Many children with ADHD will exhibit a controlling, aggressive interaction pattern with others, resulting in low acceptance or overt rejection by their classmates (Stormont, 2001). Teacher interview data are used to identify possible social skills deficits that could be targeted for further assessment and intervention as well as to delineate those settings and/or times of the school day where social relationship difficulties are most likely to be exhibited.

Review of School Record. The student's school record should be reviewed to obtain data that may be helpful in pinpointing the onset and course of classroom ADHD-related difficulties. For instance, teachers often grade the quality of a child's work habits and conduct on report cards. Not surprisingly, most students with ADHD are found to obtain below-average rankings in these areas across grade levels. These below-average grades are often supplemented with teacher comments regarding poor task completion, high degrees of restlessness, or frequent talking to peers without permission. The specific grade level where such grades and comments first appear is important to note so that it can be cross-referenced with the age of onset of ADHD as reported by the parents.

A more structured approach to reviewing school records is provided by the School Archival Records Search (SARS; Walker, Block-Pedego, Todis, & Severson, 1998). The SARS provides a standardized format for gathering information regarding 11 variables that are predictive of behavior disorders and/or school dropout. Variables include number of different schools attended, days absent, low achievement, grades retained, academic/behavioral referrals, current individualized education plan, nonregular classroom placement, receiving Chapter 1 supplemental instruction, referral for outside services, negative narrative comments, and school discipline contacts. These individual variables load on to three factors, Disruption, Needs Assistance, and Low Achievement. Walker and colleagues (1998) have established cutpoints for each individual variable and factor score that are predictive of school difficulties. As might be expected, children with behavior disorders (presumably including ADHD) are more likely to receive positive scores (i.e., below established cutpoints) for Disruption and Low Achievement. The primary advantage of the SARS is that it pinpoints key predictor variables in a standardized structured fashion, thereby providing a reliable account of a student's past academic and behavioral history.

Parent Interview. A brief (i.e., 30–45 minutes) interview with the student's parent(s) should be conducted either in person or by telephone. Although discussion of the child's past and current functioning across a variety of areas (e.g., medical history) is possible, the most important lines of questioning are as follows. First, the presence and frequency of behavior control difficulties at home should be identified. This is best accomplished by reviewing the current DSM diagnostic criteria for ADHD and related disruptive behavior disorders (oppositional defiant disorder, conduct disorder) with the parent. In addition, the presence of symptoms associated with internalizing disorders (e.g., anxiety disorders) that could be causally related to a child's inattention and overactivity should be identified. As with the teacher interview, a review of DSM criteria will aid in ruling out the presence of other disorders that may be causally related to the exhibition of ADHD symptoms.

A second area of discussion for the parent interview is information regarding the child's early childhood development. It is important to pinpoint the onset of the ADHD-related behaviors as well as to gather information about their chronicity over time. The early childhood behavior of children with ADHD typically is characterized as highly active and difficult to control (DuPaul, McGoey, Eckert, & VanBrakle, 2001). In some cases, however, the child's behavior is not seen as problematic until school entry, when independent task demands increase. This is particularly the case when the parents have little previous experience with children (e.g., the child being assessed is an only or oldest child) and/or have unrealistic expectations regarding child behavior.

A third area of investigation is the child's family history of behavioral, emotional, and learning problems. Although this may be uncomfortable for a parent and professionals to discuss, it is important for two reasons. First, research indicates that ADHD may have a genetic or familial component (Faraone, 2000), and thus tends to run in families. The presence of ADHD in the family increases the odds that the identified child has ADHD as well. Second, in 27–32% of cases, the child's mother may be depressed or have a history of depression (Biederman et al., 1987). There also is a greater incidence of paternal antisocial behavior in the families of children with ADHD (Lahey et al., 1988). The presence of such difficulties in the family has direct implications for treatment: home-based interventions for ADHD are more likely to be successful when implemented following amelioration of parental psychopathology and problems related to family functioning. For example, depressed mothers of children with behavior disorders evidence a higher failure rate in response to training in behavior modification strategies relative to mothers who are not depressed (Patterson & Chamberlain, 1994).

Parent Ratings. One or both parents should complete several questionnaires to determine the developmental deviance of the child's ADHD-related behaviors as well as to establish the pervasiveness of problem behaviors across settings. Several general, or "broad-band," behavior rating scales with adequate normative data and sound psychometric properties (for a review, see Anastopoulos & Shelton, 2001; Barkley, 1998) can serve this purpose well. Chief among these questionnaires are the Child Behavior Checklist (CBCL; Achenbach, 1991b), the Behavior Assessment System for Children (BASC; Reynolds & Kamphaus, 1992), and the Conners Parent Rating Scale (CPRS; Conners, 1997).

Each of these behavior rating scales have specific advantages that should be considered when selecting measures. Specifically, the CBCL and the BASC contain large item pools, and hence provide wide coverage of both internalizing and externalizing disturbances. This broad coverage facilitates differential diagnosis because competing hypotheses (e.g., presence of other disorders) for the exhibition of ADHD symptoms can be explored. Because the item pool and factor structure of the parent and teacher versions of the CBCL are quite similar, cross-informant agreement can be specifically examined. This information may be invaluable given that parent and teacher agreement (i.e., about the child's cross-situational exhibition of symptoms) is important in making a diagnosis of ADHD. Alternatively, the Conners Rating Scale provides extensive coverage of externalizing symptoms while still being relatively brief. The latter scale is particularly advantageous in situations where parents may be reluctant to spend extensive time completing questionnaires.

In addition to one of the broad-band rating scales, the parent(s) should complete two "narrow-band" questionnaires containing items more specific to ADHD-related behaviors: the ADHD Rating Scale–IV and the Home Situations Questionnaire (HSQ; Barkley, 1990). The ADHD Rating Scale–IV provides information regarding the frequency of occurrence of each of the 18 symptoms of this disorder in the home setting. The number of items rated as occurring "pretty much" or "very much" of the time is tallied. Scores on the Inattention and Hyperactive–Impulsive factors can be compared to normative data to determine the developmental deviance of ADHD symptomatology (DuPaul et al., 1998). Parental responses on the HSQ allow determination of the number of home settings in which behavior problems are exhibited by the child. In addition, the severity of behavior problems within each situation is rated on a 1 (mild) to 9 (severe) Likert scale. The revised version of the HSQ (HSQ-R; DuPaul & Barkley, 1992) provides more specific information regarding the pervasiveness of attention problems across home situations. Thus, the HSQ will be helpful in determining the situational specificity and severity of conduct problems, while the HSQ-R provides data regarding these same variables for attentional difficulties, which may be particularly helpful if the child is suspected of having the inattentive subtype. For example, a child who is reported to display attentional difficulties in one or two situations may be less likely to have ADHD predominantly inattentive type than a child whose attentional difficulties are evident across many situations.

Many children with ADHD symptoms will exhibit significant difficulties with homework completion and study skills. When such problems are reported by the parents or teacher, additional assessment is necessary to determine which homework-related behaviors need to be addressed. Initially, the parent would be asked to complete either the Homework Problem Checklist (Anesko, Shoiock, Ramirez, & Levine,

1987) or the Homework Performance Questionnaire (Power, Karustis, & Habboushe, 2001). These measures provide data regarding the frequency or severity of various problems (e.g., the child denies having homework assignment, fails to complete homework) related to homework. Parent responses on these questionnaires can lead to further inquiry as to the specific problems that may be present at each step of the homework completion process.

The Impairment Rating Scale (IRS; Fabiano et al., 1999) can be used to determine the degree to which parents perceive a child's ADHD symptoms to cause impairment in functioning. The IRS contains seven items related to various areas of functioning (e.g., the child's relationships with siblings) that could be affected by ADHD symptoms.

Teacher Ratings. As is the case with parent questionnaires, there are a plethora of well-standardized, broad-band teacher rating scales available. The three most prominent of these questionnaires are the Teacher Report Form (TRF; Achenbach, 1991c), the Behavior Assessment System for Children (BASC; Reynolds & Kamphaus, 1992), the Devereux Scales of Mental Disorders (Naglieri, LeBuffe, & Pfeiffer, 1994), and the Conners Teacher Rating Scale (Conners, 1997). As mentioned above, these broad-band measures have many advantages, including a wide coverage of possible problem areas and extensive standardization samples facilitating normative comparisons by gender and age.

In conjunction with one of these broad-band rating scales, inclusion of two or more additional measures should be considered. First, if the teacher has not already done so during the screening process, a narrow-band measure of ADHD symptoms, like the ADHD Rating Scale–IV (DuPaul et al., 1998) should be used to determine the specific frequency of ADHD-related behaviors from the teacher's perspective. Second, the School Situations Questionnaire (SSQ; Barkley, 1990) and/or the School Situations Questionnaire—Revised (SSQ-R; DuPaul & Barkley, 1992) should be completed. The SSQ and the SSQ-R provide information regarding the pervasiveness across situations and severity level of conduct and attention problems, respectively.

In many cases, students referred for a diagnostic evaluation also are reported to evidence social relationship and academic performance difficulties. Thus, teacher perceptions of student functioning in these areas may need to be assessed as well. There are a number of psychometrically sound social skills questionnaires that are available, including the Social Skills Rating System (Gresham & Elliott, 1990) and the Walker–McConnell Scale of Social Competence and School Adjustment (Walker & McConnell, 1988). Where indicated, teacher ratings of social competence should be supplemented by peer ratings and/or sociometric data.

Teacher ratings of academic achievement difficulties can be obtained through use of the Academic Performance Rating Scale (DuPaul, Rapport, & Perriello, 1991) or the Academic Competency Evaluation Scale (DiPerna & Elliott, 2000). Ratings on one of the latter questionnaires may indicate the need for further assessment of academic skills deficits. Finally, a teacher version of the Impairment Rating Scale (IRS; Fabiano et al., 1999) is available to determine teacher perceptions of the degree to which ADHD symptoms impair functioning. The IRS contains six items related to potential areas of impairment of school functioning.

Direct Observations of Behavior. Interview and rating scale data are subject to a number of limitations, including the inherent biases of those answering the interview questions and completing the questionnaires (Barkley, 1998). Thus, these data should be supplemented with assessment of child behavior that is potentially less subject to such biases. Direct observation of student behavior on several occasions and across settings and situations is one of the best methods to achieve this goal. In many cases, direct observations will provide the most fruitful data when conducted during independent seatwork situations. Typically, observation sessions are 10–30 minutes in length and are repeated across several days to establish a consistent estimate of behavioral frequency. Furthermore, observations are conducted on a repeated basis in several situations (e.g., math work time, language arts instruction) in the classroom, as well as in other school settings such as the playground and cafeteria. The latter provides the opportunity to observe interactions between the referred child and his or her peers.

A number of behavior observation coding systems have been developed for use in determining the frequencies of various ADHD-related behaviors during classroom task periods (for a review, see Barkley, 1998; Platzman et al., 1992). These include the ADHD Behavior Coding System (Barkley, 1998; Barkley, Fischer, Newby, & Breen, 1988), the Hyperactive Behavior Code (Jacob, O'Leary, & Rosenblad, 1978), the Classroom Observation Code (Abikoff et al., 1977), the Behavior Observation of Students in Schools (BOSS; Shapiro, 1996), and the ADHD School Observation Code (ADHD SOC; Gadow, Sprafkin, & Nolan, 1996). Each of these systems requires observers to classify behaviors into a variety of categories (e.g., off-task, fidgets) using interval recording procedures. In our research, we use an observation system (School Hybrid Observation Code for Kids [SHOCK]) that combines aspects of the BOSS and the ADHD SOC. Appendix 2.1 includes a description of coding categories, a sample observation sheet, and a sample observation summary sheet for the SHOCK.

Platzman and colleagues (1992) reviewed the various observational methods that have been developed to aid in the assessment of ADHD. Several of their findings are noteworthy for practitioners. First, they found that observations conducted in the classroom provided data that were better at discriminating children with ADHD from controls than were observations conducted in clinic analog settings. This finding further attests to the need for school-based practitioners to be involved in ADHD evaluations. Second, three categories of behavior were found to consistently discriminate between ADHD and non-ADHD samples: off-task behavior, excessive gross motor activity, and negative vocalizations (e.g., refusal to obey commands). Thus, observation systems that include these categories of behavior are most likely to provide sensitive diagnostic data. Third, they found very few studies that included female participants. Because a smaller percentage of girls with ADHD are defiant and aggressive (Barkley, 1998), certain observation categories (e.g., negative vocalization) may be less discriminatory between girls with and without ADHD. As a result, practitioners may need to emphasize differences in off-task behavior when evaluating girls suspected of having this disorder.

Because normative data based on large representative samples are lacking for most of these observation codes, the behavior of the referred student should be compared to one or two classmates who have been identified as "typical" or "average" by the classroom teacher. In this fashion, each child would be evaluated relative to a classroom-based standard of behavior. If possible, another person (e.g., classroom aide) should simultaneously conduct these observations every so often to ensure adequate levels of interobserver reliability. Regardless of the coding system used, the two goals of this phase of the assessment process are to (1) establish the frequency of inattentive, impulsive, and/or restless behaviors relative to classmates; and (2) to obtain stable unbiased estimates of these frequencies by conducting observations on several occasions in the same classroom setting.

In addition to coding the child's behavior during task situations, it is sometimes helpful to collect supplemental observation data. For instance, teacher behaviors (e.g., prompts, reprimands, feedback) could be coded as possible antecendent and/or consequent events for child behavior (Whalen, Henker, & Dotemoto, 1981). Such data are critical to determining the function of the challenging behavior, and therefore are important for treatment planning purposes. The specific teacher or classmate behaviors to be observed might be identified in the course of the teacher interview discussed above. An example of a coding system (adapted from Saudargras & Creed, 1980) that incorporates observation of teacher behavior is included in Appendix 2.2. Usually, teacher behaviors such as positive attention and/or negative reprimands are coded on an interval recording basis simultaneously with observations of child behavior, as displayed in the sample coding form in Figure 2.2. Such recording makes it possible to determine the percentage of observation intervals where specific teacher and child behaviors have occurred contiguously. For example, one might find that teacher positive attention occurred during a very low percentage of intervals where the child was on-task, while negative reprimands from the teacher were quite frequent when the child was off-task. In such cases, it might be hypothesized that teacher attention is reinforcing off-task rather than on-task behavior. Suggestions for modifications in teacher behavior (e.g., increasing positive attention to on-task behavior) can be generated readily from observations of this type.

If social relationship difficulties are identified, then observations of the child's interpersonal behaviors should be conducted in the settings of concern. An example of an observation system that can be used to determine the frequency of specific social behaviors (e.g., aggressive, negative, and positive) in settings such as the playground and cafeteria is provided in Appendix 2.3. Another observation system that has been found useful for collecting data regarding social behaviors in lunchroom and playground settings is the ADHD SOC (Gadow et al., 1996). Typically, children with ADHD exhibit higher than average frequencies of aggressive and negative behaviors (Barkley, 1998). In most cases, their rates of positive social behavior are not substantially different from their normal counterparts (Stormont, 2001). Results of these types of observations can be used not only to document the type and severity of social relationship difficulties, but also to target specific behaviors for intervention.

Assessment of Academic Performance. Although children with ADHD usually perform within the average range on traditional, individually administered achievement tests (e.g., Barkley, DuPaul, & McMurray, 1990), their day-to-day performance on classroom tasks and homework is often inconsistent and inferior relative to that of their classmates (Barkley, 1998). It is helpful to obtain relatively direct measurements of academic behavior prior to intervention, as changes in scholastic status can be considered one of the more socially valid outcomes of treatment. Important academic behaviors to assess include the completion and accuracy of independent classwork, completion and accuracy of homework, acquisition of skills being taught in the curriculum, and organizational skills.

Completion and accuracy rates on assigned work should be calculated. First, the amount of written work (i.e., percentage of items) completed relative to the amount of work assigned (Rapport, DuPaul, Stoner, & Jones, 1986) or relative to "typical" classmates during obser-

Phase _____

Day _____

CLASSROOM INTERACTIONS
OBSERVATION SHEET

Observer _____ Rel.? Y   N

Date _____

Classroom _____

	1	2	3	4	5	6	7	8	9	10	11	12	Total A
TA/On	p n o	p n o	p n o	p n o	p n o	p n o	p n o	p n o	p n o	p n o	p n o	p n o	I I
TA/Off	p n o	p n o	p n o	p n o	p n o	p n o	p n o	p n o	p n o	p n o	p n o	p n o	I I
C/App	p n o	p n o	p n o	p n o	p n o	p n o	p n o	p n o	p n o	p n o	p n o	p n o	I I
C/Inapp	p n o	p n o	p n o	p n o	p n o	p n o	p n o	p n o	p n o	p n o	p n o	p n o	I I

	13	14	15	16	17	18	19	20	21	22	23	24	Total B
TA/On	p n o	p n o	p n o	p n o	p n o	p n o	p n o	p n o	p n o	p n o	p n o	p n o	I I
TA/Off	p n o	p n o	p n o	p n o	p n o	p n o	p n o	p n o	p n o	p n o	p n o	p n o	I I
C/App	p n o	p n o	p n o	p n o	p n o	p n o	p n o	p n o	p n o	p n o	p n o	p n o	I I
C/Inapp	p n o	p n o	p n o	p n o	p n o	p n o	p n o	p n o	p n o	p n o	p n o	p n o	I I

	25	26	27	28	29	30	31	32	33	34	35	36	Total C
TA/On	p n o	p n o	p n o	p n o	p n o	p n o	p n o	p n o	p n o	p n o	p n o	p n o	I I
TA/Off	p n o	p n o	p n o	p n o	p n o	p n o	p n o	p n o	p n o	p n o	p n o	p n o	I I
C/App	p n o	p n o	p n o	p n o	p n o	p n o	p n o	p n o	p n o	p n o	p n o	p n o	I I
C/Inapp	p n o	p n o	p n o	p n o	p n o	p n o	p n o	p n o	p n o	p n o	p n o	p n o	I I

	37	38	39	40	41	42	43	44	45	46	47	48	Total D
TA/On	p n o	p n o	p n o	p n o	p n o	p n o	p n o	p n o	p n o	p n o	p n o	p n o	I I
TA/Off	p n o	p n o	p n o	p n o	p n o	p n o	p n o	p n o	p n o	p n o	p n o	p n o	I I
C/App	p n o	p n o	p n o	p n o	p n o	p n o	p n o	p n o	p n o	p n o	p n o	p n o	I I
C/Inapp	p n o	p n o	p n o	p n o	p n o	p n o	p n o	p n o	p n o	p n o	p n o	p n o	I I

	49	50	51	52	53	54	55	56	57	58	59	60	Total E
TA/On	p n o	p n o	p n o	p n o	p n o	p n o	p n o	p n o	p n o	p n o	p n o	p n o	I I
TA/Off	p n o	p n o	p n o	p n o	p n o	p n o	p n o	p n o	p n o	p n o	p n o	p n o	I I
C/App	p n o	p n o	p n o	p n o	p n o	p n o	p n o	p n o	p n o	p n o	p n o	p n o	I I
C/Inapp	p n o	p n o	p n o	p n o	p n o	p n o	p n o	p n o	p n o	p n o	p n o	p n o	I I

	61	62	63	64	65	66	67	68	69	70	71	72	Total F
TA/On	p n o	p n o	p n o	p n o	p n o	p n o	p n o	p n o	p n o	p n o	p n o	p n o	I I
TA/Off	p n o	p n o	p n o	p n o	p n o	p n o	p n o	p n o	p n o	p n o	p n o	p n o	I I
C/App	p n o	p n o	p n o	p n o	p n o	p n o	p n o	p n o	p n o	p n o	p n o	p n o	I I
C/Inapp	p n o	p n o	p n o	p n o	p n o	p n o	p n o	p n o	p n o	p n o	p n o	p n o	I I

	73	74	75	76	77	78	79	80	Total G
TA/On	p n o	p n o	p n o	p n o	p n o	p n o	p n o	p n o	I I
TA/Off	p n o	p n o	p n o	p n o	p n o	p n o	p n o	p n o	I I
C/App	p n o	p n o	p n o	p n o	p n o	p n o	p n o	p n o	I I
C/Inapp	p n o	p n o	p n o	p n o	p n o	p n o	p n o	p n o	

Data Summary Chart

Total # of Intervals Observed: _____

	A	B	C	D	E	F	G	Total	% Int.
TA/On	I I	I I	I I	I I	I I	I I	I I	I I	I I
TA/Off	I I	I I	I I	I I	I I	I I	I I	I I	I I
C/App	I I	I I	I I	I I	I I	I I	I I	I I	I I
C/Inapp	I I	I I	I I	I I	I I	I I	I I	I I	I I

FIGURE 2.2. Sample observation coding form for recording teacher–student interactions. From *ADHD in the Schools* (2nd ed.) by George J. DuPaul and Gary Stoner. Copyright 2003 by The Guilford Press. Permission to photocopy this figure is granted to purchasers of this book for personal use only (see copyright page for details).

vation sessions should be calculated. Second, the percentage of items completed correctly (i.e., academic efficiency score; Rapport et al., 1986) is calculated to determine task accuracy. In many cases students with ADHD will complete significantly less work or complete tasks in a less accurate fashion due to their problems with inattention and/or carelessness. Such data are relatively straightforward to collect in conjunction with observations of the student's classroom behavior, discussed above. Similar data regarding homework completion and accuracy could be collected by the teacher over a short time interval (e.g., 2–3 weeks) contemporaneous with the ADHD evaluation. Parents also can be asked to record the frequency of completion of various steps in the homework process over a similar time period. Furthermore, items indicated to be problematic on the Homework Problem Checklist can be used to generate possible targets for intervention.

Brief probes of a child's acquisition of skills being taught in the curriculum (i.e., curriculum-based measurement [CBM]; Shinn, 1998) can be very helpful in at least two ways. First, CBM data can pinpoint the instructional level of a child within a given subject area. It is possible that a child's attention and behavior difficulties may result from the frustration of being asked to do academic work that is beyond the child's capabilities. Stated differently, it is possible that the child is being instructed at a *frustrational* rather than at an *instructional* level. It also could be that a child is consistently being asked to complete work that is too easy (e.g., mastery level material), resulting in attentional problems. Second, because CBM probes are relatively brief (2–3 minutes), these data can be collected periodically once instructional changes are made, thus providing valuable information regarding intervention effects.

Finally, the organization of the child's desk (i.e., neatness and preparedness) can be examined directly on a regular basis over a short time interval (e.g., 2–3 weeks) and compared to classmates' desks (Atkins, Pelham, & Licht, 1985). A frequent complaint of teachers is that children with ADHD have unorganized, messy desks, with a resultant loss of task and text materials. Here too information may be gleaned that helps to pinpoint the source(s) of a student's academic difficulties, as well as to identify potential foci for instructional support.

Stage III: Interpretation of Results (Diagnosis/Classification)

Questions to Be Addressed

Data from the multimethod assessment are used to determine the diagnostic status of the referred child by reviewing the following questions:

1. Does the child exhibit a significant number of behavioral symptoms of ADHD according to parent and teacher report?
2. Does the child exhibit ADHD symptoms at a frequency that is significantly greater than that demonstrated by children of the same gender and chronological age?
3. At what age did the child begin demonstrating significant ADHD-related behaviors, and are these behaviors chronic and evident across many situations?
4. Is the child's functioning at school, at home, and/or with peers significantly impaired?
5. Are there other possible problems (e.g., learning disabilities) or factors (e.g., teacher intolerance for active behavior) that could account for the reported display of ADHD symptoms?

Interpretation Process and Procedures

The data obtained with the previously described techniques can be used to address the above questions. Although each of the assessment techniques has limitations, the advantage of using a multimethod approach is that each of their strengths and weaknesses will be balanced out as part of the larger evaluation package. The overriding goals are to derive accurate data regarding the frequency and severity of ADHD-related behaviors across caregivers and settings, as well as to determine possible causes for these difficulties. To the extent that these goals are achieved, relative confidence can be placed in conclusions drawn as a result of the assessment. The interpretation of evaluation data is discussed relative to each of the major assessment questions.

Number of ADHD Symptoms? The number of ADHD symptoms is determined based on parent and teacher interview data in conjunction with ADHD Rating Scale–IV results. When six or more inattention symptoms or six or more hyperactive–impulsive symptoms are reported by each caregiver (particularly during the interviews), this is considered diagnostically significant for one of the three subtypes of ADHD according to DSM-IV guidelines (American Psychiatric Association, 1994). Specifically, to receive a diagnosis of ADHD combined type, the child should be reported to evidence at least six of the nine inattention symptoms *and* six of the nine hyperactive–impulsive behaviors (see Table 2.1). For a diagnosis of ADHD predominantly inattentive type, six of the nine inattention symptoms must be reported combined with a *maximum* of five hyperactive–impulsive behaviors. Finally, a diagnosis of ADHD predominantly hyperactive–impulsive type would be warranted for children who are reported to exhibit at least six hyperactive–impulsive symptoms and a *maximum* of five inattention symptoms.

Frequency of ADHD-Related Behaviors? The parent and teacher questionnaires discussed above all contain at least one factor related to ADHD (e.g., labeled "Hyperactivity," "Attention Problems," "Overactive-Restless"). When a child's score on factors related to ADHD is greater than 2 standard deviations above the mean for his or her gender and chronological age, this result is considered significant for ADHD (Barkley, 1998). Scores on these same factors that are between 1.5 and 2 standard deviations above the mean are considered to be in the borderline significant (i.e., mild) range for ADHD. Thus, children receiving scores in the upper 2–7% of ADHD symptoms for their age and gender may be identified as having ADHD (depending upon other assessment findings).

When determining whether scores are diagnostically significant, it also is important to consider the child's ethnicity. Parent and teacher ratings of ADHD symptoms may vary across ethnic groups, with African American children receiving significantly higher scores than white and Hispanic children (DuPaul et al., 1998; Reid, DuPaul, Power, Anastopoulos, & Riccio, 1998). Although ethnic group differences are partially accounted for by socioeconomic status, even when the effects of the latter are removed systematic differences remain. These group differences could potentially result in overidentification of ADHD among African American children. Thus, practitioners must be especially cautious when evaluating children from different cultural backgrounds and should rely on multiple measures when assessing ADHD symptoms. Furthermore, it is imperative to use rating scales that include normative data that are representative of the U.S. population in terms of ethnic diversity.

Behavioral observation data are used to determine the frequencies of ADHD-related behaviors displayed by the referred student as compared to his or her classmates. If a large enough sample of observations is collected, the difference in behavioral frequencies between the referred and the nonreferred students could be tested statistically using a *t*-test, for example. The child with ADHD should be exhibiting inattentive, impulsive, and/or restless behaviors at a significantly higher frequency than classmates. When similar rates of behavior are observed across referred and nonreferred students, then other lines of investigation (e.g., inadequate methods of behavior management) may need to be pursued.

Age of Onset and Chronicity of Problem Behaviors? Parent report of the onset of ADHD symptoms is obtained during the interview. Typically, the age of onset is reported to be when the child begins formal schooling (i.e., kindergarten or first grade) or earlier. The consistency of ADHD-related behaviors across grades or time can be confirmed through inspection of the child's previous report cards in the school record. The onset of ADHD symptoms should be reported to be prior to age 7 (American Psychiatric Association, 2000) and must be occurring on a daily basis for at least 1 year (Barkley, 1998). It should be noted that the age cutoff of 7 years old is not empirically based and that it may be more appropriate to use childhood onset (i.e., prior to 18 years old), as is the practice with conduct disorder (Barkley & Biederman, 1997). Longitudinal investigations consistently have found that ADHD symptoms typically begin early in life and, in many cases, are present throughout the life span (Barkley, Fischer, et al., 1990; Biederman et al., 1996).

Under some circumstances, the child's ADHD symptoms will not be problematic until the fourth or fifth grade. This may be the case when a child is bright enough to "compensate" for his or her behavior regulation difficulties during the earlier grades and encounters more problems when demands for independent task completion increase. Alternatively, students with academic problems may develop ADHD-like "symptoms" as a function of continued frustrations in educational settings. In the latter situation, a student would not be diagnosed and treated as a child with "true" ADHD, as the academic skills deficit or learning disability would be the primary focus of intervention (Barkley, 1998).

Are Problem Behaviors Occurring Across Situations? At a general level, if both the parent(s) and teacher(s) are reporting significant display of ADHD-related behaviors across home and school environments, then this criterion is met. The pervasiveness of inattentive behaviors and/or conduct problems across situations *within* home and school environments can be determined using the original and revised versions of the HSQ and the SSQ. A finding of attention or conduct problems being reported in 50% or more of identified situations is considered significant (Barkley, 1990). In addition, if scores on these rating scales are 1.5–2 standard deviations above the mean using normative data (see Barkley, 1990), a more stringent criterion is reached.

To the degree that significant ADHD-related behaviors are reported to occur across home and school settings, relative confidence can be placed in the conclusion that within-child variables (i.e., presence of ADHD) account for the behavioral control difficulties to a large degree. When inconsistencies between parent and teacher report are obtained, confidence in the diagnosis of ADHD is reduced. In general, teacher ratings are given more credence because the school is the more problematic setting for most children with ADHD and teachers have greater exposure to children within a specific age range.

Functional Impairment? The degree to which the child's academic, social, and emotional functioning is impaired is determined through examination of all of the measures discussed above. The most frequently encountered signs of impairment associated with ADHD are academic achievement below expectations for the child and poor acceptance by peers (American Psychiatric Association, 2000; Barkley, 1998). Thus, a child with ADHD would be expected to produce less complete and less accurate schoolwork than classmates based on observational data and teacher ratings. Furthermore, ratings for the child on scales of social competence and peer relationships would be below average for his or her age and gender. Observational data may confirm the latter, as the child may exhibit high rates of aggressive behavior on the playground or may be ignored by classmates during free-play periods.

Other Factors Accounting for ADHD-Like Behavior? The ADHD diagnosis is usually arrived at by establishing the developmental deviance and pervasiveness of symptoms by addressing the previous questions. At the same time, it is crucial to consider alternative causes for the child's inattention, impulsivity, and motor restlessness. One possibility is that these behaviors are secondary to the frustrations encountered due to a child's academic difficulties, as discussed above. If, for instance, the child begins to exhibit ADHD symptoms later in childhood after several years of learning difficulties or only exhibits problem behaviors during academic instruction in his or her weaker subjects, then this possibility must be entertained strongly. Alternatively, if ADHD symptoms began early in life and are pervasive across settings, then a more plausible conclusion is that the child has both ADHD and a learning disability (see Chapter 3 for additional details).

A second possibility is that the child is encountering emotional and/or adjustment difficulties that have led to inattentive, impulsive, and/or restless behaviors. If this were the case, then interview and questionnaire data would indicate significant symptoms of an alternative disorder (e.g., anxiety disorder, conduct disorder) or a difficult situation (e.g., recent parental divorce) in addition to or in lieu of ADHD symptoms. Furthermore, the symptoms of emotional disturbance would predate the onset of ADHD-related behaviors. The latter would be of relatively recent onset and would probably not be exhibited on a chronic and cross–situational basis. In the case of adjustment problems, there typically will be a clear onset of symptoms in relation to an identifiable event or set of events of importance to the child/family. The practitioner should carefully consider differential diagnostic guidelines as per the DSM-IV (also see Anastopoulos & Shelton, 2001).

Poor or inconsistent academic instruction and/or behavior management practices are other possible causes of apparent ADHD symptoms. This hypothesis should be explored whenever assessment data are inconsistent across sources and settings—for example, parents and teachers disagree about the severity and frequency of ADHD symptoms. This is particularly true when there are discrepancies among several teachers regarding the presence or absence of ADHD symptoms. If the latter are reported by a single teacher in the absence of a developmental history of ADHD-related difficulties and other data supporting the diagnosis of ADHD, then closer inspection of instructional and management variables is necessary. Rather than classifying the problem behaviors as resulting from "within-child" variables (i.e., ADHD), it may be that faulty teaching practices warrant modification.

Once a diagnostic decision is reached, the findings and resultant treatment recommendations must be communicated to the student's teachers and parents, as well as to any community-based professionals (e.g., pediatrician) who may be working with the child. Typically, a written report is generated and results and recommendations are orally reviewed with pertinent school personnel and parents. Issues and procedures related to communication of assessment results are discussed in greater detail in Chapter 8.

Stage IV: Designing the Treatment Plan

Questions to Be Addressed

The following questions should be addressed when designing an intervention program for students with ADHD:

1. What are the possible functions for the child's ADHD-related behaviors?
2. What are the student's strengths and weaknesses (e.g., motivation and skills)?
3. What are the behavioral objectives for intervention?
4. What are the optimum intervention strategies?
5. What additional resources are available to address the child's ADHD-related problems?

Intervention Planning Process and Procedures

The assessment process does not conclude with a diagnosis, for the diagnosis is just one step in the process of determining which intervention strategies are most likely to be successful. Thus, the assessment data are used to generate an appropriate treatment plan. The intervention strategies that have the greatest research support in the treatment of ADHD are the prescription of psychostimulant medication (e.g., Ritalin) and behavior modification procedures (Barkley, 1998; MTA Cooperative Group, 1999; Pelham, Wheeler, & Chronis, 1998). The specifics of these interventions are reviewed in greater detail in Chapters 5, 6, and 7; further information regarding these interventions can be obtained through several recent reviews (e.g., Barkley, 1998; Goldstein & Goldstein, 1998; Pelham et al., 1998).

Interventions for ADHD typically are designed to impact target behaviors across academic and social domains. Because ADHD symptoms are, by definition, exhibited across settings, then treatment strategies must be outlined for multiple caretakers (e.g., parents and teachers) to be used across a number of situations. Although an explicit goal of the intervention program is to decrease the frequency of various ADHD-related behaviors (e.g., inattention to task materials), the primary emphasis is on enhancing competencies in a number of areas, and improving behavioral, academic, and social adjustment. Thus, treatment targets are behaviors that should increase in frequency as a function of treatment, such as completion of independent work, compliance with teacher directives, accuracy of academic responding, and positive interactions with peers. Behavioral objectives must be designed on an individual basis using data from direct observations of classroom behavior, as well as the results of parent and teacher ratings. Assessment results also will identify behavioral competencies (e.g., adequate peer relations) that possibly could aid in the amelioration of the child's deficits. Those behaviors occurring at the lowest frequencies and/or deemed most crucial to classroom functioning by the teacher usually serve as initial intervention targets.

A number of factors are considered in the process of choosing appropriate interventions for an individual child with ADHD. First, the severity of the child's ADHD should be categorized into one of four levels (i.e., borderline, mild, moderate, severe) based upon the number of symptoms reported on the ADHD Rating Scale–IV and the degree of functional impairment evidenced (American Psychiatric Association, 2000). The greater the severity of ADHD symptoms, the more likely a referral to a physician for a medication assessment will be warranted.

In general, the treatment of first resort will be the implementation of a behaviorally based intervention involving changes in antecedent conditions and/or application of positive reinforcement techniques designed to increase task-related attention and completion of assigned work (DuPaul & Stoner, 2002; DuPaul, Stoner, & O'Reilly, 2002). Observation results will aid in this process by providing baseline data and helping to identify antecedent and consequent events that could be manipulated as part of the intervention.

In fact, a second important factor to consider in designing psychosocial interventions for children with ADHD is the function that their ADHD-related behaviors serve (DuPaul & Ervin, 1996; also see Chapter 5 for more details). The most likely function for ADHD-related behavior is to avoid or escape effortful tasks, such as independent seatwork or homework. A second possible function is to gain adult or peer attention. A frequent consequent event for ADHD-related behavior is a verbal reprimand from the teacher as well as nonverbal (e.g., smiles) and verbal reactions (e.g., laughter) from the student's classmates. An additional possible function is for ADHD-related behavior to result in access to an object or activity that appears more reinforcing than the stimuli that the child is expected to attend to. For example, when presented with a set of written math problems to complete, the student begins playing with a toy that he keeps in his desk. Finally, ADHD-related behavior may result in sensory stimulation, such as accessing pleasant thoughts (e.g., daydreaming).

The specific function that is operational for a child's behavior in the classroom setting can be determined through descriptive assessment, experimental analysis, or both (Gresham, Watson, & Skinner, 2001; Nelson, Roberts, & Smith, 1998). Most typically, teacher interview and behavior observation data are used to develop a working hypothesis as to the function(s) of a particular behavior. Rarely are full-scale experimental analyses conducted in classroom settings (Ervin, Ehrhardt, & Poling, 2001). Interventions are then designed to promote functionally equivalent behavior (e.g., vis-à-vis the hypothesized function) through changes in antecedent and/or consequent conditions (see Chapter 5).

In addition to behavioral function, the specific settings where intervention procedures are to be implemented are identified based on observation data or the use of a scatter plot (Touchette, MacDonald, & Langer, 1985). For example, a student with ADHD may be found to exhibit the lowest frequencies of desired behaviors in classroom rather than in playground settings. Furthermore, task-related attention and work completion rates may be different across academic subject areas. Initial interventions may be designed to increase attention and work completion frequencies during instruction in those academic areas where the child exhibits the greatest ADHD-related difficulties and in the classroom setting only. As progress is achieved, target behaviors in other academic settings may be addressed.

A third factor to consider in developing treatment strategies is the presence of additional behavior or learning disorders. For example, many children with ADHD also are oppositional and defiant in response to authority figure commands (American Psychiatric Association, 2000). Noncompliant and aggressive behaviors would then become additional targets of the classroom intervention program. A referral to a community-based professional (e.g., clinical child psychologist) may be necessary so that parents could receive training in appropriate behavior management strategies at home.

An additional consideration in designing the treatment plan is a child's response to previous interventions. If, for example, a behavioral program has been implemented in a general education classroom, yet the child continues to exhibit a high frequency of ADHD-related behaviors, then other treatment modalities (e.g., prescription of stimulant medication or provision of special education services) may need to be recommended. As is the case for most children with special needs, the preference is for placement and treatments considered to be least restrictive. In fact, most children with ADHD are placed primarily within regular classroom settings (Pastor & Reuben, 2002; Pfiffner & Barkley, 1998). Thus, resistance to previous intervention should be the major criterion in determining whether a child's behavior control problems are severe enough to warrant special education eligibility (Gresham, 1991; see Chapter 3 for further discussion of this issue).

A final factor to consider is the availability of treatment resources in the community. For instance, this availability will determine whether the child and his or her family are referred to a community-based professional such as a clinical child psychologist or whether home-based interventions are to be designed by the school psychologist. When both parents and teachers are actively involved in the treatment process (e.g., through implementation of behavior modification strategies), there is a greater probability of success. Thus, in most cases, parents will be referred for training in behavior management strategies when such services are available.

Stage V: Program/Intervention Evaluation

Questions to Be Addressed

Once the intervention program is designed and implemented, ongoing assessment is conducted to answer the following questions:

1. Are changes occurring in the target and collateral behaviors?
2. Are the treatment changes socially valid and clinically significant?
3. Are target behaviors normalized?

Intervention Evaluation Process

The assessment of the child with ADHD does not conclude with the diagnosis, but continues on an ongoing basis as intervention procedures are implemented. In this context, the initial evaluation data not only contribute to diagnostic decisions but also serve as baseline or preintervention measures. If outcome assessment data are not collected once treatment begins, one can never be sure that the intervention is successful or whether it requires adjustments. Single-subject design methodology should be employed to evaluate treatment-related changes in target behaviors (DuPaul & Stoner, 2002; Morgan & Morgan, 2001). More details regarding the use of single-subject methodology to evaluate behavioral change can be obtained by consulting several excellent texts on this topic (e.g., Hersen & Barlow, 1982; Kazdin, 1992).

Throughout the treatment process, the student serves as his or her own "control," and behavioral change is evaluated in comparison to baseline or nonintervention conditions. This process requires the repeated acquisition of assessment data across settings and caretakers at various points in the intervention program. In addition, treatment integrity is evaluated to ensure the accurate application (e.g., treatment compliance) of the prescribed intervention. If the intervention is implemented as designed and reliable behavior change occurs, then one can assume that the treatment is working as planned. If not, then changes to either the intervention or the manner in which it is implemented by teachers or parents must be made. Thus, ongoing assessment is crucial to the treatment process and the two are inexorably linked.

Intervention Evaluation Techniques

In most cases, narrow-band assessment techniques such as direct observations of behavior and academic performance data, discussed above, are used to evaluate treatment-related change. Such data contribute to addressing whether behavioral changes are occurring as planned in association with intervention. For example, direct observations and performance data are collected on a daily or weekly basis in the context of a reversal (i.e., ABA) or multiple baseline across settings design. Changes in the mean, intercept, and trend of the data are used to determine whether the intervention has led to increases in task-related attention, compliance with classroom rules, and academic productivity and accuracy (see Chapter 5 for a specific example of the evaluation of a classroom intervention program). Occasionally, interobserver agreement is assessed by having a classroom aide, teacher, or other observer present when data are collected. Interobserver agreement should be assessed at least several times per treatment phase to ensure that observation and performance data are reliable.

Several additional assessment techniques are used to determine whether reliable behavior change has occurred as a function of the intervention. First, teacher ratings on the CBCL, BASC, or Conners Rating Scales are collected at several points, including prior to the intervention, during the treatment phase, following the return to baseline phase (if applicable), and approximately 1 month after the formal intervention has ceased. Thus, general behavior ratings are obtained at least once per treatment phase. Even though these ratings were collected during the initial evaluation, it is important to obtain them on an additional occasion prior to treatment implementation, as "practice effects" on these measures have been found (Barkley, 1998). A second administration of teacher ratings during baseline would reduce the possibility of attributing change to the treatment when it was actually due to a regression to the mean artifact. Teacher ratings that contain fewer items, such as the ADHD Rating Scale–IV or the APRS, can be collected on a weekly basis throughout all treatment phases. Typically, the means of the various teacher ratings are compared across phases to determine whether the teacher perceives any treatment-induced improvements in performance and behavior control.

A second assessment component necessary to document treatment-related change is a method to determine whether the intervention has been implemented as prescribed (Gresham, 1989; Hayes, Barlow, & Nelson-Gray, 1999; Peterson, Homer, & Wonderlich, 1982). If medication effects are being assessed, then pill counts are conducted on a regular basis (e.g., weekly) to ensure that the medicine has been administered. Alternatively, when a parent or teacher is carrying out the intervention (e.g., classroom-based token reinforcement program), treatment integrity is more difficult to determine. Ideally, direct observations of teacher behavior would be conducted occasionally throughout treatment to assess whether the intervention steps are being carried out as planned. Of course, there would then be no way to ensure that treatment integrity was intact during intervention sessions where an observer was not present. In such cases, observations of teacher behavior would be supplemented by checklists outlining the intervention steps. The teacher or treatment agent would be expected to complete the checklist every time the intervention was being implemented in an effort to promote compliance. Such checklists also could be completed by someone other than the treatment agent (e.g., classroom aide) on a regular basis. Another option is to audiotape intervention sessions for later review regarding implementation integrity (Power, DuPaul, Shapiro, & Kazak, 2003). Without at least occasional treatment integrity checks, one cannot be sure that the intervention is being applied as designed.

Although it is important to demonstrate that an intervention has led to reliable changes in the student's behavior and performance, it is crucial to determine whether such changes are socially valid and clinically meaningful. For example, a mean increase in the percentage of on-task behavior from 50% to 65% during independent work may be statistically significant, but the end result is that the student still spends too much time off-task and is not any more productive academically. Interventions that lead to behavior changes that do not meaningfully impact on the student's classroom performance are usually abandoned quite readily by the child's teacher.

The clinical significance and social validity of behavioral change can be assessed in a variety of ways (for details, see Kazdin, 2000; Schwarz & Baer, 1991). First, consumer satisfaction ratings could be completed by the student, teacher, and/or parents at the conclusion of treatment or at various points during the intervention. Each participant's views on specific components of the intervention could be obtained in this manner. A second related technique is to have the teacher complete treatment acceptability ratings of various possible intervention strategies (for a review, see Finn & Sladeczek, 2001). The acceptability of interventions may actually be assessed prior to treatment as an aid in the consultation and treatment design process (Bergan & Kratochwill, 1990).

A third way of determining the clinical significance of an intervention is to assess whether it has led to the "normalization" of behavior. Stated differently, does the intervention enhance the student's attention span, academic productivity, and social behaviors to the point where his or her performance and behavior in the classroom is indistinguishable from those of his or her peers? This particular outcome can be evaluated by collecting concurrent assessment data on one or more classmates during various points in the intervention. In this way, the treated child's performance can be compared directly to that of his or her normal counterparts. If ethical or practical considerations preclude the assessment of normal classmates, several statistical procedures can be used to determine whether clinically meaningful change has occurred. For example, if normative data are available for a specific measure, then a reliable change index (Jacobsen & Truax, 1991) can be calculated to evaluate whether the treatment has led to statistically reliable improvements in behavior. Furthermore, Jacobsen and Truax (1991) have provided several formulas for determining whether an intervention has led to normalization of performance. For example, methylphenidate (Ritalin) has been found to "normalize" the task-related attention and academic productivity of a large percentage of children with ADHD who participated in a 6-week medication trial (DuPaul & Rapport, 1993; see Chapter 6 for details). Although normalization of classroom performance is not always possible, it is one of the more important considerations in determining the value of obtained treatment effects.

DEVELOPMENTAL CONSIDERATIONS
IN THE ASSESSMENT OF ADHD

Developmental factors may alter the content and, to some degree, the process of conducting an ADHD evaluation, especially when the referred student is a preschooler or an adolescent (Anastopoulos & Shelton, 2001). We will address issues related to the identification of young children at risk for ADHD in Chapter 4. With regards to assessing ADHD in adolescents, there are several reasons why evaluation procedures may differ relative to assessment of children. First, the overall functioning of the teenager with ADHD can be more impaired than during the childhood years, given a higher risk for conduct disturbance or antisocial behavior (Barkley, Fischer, et al., 1990; Biederman et al., 1996), and academic underachievement (Barkley, Fischer, et al., 1990; Mannuzza, Gittelman-Klein, Bessler, Malloy, & LaPadula, 1993). In addition, several empirical investigations have indicated a higher frequency of substance abuse (Biederman et al., 1997) among adolescents with ADHD, especially when antisocial behavior problems (e.g., stealing, vandalism) are present. Thus, in addition to the core deficits of ADHD, teenagers with this disorder may exhibit a variety of behavioral and/or emotional disturbances, and therefore procedures designed to screen for these associated difficulties must be incorporated into the evaluation of adolescents with ADHD.

When evaluating an adolescent referred for ADHD-related difficulties, it is very important that a reliable history of the problem behaviors is obtained because, by definition, ADHD symptoms should be evident prior to the age of 7. Because the reliability of historical information provided by parents is often quite low, even for younger children, care should be taken to obtain "reliability checks" of parental verbal reports (Cantwell, 1986). A possible source of such information would be the student's school record, including report cards, previous psychological evaluations, and disciplinary history.

A third factor to consider in the assessment of adolescents suspected of having ADHD is the input of the students themselves. The teenager's perception of current adjustment difficulties must be obtained in addition to parent and teacher reports. Adolescent self-report of ADHD symptoms has been found to correlate highly with parental report (Gittelman et al., 1985), although this is equivocal across studies (see Barkley, Fischer, et al., 2002). Regardless of the relationship between self-report and other measures, the former may provide critical information (e.g., presence of depressive symptoms) not available from other sources. Moreover, adolescents are likely to agree more fully with the results of evaluations in which their own opinions were given greater attention, and hence may be more willing to participate with treatment recommendations (DuPaul, Guevremont, & Barkley, 1991). Thus, the major change to the ADHD evaluation when assessing an adolescent is the inclusion of several self-report measures, such as a diagnostic interview with the student and the completion of behavior rating scales, in the multimethod assessment stage. The student may also play a more active role in the formulation, implementation, and assessment of the treatment plan. At the very least, self-report and consumer satisfaction data should be obtained from the student during the treatment evaluation stage on an ongoing basis.

The content of the ADHD evaluation is somewhat different when assessing an adolescent, relative to assessment of younger children. First, as mentioned above, a diagnostic interview with the student should be conducted that incorporates DSM criteria for the same disorders reviewed with the adolescent's parent and teacher. Second, various self-report questionnaires are completed by the student including the Youth Self-Report (YSR) version of the Child Behavior Checklist (Achenbach, 1991c), the Youth Inventory–4 (Gadow et al., 2002), and/or the Conners–Wells Adolescent Self-Report of Symptoms (Conners et al., 2000). Normative data are available for both measures. Given the higher risk of affective or emotional disturbance among adolescents with ADHD relative to their normal counterparts, it is often necessary to include questionnaires tapping internalizing symptomatology such as the Reynolds Adolescent Depression Scale (Reynolds, 1987).

A final change in the ADHD evaluation is the inclusion of behavior ratings from multiple teachers. The interpretation of the resultant ratings can be problematic given the limited sample of student behavior that each teacher observes. It is often helpful to obtain ratings from several individuals, including nonteachers (e.g., guidance counselor) with whom the teenager has the greatest amount of contact. Rather than relying on the analysis of any single teacher rating (as with younger children), consistencies among the resultant profiles (e.g., elevations on factors related to ADHD) are used to document the pervasiveness or lack thereof of behavioral control difficulties across settings. Further details regarding the content of ADHD evaluations with adolescents are available in several recent texts (Anastopoulos & Shelton, 2001; Barkley, 1998).

IMPLEMENTATION OF THE ASSESSMENT MODEL

The assessment model proposed in this chapter represents what we believe to be a state-of-the-art evaluation process for identifying students with ADHD and designing classroom interventions for this population.

As such, it is an idealized model that must be adapted for practical application at the local level. Some assessment components or processes (e.g., parent interview) may be less feasible for some school personnel. Therefore, changes to the assessment model will be necessary.

As an example of a local adaptation of this assessment model, the Carroll County (MD) Public Schools have developed ADHD procedural guidelines for teachers and school psychologists (Carroll County Public Schools, 1997). These guidelines structure the ADHD identification and treatment process into four, rather than five, stages: screening, multimodal assessment of ADHD, interpretation of results, and treatment. Although the screening stage is virtually identical to the content and process of this stage as described in this chapter, some adaptations have been made to the multimethod assessment protocol. For example, parents are asked to complete a questionnaire rather than an interview that outlines current behavioral concerns as well as developmental, medical, and family histories. Nevertheless, this second stage of the Carroll County guidelines includes the core components of the multimethod protocol proposed in this chapter such as parent and teacher behavior questionnaires, direct observation, and review of school records.

Although our assessment model may include some components that are impractical for some school districts, it is possible to adapt this process to meet the needs and practical limitations of a local school district. The overall objective would be to retain core features of this model. First, the assessment process should utilize a data-based problem-solving model wherein psychometrically sound measures are used to make identification and treatment decisions. Second, a triage system should be used wherein students are screened to determine who will require more involved assessment and/or treatment. Third, the input of multiple respondents using more than one type of measure should be sought to obtain a comprehensive picture of a child's home and school functioning. As is the case for evaluating learning disabilities, practitioners should never rely on a single instrument or questionnaire to make ADHD identification decisions. Fourth, assessment data (e.g., functional behavioral assessment and/or curriculum-based assessment) that are useful for treatment planning should be collected routinely. Fifth, some subset of assessment measures should be collected periodically to determine the success of intervention plans and to guide ongoing changes in treatment.

CASE EXAMPLES

Case Example 1

Arthur was a 7-year-old second grader referred to the school psychologist by his regular classroom teacher due to problems completing independent seatwork, talking without permission, and noncompliance with school rules. The teacher indicated that the quality of Arthur's academic work was similar to that of his classmates when she worked with him individually. Alternatively, due to his inconsistent completion of assigned work and frequent inattention during tests, Arthur was reported to achieve below his presumed potential.

After briefly discussing the case, the school psychologist asked the teacher to complete a screening instrument (i.e., the ADHD Rating Scale–IV). Arthur's ratings were beyond the 93rd percentile for the total score as well as the Inattention and Hyperactivity–Impulsivity factor scores. Also, six inattention and six hyperactivity–impulsivity symptoms (using DSM-IV criteria) were reported to be present at least "pretty much" of the time. Based on this screening information and the nature of the referral, a multimethod assessment of ADHD appeared warranted.

As a first step in the assessment process, an interview with Arthur's classroom teacher was conducted. In the course of the interview, it was reported that he displayed frequent problems with inattention, impulsivity, overactivity, and noncompliance across most school settings and classroom activities. These problems were most evident when independent seatwork was assigned and when the teacher was instructing the whole class or small groups. There did not appear to be any differences in this behavior across academic subject areas. Arthur was reported to evidence six of the nine inattention symptoms and seven of the nine hyperactivity–impulsivity symptoms of ADHD on a frequent basis. These symptoms had been exhibited on a daily basis over the past 6 months (i.e., since the beginning of the school year). Furthermore, a significant number (i.e., five out of nine) of symptoms of oppositional defiant disorder were reported to occur on a frequent basis. The latter included noncompliance with teacher commands, frequent losses of temper, and deliberate annoyance of others. Problems associated with other disorders (e.g., conduct disorder, depression) were not reported to occur frequently.

As a result of his attention and behavior problems, Arthur was not achieving at a level commensurate with his classmates in either mathematics or reading skills. Nevertheless, his teacher did not feel that he had learning problems in either subject area. She reported that when she worked with him on an individual basis, he was able to demonstrate adequate knowledge in both skill areas (e.g., he was able to read high-interest material). When he was asked to complete independent work, particularly material that did not capture his interest, he was not able to demonstrate his abilities due to a lack of work completion.

Arthur had few friends in the classroom and was rejected by many of his peers. He did not follow the rules of games and frequently was verbally and physically aggressive in unstructured settings (e.g., on the playground). His teacher felt that many of his disruptive behaviors (e.g., talking out in the classroom) were an attempt to elicit attention from his peers. Unfortunately, these efforts to promote peer interaction resulted in further ostracism by his classmates.

The teacher reported a great deal of frustration in trying to manage Arthur's behavior. Her interventions had included ignoring his disruptive behavior, making public reprimands to get back on task, sending notes to his parents following misbehavior, giving him a reward (e.g., access to classroom computer) for a week of appropriate behavior, and reducing the number of items he is expected to complete for seatwork. None of these strategies resulted in consistent behavioral improvement.

Arthur's report cards from previous school years were reviewed. The written comments of his kindergarten and first-grade teachers indicated that he displayed similar problems with behavior control, albeit less severe, as reported by his current teacher. A pattern of attention and behavior control problems beginning at an early age and occurring across school years was evident.

Arthur's mother was interviewed briefly by telephone. She corroborated the teacher's report of significant problems with inattention, impulsivity, and overactivity. In fact, nearly all of the symptoms of ADHD were reported to occur on a frequent basis at home. These had been evident since he was 3 years old and attended a nursery school program. She reported that Arthur was very defiant and uncooperative at home, especially in response to maternal commands. He did not sustain his attention to most household chores unless he was interested in completing them. A majority of the symptoms of oppositional defiant disorder were indicated to be present. No further DSM-IV symptomatology was reported. He did not have a history of significant medical difficulties or developmental delays. Arthur's father was reported to have had similar attention and behavior problems as a child, but was now a successful businessman. No other significant problems were reported for immediate family members. Finally, she stated that she was very interested in receiving help in managing Arthur's behavior as the stress level in the household was directly related to the degree to which he behaved in an appropriate manner. Previous attempts at intervention, including family therapy, had failed.

Maternal responses on the Child Behavior Checklist resulted in significant elevations on three subscales: Attention Problems, Aggression, and Delinquent. T-scores on these scales were above 67, or greater than the 95th percentile. All remaining subscales were below the 93rd percentile (i.e., in the normal range). Ratings on the ADHD Rating Scale–IV were two standard deviations above the mean for the total score and both subscales. Arthur's attention problems were reported to occur in almost all home situations identified on the HSQ-R and their average severity was 2 standard deviations above the mean.

Teacher ratings were consistent with those provided by Arthur's mother. On the Teacher Report Form of the Child Behavior Checklist, significant elevations were obtained on the Attention Problems and Aggression subscales. T-scores were above 70, or greater than the 98th percentile for both dimensions. Remaining subscale scores were in the normal range. On the SSQ-R, Arthur was reported to exhibit attention problems in every school setting at a severity level that was 2 standard deviations above the mean. Teacher ratings on the SSRS resulted in a below-average score (T-score of 85) for social skills. Finally, ratings on the Academic Performance Rating Scale were in the clinically significant range (i.e., 1.5 standard deviations below the mean) for the Academic Productivity factor only.

Arthur's behavior was observed on several occasions in both the classroom and on the playground. Classroom observations (using the coding system described in Appendix 2.1) were conducted for 20 minutes on three occasions (once during math seatwork, twice while working on a phonics worksheet). Arthur was noted to display high rates of off-task verbal and motor behaviors. Specifically, he displayed off-task verbal behavior during an average of 20% of the observation intervals, while exhibiting off-task motor behavior approximately 15% of the time. In contrast, randomly selected classmates were observed to exhibit off-task verbal behavior only 4% of the time and were engaged in off-task motor behavior during less than 8% of the observation intervals. Arthur's playground behavior was observed on two occasions using the SOC. He was noted to be more verbally and physically aggressive than randomly selected classmates. Thus, direct observations were consistent with both parent and teacher report of significant behavior control difficulties.

Academic performance data were collected in conjunction with observations of Arthur's behavior during independent seatwork. He completed an average of 60% of the work assigned over these three occasions. This is in contrast to an average completion rate of 95% for his classmates. On a positive note, the accuracy of his work was uniformly high (i.e., M = 93% correct). This corroborates the teacher's contention that Arthur's abilities were commensurate with those of his classmates, but that he simply did not finish the assigned work.

The next step in the evaluation process was to interpret the results. Arthur's teacher and mother independently reported at least six inattention and six hyperactivity–impulsivity symptoms to be evident on a frequent basis. According to his mother, he began exhibiting ADHD-related difficulties at the age of 3 with no diminishment of severity. Thus, these symptoms were evident at an early age and were chronic. Maternal and teacher ratings indicated Arthur's problems with inattention, impulsivity, and overactivity were more frequent and severe than those of the vast majority of other boys his age. This was corroborated by direct observations of his classroom behavior. Furthermore, attention problems were reported to be pervasive across numerous school and home situations. Finally, Arthur's ADHD-related behaviors had compromised his peer relationships and academic performance to a significant degree.

Although Arthur also was reported to display a significant number of oppositional defiant disorder symptoms, the presence of the latter could not fully account for his attention difficulties. It was particularly noteworthy that his symptoms of ADHD predated the onset of his problems with noncompliance and defiance. Specifically, the former were reported to occur as early as age 3, while the latter were not evident until Arthur was 6 years old. There were no indications of any emotional or learning difficulties that could account for his ADHD symptoms. Thus, he was determined to have both ADHD and oppositional defiant disorder.

Arthur's teacher was interviewed regarding the antecedents and consequences surrounding his off-task disruptive behavior in the classroom. In addition, the school psychologist recorded the frequency of antecedent (e.g., task presentation) and consequent (e.g., peer laughter) events during various classroom situations. Interview and observation data indicated that Arthur's disruptive behavior was most likely to occur when he was asked to complete independent seatwork and that this behavior was followed by frequent teacher reminders for him to focus on his work. It appeared that the function of his off-task behavior was to avoid and escape classwork.

Several interventions were implemented based on this evaluation. First, the school psychologist and teacher designed a classroom intervention program that included modifying task demands, token reinforcement, response cost, and a home–school communication program (see Chapter 5 for details of classroom programming). These interventions were designed to reduce Arthur's desire to avoid work by enhancing the positive aspects of the latter while providing greater motivation for him to complete assigned tasks. Second, referrals were made to a clinical child psychologist and Arthur's pediatrician for provision of parent training and a medication assessment, respectively. Parent training was necessary due to his high level of defiance and inattention at home. A medication assessment was recommended due to the severity of Arthur's ADHD and the high likelihood of continued impairment in functioning in a number of key areas. The chronicity and severity of his behavior problems may require special education programming, which Arthur's family would like to avoid if possible. The probability of special education placement may be reduced if Arthur is a positive responder to medication. Finally, a social skills intervention was designed to address Arthur's playground behavior. Specifically, a peer-mediated procedure was used wherein several of his classmates were trained to prompt and reinforce appropriate social behavior. It was felt that this combination of interventions would be necessary over the long term given the chronicity and severity of Arthur's ADHD.

Continued assessment of Arthur's classroom performance was conducted by the school psychologist to evaluate his progress and to determine whether changes were warranted in his intervention program. Teacher ratings and classroom observations were obtained on at least a weekly basis during the initial stages of implementing the multicomponent behavioral intervention. Adjustments were made to the timing and frequency of reinforcement as a result. These same measures were used on a daily basis over several weeks of evaluating three different doses of Ritalin (i.e., 5 mg, 10 mg, 15 mg). Over the course of the school year, these measures were periodically readministered to ascertain whether further adjustments in behavioral procedures or medication dosage were necessary.

Case Example 2

Keesha was a 10-year-old African American girl participating in a fifth-grade general education classroom in an urban school setting. She had experienced some difficulties with reading and math throughout her school years, although she had never been referred for special education services. Her current teachers became concerned that she might have ADHD because she frequently had difficulties concentrating on her work, often forgot class materials and assignments, and frequently appeared distracted. Teacher ratings on the Inattention subscale of the ADHD Rating Scale–IV were above the 85th percentile, indicating a need for further assessment of possible ADHD.

Parent and teacher ratings on the BASC resulted in clinically significant scores in the Inattention and Anxiety domains, with only borderline ratings of hyperactivity–impulsivity and conduct problems. Her mother's and teacher's responses to diagnostic interview questions revealed that although Keesha exhibited seven of the nine inattention symptoms of ADHD, she did not evidence many hyperactive–impulsive symptoms. Furthermore, her inattention problems were relatively recent (i.e., began occurring at the beginning of the school year). Keesha also was reported by both her mother and her teacher to exhibit symptoms of generalized

anxiety disorder (e.g., excessive concerns regarding the quality of her social and academic performance) that appeared to be worsening as the
school year went on. Significant symptoms of oppositional defiant disorders or conduct disorder were not reported by Keesha's mother or
teacher.

The school psychologist observed Keesha's behavior during reading
and math class activities (e.g., teacher-led instruction, independent
seatwork, small-group work). Keesha displayed off-task behavior (e.g.,
looking away from task or activity, talking with classmates) during approximately 15% of the observation intervals, whereas her classmates
exhibited similar behavior during only 6% of those intervals. Keesha
also was noted to complete far less written seatwork than her peers.

An interview with Keesha revealed that she "felt stupid" and frequently felt frustrated by her inability to read material at the same pace
as her classmates. She recognized that she often did not get her work
done and stated that she was worried that she would not pass fifth
grade. She also indicated a concern about her mother's welfare as the latter had been ill frequently during the present school year. Finally, Keesha
reported that she did not have many friends and that she felt embar-
rassed when she had to speak in front of a group of her peers. Self-report
ratings on the RCMAS also were elevated.

Given that Keesha's attention problems were relatively recent, were
not associated with hyperactivity–impulsivity symptoms, and appeared
to be associated with significant anxiety disorder symptoms, the school
assessment team concluded that she probably did not have ADHD. The
school psychologist suggested that she receive individual counseling at
school for her anxiety symptoms and that further evaluation by a clinical
psychologist might be necessary. Furthermore, because of her chronic academic difficulties, assessment of possible learning disabilities should be
conducted by the school team.

INVOLVEMENT OF SCHOOL PROFESSIONALS
IN THE ASSESSMENT PROCESS

In recent years, there has been controversy as to the role of school professionals in the diagnostic assessment of ADHD. For example, legislation in several states have limited school-based identification of students
with ADHD, particularly for the purpose of referring them for possible
medication treatment. Opponents of schools being involved in the diagnostic process point out that ADHD is a "medical diagnosis" given its
inclusion in the DSM-IV, and therefore evaluations of this disorder
should be conducted by medical professionals. Yet when one examines

the assessment methods that are empirically supported for identification of ADHD, it is clear that school psychologists and other educational professionals have the training and expertise to be involved in this process. In fact, recent survey data indicate that school psychologists were as likely to use empirically supported assessment methods as clinical psychologists (Handler & DuPaul, 2002). School psychologists also have more opportunities—to conduct observations in classroom and playground settings than do other professionals. Furthermore, very few medical professionals have that same background, expertise, and opportunities—at least as far as administration of rating scales and behavioral observations is concerned. Also, the mere inclusion of ADHD in the DSM-IV does not delegate this diagnosis solely to medical professionals, as diagnostic criteria for mental retardation and learning disabilities (entities that are assessed routinely by school psychologists) also are included in the DSM. Finally, because children with ADHD arguably experience their greatest difficulties in school settings, for school professionals to not be involved in identification is tantamount to malpractice.

To be clear, we are not advocating for school psychologists and other educators to be the only professionals identifying children with ADHD. On the contrary, we strongly believe that the diagnosis and treatment of students with this disorder requires collaboration among parents, school professionals, physicians, and other community-based professionals (e.g., clinical psychologists). A comprehensive assessment of ADHD requires the collection of reliable and valid data regarding child functioning across settings. All too often, community-based evaluations of children suspected of having ADHD do not include detailed information from the school. Alternatively, school-based evaluations may neglect parental input. Thus, school-based professionals should seek to collaborate with others, such that school-based data can be communicated in a systematic fashion to physicians and clinical psychologists so that informed diagnostic decisions are made (see Chapter 8).

SUMMARY

The school-based evaluation of ADHD is comprised of multiple assessment techniques utilized across a variety of settings and sources of information. Following a teacher referral for possible ADHD, five stages of assessment are conducted: (1) screening for ADHD symptoms, (2) multimethod assessment, (3) interpretation of results to reach a classification decision, (4) development of the treatment plan, and (5) ongoing assessment of the intervention program. The goal of the evaluation is not simply to arrive at a diagnosis of ADHD, but to determine an intervention plan that is likely to succeed based upon the information gathered. The use of a behavioral assessment approach incorporating parent and teacher interviews, parent and teacher rating scales, direct observations of behavior, and academic performance data is the optimal methodology for addressing both goals of the evaluation process. Importantly, assessment data are collected on an ongoing basis throughout treatment to determine the efficacy and/or limitations of the intervention program.

APPENDIX 2.1

♦

School Hybrid Observation Code for Kids (Volpe & Lorah, 2000)

The School Hybrid Observation Code for Kids (SHOCK) is a combination of two existing observation codes: the ADHD School Observation Code (ADHD SOC; Gadow, Sprafkin, & Nolan, 1996) and the Behavioral Observation of Students in Schools (BOSS; Shapiro, 1996). Behavior codes from the BOSS include Active Engaged Time (AET), Passive Engaged Time (PET), Off-Task Motor (OFT-M), Off-Task Verbal (OFT-V), Off-Task Passive (OFT-P), and Teacher-Directed Instruction (TDI). The category Noncompliance (NonC) from the ADHD SOC is also coded. With the exception of AET and PET (which are coded on a momentary time sampling basis), all behaviors will be scored using partial (15-second) intervals. Readers interested in this observation code should consult Gadow and colleagues (1996) and Shapiro (1996) to obtain the specific definitions of each observation category.

Appendix 2.1

SHOCK Summary Sheet

Child: _____ Academic Subject: _____

Date: _____ Setting:

Observer: _____
ISW: TPsnt   SmGp: TPsnt
ISW: TSmGp   LgGp: TPsnt

Time of Observation: _____ Other: _____

Summary

Target Student

	Σ AET	____	% AET	____
	Σ PET	____	% PET	____
	Σ OFT-M	____	% OFT-M	____
	Σ OFT-V	____	% OFT-V	____
Total Intervals	Σ OFT-P	____	% OFT-P	____
Observed	Σ NPAg	____	% NPAg	____
	Σ NonC	____	% NonC	____
____		____		____

Peer Comparison				Teacher	
Σ AET		% AET	____	Σ TDI	____
Σ PET	____	% PET	____	% TDI	____
Σ OFT-M	____	% OFT-M	____		____
Σ OFT-V	____	% OFT-V	____		
Σ OFT-P	____	% OFT-P	____	Total Intervals	
Σ NPAg	____	% NPAg	____	Observed	
Σ NonC	____	% NonC	____		
	____		____		____

SHOCK Observation Form

Moment	1	2	3	4	5	6	7	8	9	10	11	12	13	14	15	S	P	T
AET																		
PET																		
Partial																		
OFT-M																		
OFT-V																		
OFT-P																		
NonC																		
TDI																		

Moment	16	17	18	19	20	21	22	23	24	25	26	27	28	29	30	S	P	T
AET																		
PET																		
Partial																		
OFT-M																		
OFT-V																		
OFT-P																		
NonC																		
TDI																		

Moment	31	32	33	34	35	36	37	38	39	40	41	42	43	44	45	S	P	T
AET																		
PET																		
Partial																		
OFT-M																		
OFT-V																		
OFT-P																		
NonC																		
TDI																		

Moment	46	47	48	49	50	51	52	53	54	55	56	57	58	59	60	S	P	T
AET																		
PET																		
Partial																		
OFT-M																		
OFT-V																		
OFT-P																		
NonC																		
TDI																		

♦

Criteria for the Teacher–Student Behavior Coding System

The first observation categories pertain to who (teacher or student) initiated the interaction and how it was initiated (by teacher when student was on- or off-task, or by student in an appropriate or inappropriate manner.

TA/ON = Teacher Approaches Student Engaged in On-Task Behavior
Teacher verbally or physically initiates an interaction with student, who at moment of contact is engaged in on-task behavior (see above). Not coded if student has raised hand or called out to get teacher's attention.

TA/OFF = Teacher Approaches Student Engaged in Off-Task Behavior
Teacher physically or verbally initiates an interaction with student who is off-task at that moment (see above definition of off-task). TA/OFF is coded regardless of what happens after the interaction (e.g., a redirection back to work results in student going back on-task).

SA/APP = Student Approaches Teacher in an Appropriate Manner
Student physically or verbally initiates an interaction with the teacher in an "appropriate" manner including:
- Raising hand
- Asking questions without raising hand when classroom rules are specifically relaxed (must be specified by the teacher, for example, during small-group instruction)
- Approaching teacher at desk during independent seatwork

SA/INAPP = Student Approaches Teacher in an Inappropriate Manner
Student physically or verbally initiates an interaction with teacher in an "inappropriate" manner, including:
- Calling out without permission
- Getting out of seat (unless during independent seatwork or similar activity when that is acceptable in the classroom)
- The second category of teacher observation codes is a determina-

tion of whether the teacher–student interaction was positive, negative, or other.

POSITIVE = Interaction included any type of positive verbal comment regarding appropriate social or academic behavior. May also include physical contact (e.g., pat on shoulder) as long as it is not for discipline. Positive comments may be directed at the target student or the group if the student is part of it.

NEGATIVE = Interaction includes verbal comments of disapproval such as criticism, negative reprimands, or if teacher threatens to punish the student. May include physical contact (e.g., leading student by hand to his or her desk) if it occurs in response to inappropriate behavior on the part of the student. Student may be either directly targeted by the teacher or part of a group to whom the teacher makes a negative statement.

OTHER = Any other teacher–student interaction that is not coded as positive or negative, such as:
- Instructing the class
- Answering questions (unless the teacher adds "good job" or other approval statement)
- Conversing with student
- Giving directions to class (e.g., to change activities).

CHAPTER 3

◆ ◆ ◆

ADHD and Learning Difficulties: What Is the Connection?

◆

Children with ADHD frequently underachieve academically (Barkley, 1998; Forness & Kavale, 2001). Within classroom settings, these children often exhibit significantly lower rates of on-task behavior during instruction and independent work periods than those displayed by their classmates (Abikoff et al., 1977). As a result, children with ADHD have fewer opportunities to respond during academic instruction and complete less independent work relative to their peers (Pfiffner & Barkley, 1998). The latter may, at least partially, account for the association of ADHD with academic underachievement: up to 80% of children with this disorder have been found to exhibit learning and/or achievement problems (e.g., Cantwell & Baker, 1991; Frick et al., 1991; Pastor & Reuben, 2002). Furthermore, the results of prospective follow-up studies of children with ADHD into adolescence (e.g., Barkley, Fischer, et al., 1990) indicate the greatest risks for this population are chronic academic underachievement and higher rates of dropping out of school.

Given the association between ADHD and academic underachievement, it is important for school psychologists and other education professionals to be aware of the potential for learning difficulties among children diagnosed with or suspected of having ADHD. In addition, where warranted, it is incumbent upon these professionals to design and implement effective prevention and intervention strategies to enhance academic functioning (see Chapters 4 and 5). The purpose of this chapter is to provide an overview of several aspects of the relationship between ADHD and learning problems. First, we provide a review of specific learning problems found to be associated with ADHD. Second, we provide a review of empirical studies examining possible causal connections between learning difficulties and ADHD, from the first edition of this book (DuPaul & Stoner, 1994), along with a section on contemporary perspectives on the relationship between learning and attentional difficulties. The possibility of treating ADHD plus learning disabilities as a subtype of ADHD is discussed in this context. Third, suggestions for assessment and intervention to address academic performance difficulties among students with ADHD are delineated. Here, federal statutes regarding the potential eligibility of students with ADHD for special education and other services are discussed. Fourth, suggestions are offered for determining whether a student with ADHD may be eligible for special education or other support services vis-à-vis these regulations.

ASSOCIATION OF ADHD WITH COGNITIVE DEFICITS

Differences between children with ADHD and their typically developing peers have been found in several areas of cognitive functioning. First, children with ADHD often display difficulties on tasks that require complex problem-solving strategies and organizational skills (Barkley, 1998; Tant & Douglas, 1982). Interestingly, these problems are not necessarily due to a lack of problem-solving abilities per se, but rather appear to reflect either insufficient effort or inefficient use of proper strategies during the task itself (Barkley, 1990, 1998; Voelker, Carter, Sprague, Gdowski, & Lachar, 1989). A second area of deficit relative to typical peers is frequently observed on neuropsychological measures of executive functioning (Barkley, 1990; Barkley, Grodzinsky, & DuPaul, 1992). Tests that purportedly assess problem solving, response inhibition, and sustained effort have been found to reliably discriminate between children with and without ADHD (Barkley et al., 1992; Chelune, Ferguson, Koon, & Dickey, 1986; Rapport et al., 2000). Again, the strategies that children with ADHD employ on these tasks are inefficient, frequently impulsive, and poorly organized (Zentall, 1988). Thus, it is no wonder that teachers of these students frequently report difficulties with note taking, completion of long-term assignments, desk organization, and study skills.

Another area of functioning in which children with ADHD may be more likely than nondisordered children to evidence difficulties is speech and language development. Although empirical investigations have provided equivocal results regarding possible delays in the onset of speech, there is relatively consistent evidence of expressive language difficulties among many children with ADHD (Barkley, 1998). Specifically, 10–54% of children with ADHD may exhibit expressive language problems relative to 2–25% of the normal population (Barkley, DuPaul, & McMurray, 1990; Hartsough & Lambert, 1985). Furthermore, children with ADHD display a higher rate of dysfluent (e.g., misarticulations) and/or disorganized speech on tasks that require verbal explanation (e.g., responding to reading comprehension questions) (Hamlett, Pelligrini, & Conners, 1987; Zentall & Leib, 1985).

Problems with fine and gross motor coordination may be associated with attention-deficit/hyperactivity disorder. Group studies have found that approximately 52% of children with ADHD are reported to display poor fine motor coordination as compared to a maximum of 35% of nondiagnosed children (Barkley, DuPaul, & McMurray, 1990; Hartsough & Lambert, 1985; Szatmari et al., 1989). Such findings have been obtained rather consistently on tasks such as maze drawings or pegboard tests (e.g., Ullman, Barkley, & Brown, 1978). Here again these results are not surprising, as teachers frequently report students with ADHD to have significant problems with handwriting and penmanship (Barkley, 1998). Several studies also have documented a greater frequency of neurological "soft" signs, including gross motor coordination difficulties and motor overflow movements, among children with ADHD relative to their typically developing and/or learning-disabled counterparts (Denckla, Rudel, Chapman, & Krieger, 1985). For example, when asked to perform specific muscle group movements (e.g., toe tapping), children with ADHD may display unnecessary associated movements perhaps indicative of poor motor inhibition (Denckla & Rudel, 1978).

The extent to which ADHD is associated with delays in general intellectual functioning is somewhat controversial. At a group level of analysis, children with this disorder consistently score an average of 7–15 points below their own siblings or typical children on standardized tests of intelligence (Barkley, 1998). Although these differences could represent an actual discrepancy in cognitive functioning between groups, there are at least two alternative explanations for these results. First, differential IQ test performance may be due to differences in test-taking behavior such as greater levels of inattention among the ADHD group relative to their typically functioning peers (Barkley, 1998). A second possible factor accounting for these findings is the high likelihood of a greater number of children with co-occurring learning disabilities among the ADHD group. Thus, lower IQ test scores for the ADHD group as a whole may be due to the scores of a subset of children who also have learning disabilities. Supporting this contention are the results of two studies that found no differences in IQ between ADHD and normal samples when the influence of learning disabilities was partialled-out

(August & Garfinkel, 1989; Dykman & Ackerman, 1991). Regardless of obtained differences in IQ between normal and ADHD samples, it is clear that the range of intellectual functioning in groups of children with ADHD is similar to that obtained in the general population (i.e., represented by a normal distribution from significantly below-average to significantly above-average functioning; Kaplan, Crawford, Dewey, & Fisher, 2000).

Summary

Children with ADHD are at higher risk for a number of weaknesses in areas of test performance and cognitive functioning relative to their peers. Specifically, a significant percentage of children with this disorder display problems with problem-solving and organizational skills, expressive language abilities, and/or fine and gross motor control. When any one of these difficulties or their combination is exhibited by a child with ADHD, the risk for scholastic underachievement is compounded. In contrast to these concerns, there are at least two positive findings from this research literature. First, on average, children with ADHD do not differ from the rest of the school population in intellectual functioning. That is, this disorder does not appear to affect the general cognitive abilities of diagnosed children as a group. This reinforces the assumption that ADHD is not related to a lack of ability, but rather represents a performance deficit (Barkley, 1998). Second, many individual children with ADHD do not evidence the specific cognitive deficits listed above. That is, while as a group children with ADHD are at a greater than average risk for language, motor control, and problem-solving difficulties, many children with this disorder do not exhibit these problems.

ASSOCIATION OF ADHD
WITH ACADEMIC UNDERACHIEVEMENT

One of the most common and potentially debilitating difficulties exhibited by children with ADHD is chronic academic underachievement relative to their intellectual capabilities (Barkley, 1998). The clear majority of students with this disorder obtain lower academic grades than expected across one or more subject areas. Furthermore, these children typically obtain significantly lower standardized achievement test scores than do comparable groups of typical children (Barkley, DuPaul, & McMurray, 1990; Cantwell & Satterfield, 1978). Problems with academic performance are differentially associated with ADHD even among groups of children with other psychological disorders. For example, children with ADHD have been found to receive the poorest teacher ratings of academic competence on the Child Behavior Checklist among clinic-referred groups of children (McConaughy, Achenbach, & Gent, 1988). This academic underachievement presumably is due to the exhibition of the core symptoms (i.e., inattention, impulsivity, and motor restlessness) of ADHD in classroom settings, although this is a matter of some debate, as discussed in the next section.

The chronic achievement difficulties encountered by many children with ADHD increase their risk for poor scholastic outcome, as measured by a number of variables. Approximately 40% or more children with ADHD are placed in special education programs for students with learning disabilities or behavior disorders (Barkley, 1998). Furthermore, about one-third of children with ADHD in research samples have been retained in at least one grade before reaching high school (Barkley, Fischer, et al., 1990; Brown & Borden, 1986). School suspensions and expulsions occur at a higher than average frequency for students with ADHD, although this may be due, at least partially, to the higher rate of conduct disorder among children with attention deficits (Barkley, Fischer, et al., 1990). Moreover, the high school dropout rate is higher (i.e., about 10%) among students with this disorder relative to the general population (Barkley, Fischer, et al., 1990). The academic performance difficulties associated with ADHD may even persist into adulthood, as follow-up studies indicate that only about 20% of adults with a childhood history of the disorder are continuing their education at age 21 as opposed to about 50% of normal samples (Weiss & Hechtman, 1986, 1993). The educational problems and outcomes associated with this disorder thereby increase the risk of experiencing significant vocational and social difficulties in adulthood (Barkley, Fischer, et al., 1990; Weiss & Hechtman, 1986, 1993).

POSSIBLE CAUSAL CONNECTIONS
BETWEEN ADHD AND ACADEMIC PROBLEMS

Hypothesized Relationships between ADHD and Academic Problems

Given the potential for chronic academic underachievement and related learning difficulties that children with ADHD may experience, several possible connections between significant academic skills deficits (i.e., learning disabilities) and ADHD have been proposed in the research literature. At least three hypothesized causal connections have been delineated: (1) academic skills problems lead to the exhibition of ADHD-related behaviors; (2) the behavioral symptoms of ADHD (inattention, impulsivity, and overactivity) disrupt academic skills acquisition and performance; and (3) both ADHD and learning difficulties are caused by one or more third variables (e.g., neurological deficits). Each of these hypotheses is detailed below, followed by a section summarizing the results of empirical studies designed to investigate them.

Hypothesized Relationship 1: Academic Skills Problems Cause ADHD

One possible connection between learning difficulties and ADHD is that academic skills deficits eventually lead to the display of inattention, impulsivity, and related behavior problems. This hypothesis has been articulated most clearly by McGee and Share (1988). These authors posit that learning disabilities lead to chronic academic failure that over time causes a child to develop a poor academic self-concept (i.e., low self-esteem). As a result of a lack of confidence in their own academic abilities, these children are less motivated to attend to instruction and to follow classroom rules. These apparent behavioral "symptoms" of ADHD then lead to further academic underachievement, thus completing the "vicious circle." Given this scenario, McGee and Share argue that the learning difficulties of children with apparent ADHD should be the primary focus of treatment rather than the behavioral symptoms of ADHD per se.

McGee and Share (1988) cite several lines of evidence as support for this hypothesis. First, low scholastic achievement is a significant characteristic of children with ADHD. Second, children with ADHD, as a group, exhibit deficient performance on cognitive tests that also are correlated with reading disabilities (e.g., naming tasks, tests of perceptual processing speed). Third, the attentional deficits of children with ADHD may reflect poor motivation rather than an intrinsic deficit in concentration abilities. Fourth, McGee and Share state, albeit erroneously, that there is no evidence that the primary treatment for ADHD (e.g., stimulant medication) leads to improvements in academic performance concomitant with reductions in ADHD symptomatology. Although their arguments in support of this hypothesis are quite convincing, there are important limitations to each of these, as will be delineated in the next section.

Hypothesized Relationship 2: ADHD Leads to Academic Problems

It is possible that the primary behaviors comprising ADHD (i.e., inattention, impulsivity, and overactivity) disrupt the child's ability to acquire academic skills and/or to demonstrate his or her knowledge in a consistent fashion (Silver, 1990). One of the earliest versions of this hypothesis was proposed by Keogh (1971). She stated that behaviors related to ADHD may interfere with learning in at least two ways. First, the child's high activity level could divert his or her attention from instruction and thereby minimize the *acquisition* of academic information. Second, and alternatively, because children with ADHD are impulsive, they may make decisions on academic tasks in too rapid a fashion, thus debilitating their *performance* on independent tasks.

In support of this hypothesis is the growing evidence that stimulant medication (e.g., methylphenidate) not only ameliorates ADHD symptomatology, but leads to enhancement of academic performance (DuPaul, Barkley, & Connor, 1998; Rapport & Kelly, 1991). Thus, a treatment that directly affects a child's attention span and behavior control often leads to concomitant, albeit indirect, enhancement of the child's productivity and accuracy on school tasks, thereby implicating ADHD symptoms as the primary cause of the child's academic difficulties. Nevertheless, there have been few direct studies of the causal relationship between ADHD and learning difficulties, and thus conclusions about causality are premature. Furthermore, although a minority of children with ADHD have been found to evidence learning *disabilities* (see below), most do not have specific learning *deficits* (Cantwell & Baker, 1991). Therefore, this hypothesis does not explain why some children with ADHD evidence learning disabilities while others do not.

Hypothesized Relationship 3: Unspecified Third Variable Leads to Both ADHD and Academic Problems

The two hypotheses described above have proposed direct causal relationships between ADHD and learning difficulties. It also is possible that both problems are caused by a separate and distinct third variable. The most common hypothesis is that some nonspecific neurological impairment may lead to both ADHD and learning difficulties, at least in some children (Keogh, 1971). A variety of other organismic (e.g., temperament, language difficulties) and environmental (e.g., discordant homes) variables also have been posited as causal factors for both ADHD and academic difficulties (Hinshaw, 1992b).

Research investigating this hypothesis has been plagued by the fact that groups of children identified with ADHD and/or learning deficits are typically heterogeneous. Rather than searching for a single causal factor, multiple variables may need to be investigated, thus complicating verification of this hypothesis (Cantwell & Satterfield, 1978; Hinshaw, 1992b). In fact, it may be that distinct causal mechanisms are involved for different subgroups of children (Hinshaw, 1992b). Longitudinal investigations that assess hypothesized developmental trajectories for varying subgroups of children with ADHD, learning problems, or both will be necessary to delineate the multiple variables involved.

Association between ADHD and Academic Problems: Empirical Evidence

One factor that has obfuscated conclusions about the association between ADHD and learning problems is the confusion between academic *skills* deficits (i.e., learning disabilities) and academic *performance* deficits. The former presumes a lack of *ability* to learn a specific subject matter, at least as the material is currently taught. As such, the student may show deficiencies in the actual skills being taught even under conditions of individual instruction. Alternatively, a deficit in academic *performance* would be defined as an instance where a student possesses the necessary skills but does not demonstrate this knowledge on a consistent basis under typical classroom conditions (e.g., by producing accurate independent seatwork). In the case of the child with ADHD, a lack of attention to academic materials may lead to poor performance on assigned tasks even though the child may possess the requisite skills to complete the assignment correctly. Furthermore, inattention and behavioral control difficulties could compromise the student's *availability* for learning (e.g., missing important teacher lecture points due to inattention), and thus lead to greater levels of academic underachievement (Silver, 1990). The academic performance of children with ADHD also may be deficient due to their inefficient and inconsistent problem-solving abilities (Douglas, 1980). Unfortunately, much of the work that has investigated the relationship between ADHD and academic problems has not clearly differentiated between academic skills deficits and performance decrements.

Empirical investigations of the association between ADHD and academic problems primarily have employed correlational designs. Very few studies have been conducted that have used research designs allowing for attributions of causality and specific examination of the hypotheses listed above. In contrast, much research has examined the prevalence of academic problems in populations of children with ADHD. Most of these studies defined academic problems as "learning disabilities," although there have been great inconsistencies in the definition of this construct across studies, as was discussed above. Nevertheless, the term *learning disabilities* will be used here when discussing this literature given the preference for this label by the authors of the studies reviewed. Although substantial numbers of children with ADHD have been found to evidence learning disabilities relative to the normal population, the

prevalence rates vary greatly between studies and the association between the two disorders is decidedly less than perfect. In the next two
sections, a brief overview of this research literature will be provided.
Several papers can be consulted to provide more comprehensive reviews
of this area of research (Cantwell & Baker, 1991; Hinshaw, 1992b;
Semrud-Clikeman et al., 1992).

Prevalence of Learning Disabilities in ADHD Samples

At least 17 separate studies were conducted between 1978 and 1993 that
determined the percentage of children with ADHD who also had learning disabilities in one or more subject areas (see Table 3.1 for a listing of
these studies). The obtained prevalence rates for learning disabilities
have varied widely across studies, ranging from a low of 7% (August &
Holmes, 1984) to a high of 92% (Silver, 1981). Averaging across studies,
approximately one out of every three children with ADHD was found to
have a learning disability ($M = 31.1\%$; Median = 27%). The association
between ADHD and learning disabilities was even stronger for those
children identified with both ADHD and a conduct disorder (see Table
3.1).

   As expected, the prevalence of learning disabilities among normal
controls is much lower than among their ADHD counterparts, ranging
from 0% (Barkley, 1990) to 22% (Semrud-Clikeman et al., 1992). The
mean percentage of learning disabilities in the control groups across
studies was 8.9% (Median = 3%), which corresponds to estimates of the
prevalence of this disorder in the general population. Based on these
studies, it appears that children with ADHD are roughly three to four
times more likely to exhibit learning disabilities than their peers.

   The studies summarized above have led to several important conclusions about the association of ADHD and learning disabilities. First,
investigations employing epidemiological samples are consistent in establishing a significant correlation between academic underachievement
and the display of inattention and hyperactivity (for reviews, see Hinshaw, 1992b; Semrud-Clikeman et al., 1992). This association is strongest
among children of elementary school age (i.e., 6–11 years old). Second,
although learning disabilities also are highly correlated with other disruptive behavior disorders (e.g., conduct disorder), the relationship with
academic difficulties is strongest for ADHD (Frick et al., 1991; Hinshaw,
1992b). In fact, the coexistence of ADHD with other behavior disorders
may account for the association of the latter with learning disabilities.
Third, the relationship between ADHD and learning disabilities is highly
dependent upon the criteria used to define learning disabilities. Studies
employing stringent criteria for learning disabilities (e.g., Frick et al.,

TABLE 3.1. Studies Examining the Prevalence of Learning Disabilities in Children with ADHD

Study	Sample description	Diagnostic groups	N	Rates of LD (%)
August & Garfinkel (1989)	School-based epidemiological	ADHD	50	22
		Control	47	8
Holborow & Berry (1986)	School-based epidemiological	ADHD	188	27
		Control	1,405	5
Lambert & Sandoval (1980)	School-based epidemiological	ADHD	100	14.8–42.6
		BD	44	0.0–14.6
		Control	108	2.8–11.3
		ADHD	18	19
		CD	21	19
McGee, Williams, & Silva (1984)	School-based epidemiological	ADHD+CD	24	37
		Control	426	7
Schachar, Rutter, & Smith (1981)	School-based epidemiological	ADHD	31	23
		Control	1,285	2
August & Garfinkel (1990)	Clinic-referred	ADHD	115	39
		Control	50	8
August & Holmes (1984)	Clinic-referred	ADHD	14	7
		ADHD+CD	24	8
Barkley (1990)	Clinic-referred	ADHD	42	19.0–26.2
		Control	36	0.0–2.9
Cantwell & Satterfield (1978)	Clinic-referred	ADHD	93	27.6
		Control	54	5.5
Dykman & Ackerman (1991)	Clinic-referred	ADHD	182	45
		Control	52	0
		ADHD	111	18
		ADD+H	97	17
		ADD–H	15	20
Frick et al. (1991)	Clinic-referred	CD	68	16
		Clinic control	42	2
Halperin et al. (1984)	Clinic-referred	ADHD	241	9
Levine, Busch, & Aufseeser (1982)	Clinic-referred	ADHD	220	66
Livingston (1990)	Clinic-referred	ADHD	147	>50
		Control	52	Not reported
Nussbaum et al. (1990)	Clinic-referred	Young ADHD	38	29
		Old ADHD	36	53
Semrud-Clikeman et al. (1992)	Clinic-referred	ADHD	60	23–30
		Academic	30	10–33
		Problems		2–22
		Control	36	
Silver (1981)	Clinic-referred	ADHD	95	92
		Clinic control	100	4

Note. LD, learning disability, ADHD, attention-deficit/hyperactivity disorder; BD, behavior disorder; CD, conduct disorder; ADD+H, attention deficit disorder with hyperactivity; ADD–H, attention deficit disorder without hyperactivity.

1991; Semrud-Clikeman et al., 1992) are consistent in identifying the overlap between ADHD and learning disabilities to be less than 20%. Although this represents a significant number of children, the extent of learning disabilities among students with ADHD is not as high as was once believed. Finally, the academic problems of children with ADHD are not limited to learning disabilities, as they are also at higher risk for in-grade retention, failing scholastic grades, and dropping out of high school (Hinshaw, 1992b). The use of grade retention to address ADHD-related difficulties is particularly problematic given that behavior difficulties typically persist or worsen following grade retention (Pagani, Tremblay, Vitaro, Boulerice, & McDuff, 2001).

Prevalence of ADHD in Samples of Children with Learning Disabilities

Several studies have examined the incidence of ADHD among students initially identified as having learning disabilities. Table 3.2 includes seven studies that were conducted in this area between 1982 and 1993. Prevalence rates for ADHD ranged from 18% to nearly 60%, with a mean percentage of 37.2% (Median = 38.2%) across studies (see Table 3.2). As with the studies reviewed in the previous section, the percentage of children identified as having ADHD was partially a function of the criteria used to define this disorder. For instance, Fuerst, Fisk, and Rourke (1989) used cluster analyses of the Personality Inventory for Children (Wirt, Lachar, Klinedinst, & Seat, 1977) scores to obtain a relatively low prevalence rate of 18% for ADHD in their learning disabilities sample. Alternatively, Holborow and Berry (1986) used a more liberal criterion of exceeding a cutoff score for "hyperactivity" on the Abbreviated Conners Teacher Rating Scale. As a result, they found that nearly 42% of the children with learning problems in their sample also met their criteria for ADHD. Interestingly, the latter result is commensurate with the prevalence rate obtained by Vatz (1990) who, relative to this group of studies, used the most comprehensive assessment battery (i.e., structured diagnostic interview with parents and two teacher rating scales) to define ADHD (see Table 3.2).

It is clear that a substantial proportion of students with learning disabilities also exhibit significant symptoms of ADHD. In fact, students with learning disabilities are seven times more likely to have ADHD compared to their normal counterparts. Furthermore, the prevalence of ADHD in the learning-disabled population is higher than the incidence of learning disabilities among ADHD samples. The strength of this association has led to the question of whether ADHD and learning disabilities are one and the same disorder (Silver, 1990). The empirical evidence

TABLE 3.2. Studies Examining the Prevalence of ADHD in Children with Learning Disabilities

Study	Sample description	Diagnostic groups	N	Rates of ADHD (%)
Cantwell & Baker (1991)	Sp. & Lang. impaired	Total sample LD	600 42	19 40
Felton et al. (1987)	School-based sample	RD Non-RD	45 53	57.7 24.5
Fuerst et al. (1989)	Referred for learning difficulties	LD	132	18
Holborow & Berry (1986)	School-based epidemiological	LD Non-LD	123 1,470	41.1 7.9
Levine et al. (1982)	Referred for learning difficulties	LD	646	34
McConaughy, Mattison, & Peterson (1994)	School-based epidemiological	LD	503	28.1–36.3
Vatz (1990)	School-based epidemiological	LD Random cont.	84 87	42 Not reported

Note. ADHD, attention-deficit/hyperactivity disorder; Sp. & Lang. impaired, speech and language impaired; LD, learning-disabled; RD, reading-disabled; Random cont., random control group.

suggests, however, that learning disabilities and ADHD are separate, but overlapping, dimensions, as depicted in Figure 3.1. Although these disorders share considerable variance, their association is not nearly as complete as would be expected were they identical disorders. Thus, the association between ADHD and learning disabilities is probably a function of specific characteristics exhibited by certain individuals with either disorder rather than a unitary phenomenon for all children with either disorder.

Studies of Causal Relations between ADHD and Learning Disabilities

To date, no controlled longitudinal investigations have been conducted that allow for a direct assessment of causal connections between ADHD and learning disabilities. However, the results of two studies employing structural equation modeling partially address this issue. The results of these studies imply that the predominant direction of causality is for attention deficits to influence academic achievement rather than the converse.

Fergusson and Horwood (1992) investigated possible reciprocal relationships between ADHD and reading achievement in a sample of 777 children from New Zealand. Measures of reading achievement and

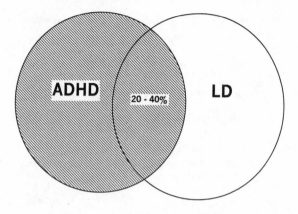

FIGURE 3.1. Venn diagram depicting the overlap between learning disabilities and ADHD.

ADHD-related behavior were collected at two points in time, when the subjects were 10 and 12 years of age. Possible causal connections between ADHD and academic functioning were analyzed using structural equation modeling procedures. These statistical techniques are designed to test the "fit" of obtained data to a theoretical model of causal relationships among specific variables. In this case, a model of reciprocal causal connections between ADHD and reading achievement was proposed and tested. The results of this study indicated that a child's degree of attention deficit at age 12 negatively influences reading achievement, while there was no evidence indicating that reading ability at this age exerted any effect on attention deficits. Thus, ADHD symptoms appeared to be, at least in part, causally related to reading achievement levels in this sample. The authors of this study are quick to point out, however, that it is possible that different relationships between attention deficits and reading achievement exist among younger or older age groups.

Similar findings were obtained by Rowe and Rowe (1992), who employed structural equation modeling to test two possible models for the relationship between reading achievement and inattentiveness in the classroom. The first model hypothesized that although several factors (e.g., family socioeconomic status, attitudes toward reading, and reading activity at home) may impact on reading achievement, there is a direct negative influence of inattentiveness on achievement. The second model proposed a reciprocal causal relationship between inattentiveness and reading achievement, while allowing for the effects of home background factors on these two variables. Subjects included 5,092 students from Australia who were divided for the study into four age groups: 5–6 years, 7–8 years, 9–11 years, and 12–14 years. Teacher ratings, self-report ratings, and achievement tests were used to measure classroom inattentiveness, home background factors (e.g., socioeconomic status), and reading achievement.

The results of this study supported both proposed models of influence between reading achievement and inattentiveness. As posited in the first model identified above, classroom inattentiveness was found to directly influence reading achievement, student attitudes toward reading, and reading activity in the home in a negative fashion. Therefore, greater levels of inattentiveness were associated with lower reading achievement scores. In fact, of the variables studied, classroom inattentiveness accounted for the most variance in reading achievement, as depicted in Figure 3.2. The amount of variance accounted for ranged from 13.4% (7–8 group) to 22.9% (12–14 group). In addition, the proposed reciprocal influence model also was supported because higher levels of reading

FIGURE 3.2. Histogram showing proportions of explained variance in reading achievement as a function of family socioeconomic status, reading activity at home, attitudes toward reading, and inattentiveness in the classroom, for four age groups of students. From Rowe and Rowe (1992). Copyright 1992 by the American Academy of Child and Adolescent Psychiatry. Reprinted by permission.

achievement were found to have a significant positive influence on classroom attention.

More recently, a series of longitudinal studies (Fergusson & Horwood, 1995; Fergusson, Horwood, & Lynskey, 1993; Fergusson, Lynskey, & Horwood, 1997) conducted with a sample of over 700 children in New Zealand has demonstrated clear linkages between ADHD behaviors in elementary and middle school (based on maternal and teacher ratings) and later levels of academic achievement (middle school through age 18). Specifically, structural equation models demonstrated that early high levels of ADHD behaviors were associated with concurrent and later lower levels of academic achievement.

Rapport, Scanlan, and Denney (1999) attempted to replicate the findings of Fergusson and colleagues by assessing ADHD symptoms and scholastic achievement in an ethnically diverse sample of 325 Hawaiian schoolchildren. The relationship between early ADHD symptoms (based on teacher ratings) and later academic achievement (based on a group-administered achievement test) was confirmed by these investigators. Further analyses indicated that the influence of ADHD behaviors on scholastic status was mediated by both cognitive (e.g., memory) and behavioral (e.g., classroom deportment) variables.

Although structural equation modeling techniques do not allow direct tests of causality, they do provide measures of relative influence among variables. It is clear from the studies reviewed that ADHD-related behavior (e.g., inattentiveness and impulsivity) directly influences academic achievement in a negative fashion, with higher levels of ADHD symptoms associated with inferior scholastic performance. The results of the Rowe and Rowe (1992) study, in particular, indicate that inattentiveness may play an even stronger role in influencing reading achievement than do other factors (e.g., family socioeconomic status) purported to have an effect on reading. It is important to note, however, that the relationship between achievement and ADHD is most likely bidirectional, although this assumption was not supported by Fergusson and Horwood's (1992) study.

Limitations to Results of Empirical Investigations

In addition to the fact that no study has directly evaluated the causal relationship between ADHD and learning disabilities, several other factors limit conclusions about the association between the two disorders based on the extant literature. One of the most ubiquitous difficulties with previous investigations in this area has been the inconsistency in definitions of learning disabilities utilized across studies (Barkley, 1990, 1998; Frick et al., 1991; Hinshaw, 1992b). Depending on the study, learning disabilities has been defined in a variety of ways, including below-average performance on an achievement test, a discrepancy of more than 1 standard deviation between IQ and achievement test scores, or teacher ratings of significant learning problems. Not surprisingly, this lack of consensus on the definition of learning disabilities has led to a wide range of prevalence rates for learning disabilities in samples of children with ADHD (see Table 3.1), and has in some cases overinflated the incidence of learning disabilities (see Semrud-Clikeman et al., 1992, for a discussion of this issue).

Another factor that limits conclusions from the available research literature has been the frequent use of a single measure to define learning disabilities and/or ADHD within a given study. For example, Holborow and Berry (1986) used cut-off scores on a teacher rating scale to determine ADHD and learning disabilities status. Even when such measures are reliable and valid, the use of a single measurement technique to "diagnose" either disorder is likely to produce erroneous classification decisions. Therefore, this practice is not recommended for either research or professional service delivery purposes.

Most of the studies conducted to date have used clinic-referred samples to investigate the degree to which learning disabilities and ADHD are associated. Use of such samples may lead to an overestimate in the prevalence rate of learning disabilities in ADHD samples and vice versa because children with multiple problems are more likely to be referred for clinic-based services (Semrud-Clikeman et al., 1992). Thus, the average prevalence rate of learning disabilities in ADHD samples reported above (i.e., 31.1%) should probably be viewed as an upper limit estimate, as is the same figure for the incidence of ADHD in samples of children with learning disabilities.

Recent Perspectives on the Relationship between ADHD and Learning Difficulties

Since the review completed for the first edition of this book, researchers have continued to investigate, speculate, and write about the relationship between attention deficits and learning difficulties. We discuss some of this work here, and note from the outset that the basic conclusions to be drawn today remain consistent with those of our previous work, as delineated in the following section of this chapter. On the topic of prevalence rates of ADHD and learning disabilities, and their co-occurrence, what is likely the largest study with this focus ever conducted was recently published (Pastor & Reuben, 2002). Here researchers from the National Center for Health Statistics reported pertinent results from the National Health Interview Survey conducted in 1997–1998. Data were gathered for more than 8,600 children between the ages of 6 and 11 within more than 78,000 households determined to be representative of the U.S. population.

From the data collected, the researchers generated national estimates of the prevalence of ADHD, the prevalence of learning disabilities, and the prevalence of the co-occurrence of these childhood disorders. A primary finding of the study was that

> in 1997–98 over 2.6 million 6–11 years of age were reported to have ever had a diagnosis of Attention Deficit Disorder (ADD) or Learning Disability (LD). Three percent of children 6–11 years had been diagnosed with only ADD, 4 percent with only LD, and 4 percent for children with both conditions. (Pastor & Reuben, 2002, p. 1)

These estimates are consistent with previous ones for prevalence of ADHD in the population of U.S. children (Barkley, 1990, 1998). Also consistent with previous research were findings that boys were three times more likely than girls to be diagnosed with ADHD (Pastor & Reuben, 2002). Of further interest, children with a sole diagnosis of learning disability were five times more likely to be participating in special education services relative to children with a sole diagnosis of ADHD. This finding is consistent with our earlier discussion suggesting that some, but not all, children diagnosed with ADHD will experience significant learning problems warranting special education services. However, in comparing children with ADHD alone, children with learning disabilities alone, and children with both diagnoses, children with co-occurring ADHD and learning disabilities were reported to have the highest rates of prescription drug use and use of mental health services during the previous year. By comparison, usage rates of these two supports were next highest for children with ADHD, and lowest among the three groups for children with learning disabilities alone.

On a related prevalence topic, but with more of an educational service delivery focus, Forness and colleagues (Forness & Kavale, 2001; Forness, Kavale, Sweeney, & Crenshaw, 1999) report that children with ADHD represent more than 40% of children in special education programs in the category of emotional disturbance. Furthermore, children with ADHD make up approximately 25% of the population of children receiving special education services for learning disabilities. These researchers go on to suggest that careful diagnosis of the presence or absence of comorbidities such as learning disabilities and conduct disorders is a crucial component to determining appropriate service delivery mechanisms and school-based interventions.

In a similar manner, other prominent researchers in the area agree with the importance of careful diagnosis (Barkley, 1997; Shaywitz, Fletcher, & Shaywitz, 1995; Shaywitz & Shaywitz, 1991) while making the case that ADHD and learning disabilities are distinct disorders with different underlying causes. In positing ADHD as a disorder of disinhibition and self-control, with neuropsychological underpinnings, Barkley (1997) suggests from his review of available research that ADHD involves demonstrated inhibitory and executive function deficits not found among children with learning disabilities. Similarly, Shaywitz and colleagues basically view learning disabilities as having their foundation in cognitive factors, but view ADHD as having behavioral foundations. They too recognize and underscore the importance of determining the occurrence of one, the other, or both in a given child who is struggling in the classroom with problems of learning and attention.

Conclusions

Despite the limitations noted, available empirical evidence indicates a consistent relationship between ADHD and significant academic skills deficits (i.e., learning disabilities). Approximately one out of every three or four children with ADHD is likely to have a specific learning disability. Furthermore, the majority of children with ADHD will be seen as underachieving academically, presumably due to inconsistent completion of assignments and/or low levels of accuracy on seatwork and tests. Nearly 40% of students with learning disabilities will display significant symptoms of ADHD as well. Thus, there is a great deal of overlap between the two disorders, as depicted in Figure 3.1. It is important to note, however, that the association between ADHD and learning disabilities is not perfect and that they are not one and the same disorder as has been asserted by some investigators (McGee & Share, 1988). In fact, most children with ADHD do *not* have a learning disability and most students with learning disabilities do *not* meet diagnostic criteria for ADHD. Nevertheless, the fact that a significant minority of children in each group can be identified with both disorders must be considered when planning school-based assessment and intervention procedures, as discussed below.

It is unclear whether ADHD "causes" or leads to learning disabilities in some children or vice versa. No study has been conducted that adequately addresses this issue. It is perhaps a nonfeasible task. Investigations employing structural equation modeling have shed some light on this question, however. These indicate that ADHD-related behaviors, specifically inattentiveness and impulsivity, exert a strong negative influence on academic achievement. This relationship may be reciprocal (i.e., level of reading achievement may influence classroom inattentiveness);

however, the effect of ADHD on achievement appears to be more clear-cut. In fact, the results of one study (Rowe & Rowe, 1992) indicate that inattentiveness is one of the most prominent factors determining reading achievement.

Although the direction of causality is presently unknown, it is clear that many children with ADHD have academic skills deficits that must be addressed. It has been speculated that certain subtypes of ADHD may be associated with a greater likelihood of learning problems. For instance, some studies have investigated whether children with ADHD-predominately inattentive type are at higher risk for learning deficits than children with ADHD-combined type. In general, these studies have not found significant differences in the prevalence of learning disabilities between ADHD subtypes (Lahey & Carlson, 1992). Conversely, certain subtypes of children with learning disabilities may be at higher risk for behavior control problems, including ADHD. Specifically, Rourke (1988) has identified children with nonverbal learning deficits to be at higher risk for such difficulties. In fact, future research into the association between ADHD and learning disabilities should divide samples into known subtypes of each disorder rather than grouping children into two heterogeneous samples. The former procedure may provide the best opportunity to identify which children with ADHD are at greatest risk for learning deficits and vice versa.

SUBTYPING OF ADHD BASED ON ACADEMIC SKILLS DEFICITS

Given the heterogeneity in functioning among children with ADHD, efforts have been made to identify possible subtypes of the disorder that may be more homogeneous within important dimensions (e.g., hyperactivity, aggression, internalizing symptoms). Because almost one-third of children with ADHD exhibit significant learning deficits, it is worth considering whether the presence of learning disabilities could represent a viable subtype of the disorder. To be practically useful, children with both ADHD and learning disabilities should differ from those with ADHD alone, with respect to etiology, developmental course, long-term outcome, and/or response to treatment (Barkley, 1990, 1998). In other words, they must differ in clinically meaningful ways beyond discrepancies specific to the measures on which the subtyping classification was made (i.e., academic achievement). In this section, we briefly review the arguments and evidence for and against a learning disabilities subtype of ADHD.

Beyond the increased risk for learning disabilities associated with

ADHD, there are at least two additional reasons for exploring the value of an ADHD + learning disabilities subtype. First, subdividing children on the basis of learning deficits could be helpful in determining the "causal mechanisms" underlying both their behavioral and their cognitive difficulties. Rather than searching for unitary causes for all children with either disorder, it may be more productive to explore the possibility of different etiologies for subtypes of both learning disabilities and ADHD (Hinshaw, 1992a; Rourke, 1988). For example, the attention deficits of children with reading disabilities may be caused by or related to a different factor or set of factors than those leading to attention deficits without reading difficulties (Felton, Wood, Brown, Campbell, & Harter, 1987; Shaywitz et al., 1995; Shaywitz & Shaywitz, 1991).

A second factor used to argue in favor of a learning disabilities subtype for ADHD relates to possible differences in long-term outcome. It is possible that children with both ADHD and some form of learning disability are at greater risk for chronic difficulties than are students with either ADHD or learning disabilities in isolation. For example, Beitchman, Wekerle, and Hood (1987) found significant expressive and receptive language deficits and visual–motor difficulties among a small group of preschoolers with both ADHD and language delays. Based on these findings, they proposed that such youngsters are at greater risk for exhibiting ADHD and reading disabilities later in life. In similar fashion, Felton and colleagues (1987) discovered differential patterns of performance on various tests of verbal skills among children with ADHD who were subdivided on the basis of the presence of reading disabilities. The fact that children with both ADHD and reading disabilities exhibited weaknesses in all areas of verbal functioning led these investigators to hypothesize that these children were at greatest risk for chronic deficits. It should be pointed out, however, that a more problematic outcome for children with both ADHD and learning disabilities remains a hypothesis, as no well-controlled longitudinal investigations specifically examining this issue have been conducted.

Children with both ADHD and learning disabilities have been found to differ from youngsters with only ADHD or only learning disabilities along several dimensions. The most prominent finding is that children identified with ADHD *and* learning disabilities are "doubly handicapped" (August & Garfinkel, 1990). In addition to displaying behaviors associated with ADHD, children with both disorders are found to display deficiencies on cognitive tests that are associated with both ADHD and learning disabilities. August and Garfinkel (1990) found children with reading disabilities alone to have difficulties on tasks requiring automatic-processing skills (e.g., rapid letter identification, naming objects). Alternatively, children with ADHD alone were found to display normal automatic-processing skills but to be deficient on tests that required sustained and the effortful processing (e.g., memorizing rote material). Children with both ADHD and reading disabilities displayed weaknesses on tasks in both the automatic and effortful processing domains. Furthermore, children with ADHD and learning disabilities have been found to be at a higher risk for separation anxiety (Dykman & Ackerman, 1991) and social rejection (Flicek, 1992) than those with either disorder in isolation. These and other findings have been used to support the differentiation of ADHD into behavioral (i.e., ADHD without learning disabilities) and cognitive (i.e., ADHD with learning disabilities) subtypes (August & Garfinkel, 1989).

Despite the above findings, it is premature to conclude that subtyping ADHD on the basis of learning deficits is a practically useful procedure. Most of the studies examining the subtyping issue have obtained differences between subtypes on measures related to academic functioning (e.g., IQ, learning tasks, academic achievement tests). These differences would be expected, as they result from measurement of the same dimension that was used to define the subtypes. Other than the isolated cases (e.g., Flicek, 1992) cited above, most studies have not obtained qualitative or quantitative differences in behavioral functioning between subtypes (August & Garfinkel, 1989, 1990; Dykman & Ackerman, 1991; Halperin et al., 1984). Furthermore, children with ADHD and learning disabilities do not differ from those with ADHD alone in response to treatment with stimulant medication (Dykman & Ackerman, 1991; Halperin, Gittelman, Klein, & Rudel, 1984). Thus, reliable evidence establishing differences between subtypes with respect to etiology, developmental course, long-term outcome, and response to treatment has not been gathered. Until further research is conducted on this issue, subtyping ADHD along other dimensions (e.g., with and without aggression) will be a more useful path for practitioners.

ASSESSMENT GUIDELINES: ADHD AND ACADEMIC PERFORMANCE DEFICITS

As previously noted, the academic achievement difficulties of children with ADHD can be divided into two categories: academic performance deficits and academic skills deficits. Thus, the school-based assessment of students referred for attention problems must include measures of academic achievement that tap potential performance and skills deficits. The assessment of ADHD is detailed in Chapter 2. The following section is intended to delineate evaluation procedures relevant to the academic functioning of referred children. First, methods to screen for academic skills deficits among children who might have ADHD are discussed. In similar fashion, procedures to screen students with academic skills difficulties (i.e., learning disabilities) for ADHD are covered. Next, because the most frequent achievement problem exhibited by children with ADHD is inconsistent academic performance (e.g., work completion), techniques to assess possible performance deficits are detailed. Finally, methods to determine whether a child's attention problems are due to a lack of academic skills, ADHD, or both are delineated. A case study is presented to further explicate this challenging discrimination.

Screening Procedures

Whenever a child is referred due to attention and behavior control problems possibly related to ADHD, several procedures should be incorporated into the evaluation to screen for academic skills deficits. First, questions related to academic difficulties should be incorporated into the parent and teacher interviews (see Chapter 2; see also Barkley, 1990, 1998). In particular, the child's teacher should be asked to provide information regarding possible difficulties in each subject matter area. Second, teacher ratings of academic achievement difficulties should be obtained through use of the Academic Performance Rating Scale (APRS; DuPaul, Rapport, & Perriello, 1991) or the Academic Competence Evaluate Scale (ACES; DiPerna & Elliott, 2000). Scores that are greater than or equal to 1.5 standard deviations below the mean for the child's age and gender for the APRS Total Score and Academic Success subscale are considered significant for screening purposes. The child's teacher should be queried about responses to specific APRS items to clarify the specific nature of possible academic difficulties.

In most cases, children with ADHD will be reported to be at or near grade level across all subject areas with no question of academic skills deficits. Ratings on the Academic Success subscale of the APRS would be expected to be within 1.5 standard deviations of the mean. These same children are typically reported to evidence problems with academic performance (e.g., poor completion and/or accuracy on independent seatwork) with below-average ratings for the APRS Total and Academic Productivity scales. Further assessment of academic performance difficulties should be conducted, as discussed below.

If interview and rating scale data indicate potential academic skills deficits, further assessment of learning abilities will be necessary. Although typically a psychoeducational evaluation incorporating IQ and achievement measures is conducted, we prefer a behavioral assessment of academic skills deficits for a number of reasons (e.g., greater relevance to teaching strategies, stronger ecological validity). A behavioral assessment usually will include curriculum-based measurement probes (Shinn, 1989, 1998), direct observations of task-related behavior, review of written products, and problem-focused interviews with the teacher (for details, see Shapiro, 1996; Shapiro & Kratochwill, 2000). The assessment of academic functioning should be conducted contemporaneously with further evaluation of ADHD, as discussed in Chapter 2.

Children referred for an evaluation of possible learning disabilities also should be screened for possible ADHD given that they are at higher risk for the latter disorder relative to their peers. This screening should be conducted even if the referral agent did not specify attention and/or behavior problems as part of the reason for the evaluation request. Screening procedures for ADHD are discussed in detail in Chapter 2. These include questioning the teacher(s) about the presence of possible ADHD-related behaviors. This is most easily accomplished by having the teacher complete the ADHD Rating Scale–IV (DuPaul, Power, et al., 1998). Using DSM criteria, if six or more of the items in either the Inattention or Hyperactivity–Impulsivity domains are rated as occurring "pretty much" or "very much" of the time, then further assessment of possible ADHD is warranted. If a lesser number of symptoms is reported, further assessment of ADHD would be pursued in cases where other assessment information warranted it.

Assessing Academic Performance Deficits

Even when children with ADHD do not demonstrate significant weaknesses in specific academic skills, they often have difficulty completing independent work in a timely fashion, obtaining accurate scores on classroom tests, studying for exams, taking notes on classroom lectures, and following through on homework assignments. In fact, behaviors related to academic performance are among the most important targets for change in any intervention program devised to address ADHD. Therefore, assessment of academic behaviors should be a standard component of an evaluation concerned with ADHD.

Some of the more important academic behaviors to assess include the completion and accuracy of independent seatwork, completion and accuracy of homework, and organizational skills (e.g., neatness of desk, accuracy of lecture notes). Methods for obtaining these data include direct observations of classroom behavior, teacher ratings, and collection of products (e.g., homework assignments, seatwork) completed by the student. These methods are discussed in greater detail in Chapter 2. It is expected that children with ADHD will complete significantly less work and/or complete tasks in a less accurate fashion than their classmates.

Differentiating between ADHD and Academic Skills Deficits

As reviewed above, there is a great deal of overlap between ADHD and academic skills deficits or learning disabilities. Thus, many youngsters referred for an evaluation concerning ADHD will be found to exhibit symptoms of both ADHD and academic skills deficits. The vast majority of children with ADHD, however, do not have problems with academic skills per se. Rather, their problems with inattention and impulsivity lead to difficulties following directions; completing tasks in a consistent, accurate fashion; and obtaining test scores that accurately represent their knowledge. Thus, one of the goals of an ADHD evaluation is to determine whether a student's academic problems are due to ADHD, learning disabilities, or both. What makes this discrimination particularly difficult is the ambiguity of the many definitions of learning disabilities, as well as the inconsistencies in learning disabilities definitions across school districts. Regardless of the definition of learning disabilities employed, the goals relative to an evaluation of ADHD are twofold. The first is to assess whether a child's apparent symptoms of ADHD meet criteria for this disorder. The second is to gather information to help judge the extent to which a student's academic problems are accounted for by difficulties with inattention, impulsivity, and overactivity.

Several factors should be considered in determining whether a child's problems with attention in school, impulse control, and activity level are due to ADHD or are secondary to academic skills deficits. These considerations are listed in the context of three possible scenarios:

1. If the data collected in the course of the evaluation, as described in Chapter 2, indicate clinically significant levels of ADHD symptoms evident across settings on a chronic basis, it is likely that the child's academic problems are secondary to ADHD. In this case, parent and teacher interview data, parent and teacher ratings, and the results of direct observations are consistent in placing the child's ADHD-related behavior in the extreme range for his or her gender and age. Further assessment of possible learning disabilities is warranted only if there is some question of below-average *ability* in one or more academic areas.

2. A second scenario is one in which the assessment data consistently indicate that few symptoms of ADHD are present and those that are observed are exhibited primarily in academic situations (e.g., classroom instruction, independent seatwork). In such cases, parent and teacher interview data, parent and teacher ratings, and direct observation data will be in the normal range for ADHD symptoms. If academic problems are present, then hypotheses other than ADHD must be explored, including the possibility of academic skills deficits.

3. Conclusions based on the above two scenarios are relatively straightforward. More difficult professional judgments must be made in cases where assessment data are inconsistent relative to the frequency, severity, and cross-situational pervasiveness of possible ADHD symptomatology. For instance, a child's teachers may report significant ADHD symptoms, while his or her parents report few, if any, attention and behavior control problems. Although the general problem of interpreting inconsistent assessment data is discussed in Chapter 2, the specific discrimination between ADHD and academic skills deficits will be aided by considering the following:

    a. Children with ADHD typically obtain clinically significant ratings on parent and teacher ratings of disruptive behavior problems in addition to ADHD (e.g., Aggression subscale on the Child Behavior Checklist). Children with learning disabilities in the absence of ADHD usually do not obtain high scores in these dimensions (Barkley, DuPaul, & McMurray, 1990). Furthermore, children with learning disabilities rarely are impulsive, disinhibited, and aggressive, while children with ADHD are more likely to display such difficulties (Barkley, 1990, 1998).

    b. Children with learning disabilities obtain average-range scores on measures that tap the situational pervasiveness of behavior (e.g., HSQ, SSQ) and attention (e.g., HSQ-R, SSQ-R) problems, while those with ADHD usually receive high scores for the number of problem situations and the mean severity of behavior problems on these measures (Barkley, DuPaul, & McMurray, 1990).

    c. Children with learning disabilities who do not have ADHD usually are observed to exhibit rates of on-task behavior and work completion that are no different from their normal counterparts when observations of independent seatwork are conducted (Barkley, DuPaul, & McMurray, 1990).

    d. Students with learning disabilities also differ from those with ADHD with respect to the onset and pervasiveness of apparent ADHD symptoms. Usually, children who are exhibiting problems with attention and behavior control due to academic skills deficits lack an early childhood history of hyperactivity and problem behavior. The latter is a hallmark of ADHD as it is typically a disorder with an early onset. In contrast, the attention problems of students with learning disabilities usually arise in middle childhood (i.e., third or fourth grade) and are exhibited only in specific situations. Usually, attention problems are reported to occur only when they are receiving academic instruction and/or completing work in their most problematic subject areas. Alternatively, children with ADHD are likely to exhibit ADHD symptoms across most, if not all, school and home situations.

e. Children with ADHD alone are likely to obtain scores on individual academic achievement tests that are similar to their peers, in contrast to the below-average scores usually obtained by students with learning deficits.

Overall, children with academic skills deficits can be differentiated from those with ADHD on the basis of the onset, severity, and situational pervasiveness of observed ADHD symptoms. In particular, the more specific the attention and behavior problems are to academic situations and tasks, the more likely it is that these difficulties are secondary to academic skills deficits rather than to ADHD.

CASE EXAMPLE

David was an 8-year-old boy referred by his second-grade teacher. Concerns were raised regarding problems with inattention and difficulties of an academic nature. David was reported to exhibit significant difficulties completing assigned work within a reasonable time period and to daydream frequently during classroom instruction. He displayed these problems on an inconsistent basis across school days. The teacher was particularly concerned that David was making very slow progress with reading skills and had difficulties comprehending material he had just finished reading.

An interview with David's mother indicated his birth, early development, and medical histories were unremarkable. His activity level as a toddler and preschooler was described as "normal for a boy." His father was reported to have evidenced learning problems and possible ADHD as a child, but no other significant problems were reported for family members. His mother reported no significant problems handling David's behavior at home and described his peer relationships as "excellent." David was not involved in special services or professional therapy at the time of the evaluation, although his mother did report recently placing him on a modified Feingold diet with resultant mild changes in behavior control. No formal behavior modification strategies were being used in either home or school settings.

A psychoeducational evaluation was conducted by the school psychologist, including intelligence testing and several individual achievement tests. Results suggested David was of average intelligence with a relative weakness in verbal abilities. Achievement testing indicated a number of deficits in language and reading functioning. Based on these results, the school team suggested that David receive academic support in reading and language arts skills several times per week with a resource room teacher.

Several measures were employed to evaluate whether David might have ADHD. A diagnostic interview with David's mother was conducted wherein only six of the 18 DSM-IV symptoms of ADHD were reported as present on a frequent basis. These included distractibility and often shifting from one uncompleted activity to another. Notably, David was reported to evidence inattention only on tasks that were school-related (e.g., reading), but was able to complete assigned household chores in a reliable fashion. No problems with impulsivity or overactivity were reported. Further reports indicated that David did not evidence behaviors related to any other behavior disorder including conduct disorder, depression, or anxiety disorder.

David's mother completed several rating scales to document the severity of his behavior control problems relative to other boys his age. Her responses on the Child Behavior Checklist resulted in a normal range profile (i.e., T-scores < 65) across all clinical scales including those related to ADHD. On the ADHD Rating Scale–IV, only five of the 18 symptoms of ADHD were reported to occur on a frequent basis. Ratings on the Home Situations Questionnaire—Revised indicated mild attention problems were present only in selected home settings (e.g., when asked to complete homework). Scores on the Social Skills Rating System (Gresham & Elliott, 1990) were in the normal range. Thus, parent ratings did not indicate ADHD symptoms to be problematic, nor were these seen as pervasive across settings.

David's second-grade teacher completed similar questionnaires. Her responses on the Teacher Report Form of the Child Behavior Checklist resulted in borderline significant ratings (i.e., T-score = 66, or greater than the 93rd percentile) on the Attention Problems subscale. Remaining scales, including those related to other disruptive behavior disorders, were in the normal range. Scores on the Social Skills Rating System did not indicate clinically significant levels of peer relationship difficulties. On the ADHD Rating Scale–IV, five of the 18 symptoms of ADHD were reported to occur on a frequent basis. On the School Situations Questionnaire—Revised, mild attention problems were reported to occur across most structured classroom settings. The most significant problems related to ADHD that were reported were with respect to concentration and completion of tasks, not with impulse control or hyperactivity. Thus, the symptoms reported by David's teacher were more consistent with ADHD-predominantly inattentive type.

David was observed in his regular classroom on several occasions using the Restricted Academic Situation Coding System (Barkley, 1990, 1998). Each observation took place during a time when David was assigned independent seatwork related to reading and language arts. Averaged over three 20-minute observations, David was observed to be on-task approximately 80% of the time, although these percentages ranged from a low of 53% to a high of 90%. Thus, his task-related attention was quite variable across days. David exhibited fidgety restless behavior during an average of only 28% of the observation intervals. David completed an average of 80% of the work assigned to him at a relatively low accuracy level (i.e., 74%). Although he did evidence some behaviors related to ADHD, his main problems were related to his understanding and accurate completion of assigned tasks.

In summary, most of the data collected in the course of this evaluation were not consistent with the conclusion that David met the criteria for a diagnosis of ADHD. In fact, only one piece of information, teacher ratings on the Child Behavior Checklist, was in the clinically significant range for this disorder. The remaining measures were in the normal range, including parent interview data, parent and teacher ratings on the ADHD Rating Scale–IV, parent ratings on the Child Behavior Checklist, and behavioral observation data. Behaviors related to ADHD were strictly in the realm of inattention and, more specifically, attention during academic tasks only. According to his parents, David was quite attentive to household chores and other nonacademic tasks assigned to him. Thus, David's problems with inattention were seen to be a reflection of his frustration in attempting tasks that were quite difficult for him rather than representing ADHD. Recommendations included further behavioral assessment of possible academic skills deficits to determine appropriate goals and procedures to increase his scholastic competencies. Although it was assumed that improving his academic skills would enhance his task-related behavior, the latter was directly targeted for change using a classroom-based contingency management program combined with a daily report card system (see Chapter 5).

IMPLICATIONS FOR INTERVENTION

The determination of whether a student's academic difficulties are due to ADHD, an academic skills deficit, or both has direct implications for classroom intervention (Cantwell & Baker, 1991). The behaviors targeted for change, the treatment settings, and the specific interventions employed will vary as a function of assessment decisions. As discussed in Chapter 5, the usual treatment targets for a student with ADHD are behaviors related to classroom deportment, such as paying attention to instruction, staying seated, and following classroom rules. To the extent that academic performance difficulties are present, then certain scholastic behaviors will be targeted as well, including timely completion of seatwork and/or accuracy of written work. For those children with academic skills deficits, achievement-related behaviors and academic skill development are the primary targets for intervention. These would include not only behaviors related to independent seatwork, but other academic survival skills as well, such as correct responding during reading group, accurate note taking during lectures, and providing correct answers to written test items. When a child is found to have both ADHD and an academic skills deficit, scholastic behaviors typically serve as the primary targets for intervention. This is due to the frequent finding that when academic performance is enhanced, classroom deportment often improves as well (DuPaul & Eckert, 1997; Hinshaw, 1992a; McGee & Share, 1988). It is not unusual, however, to find circumstances where both academic and deportment behaviors must be targeted for change to obtain consistent and durable effects. Furthermore, for those youngsters who have ADHD and learning deficits, extrinsic motivational programming must be combined with academic interventions regardless of the specific behaviors targeted for change (Hinshaw, 1992a).

Intervention programs designed to treat children with ADHD commonly are applied across a variety of settings given the cross-situational pervasiveness of symptoms of this disorder (Barkley, 1998). For instance, token reinforcement systems may be applied across a variety of situations (e.g., playground, classroom, cafeteria) in both school and home settings in an attempt to enhance compliance with rules and attention to assigned tasks. In contrast, the primary intervention setting for children with academic skills deficits is the classroom. Although a number of classroom settings may be involved, treatment of academic difficulties rarely takes place outside of the classroom, yet strong arguments for adjunctive, home–school interventions have been made in recent years (Kelley, 1990). Those children with both ADHD and academic skills deficits will require treatment in multiple settings implemented by a number of professionals. In such cases, the need for effective communication and collaboration among the individuals involved in the child's treatment is obvious (see Chapters 5 and 8).

As discussed in subsequent chapters, the two most effective interventions for ADHD are stimulant medication (e.g., methylphenidate) and contingency management procedures. Although the latter can involve changes to both antecedent conditions (e.g., more frequent prompts to pay attention) and consequences (e.g., positive reinforcement for task completion), motivational programming has received most of the emphasis in the ADHD treatment literature (DuPaul & Eckert, 1997;

Pfiffner & Barkley, 1998). Thus, behaviorally based classroom interventions for ADHD usually include token reinforcement systems combined with response cost wherein contingencies are available at school, at home, or in both settings in order to motivate the child to attend to assigned tasks and classroom rules (see Chapter 5 for details). In contrast, academic skills deficits are not directly enhanced by pharmacotherapy and are usually treated with psychoeducational programming designed to ameliorate presumed processing deficits that underlie the child's learning problems (Semrud-Clikeman et al., 1992; see also Crenshaw et al., 1999, for a meta-analytic review of psychostimulant effects on behavioral and academic outcomes). This treatment approach remains quite prevalent in this country despite a lack of evidence for its efficacy (e.g., Kavale & Mattson, 1983). Behaviorally based and instructionally based interventions for academic skills deficits that have received empirical support include modifications to both antecedent and consequent conditions (see Shinn, Walker, & Stoner, 2002). Although motivational programming similar to that employed for ADHD has been found helpful in addressing academic skills deficits, there is an equivalent emphasis in the literature on changing antecedent stimulus conditions (e.g., rate of presentation of academic material). Thus, even though both ADHD and academic skills deficits can be treated behaviorally, the specific parameters of the intervention program will vary as a function of diagnostic status.

ADHD AND SPECIAL EDUCATION

Prior to 1991, students with ADHD were not eligible to receive special education services unless they qualified for such services on the basis of existing classification categories (e.g., specific learning disability, seriously emotionally disturbed). Thus, the vast majority of children with ADHD were placed in general education classrooms and minimal alterations were made to their instruction. Due to the intense lobbying efforts of a variety of professional and parent groups, a change in the interpretation of federal guidelines was issued by the U.S. Department of Education in 1991 (see Hakola, 1992). In this section, we provide a synopsis of these changes in federal regulations and offer suggestions to school psychologists on how to determine whether a specific child with ADHD requires special education services.

In a memorandum to chief state school officers issued on September 16, 1991, officials from the U.S. Department of Education provided clarification of the department's policy to address the educational needs of children with ADHD (Davila, Williams, & MacDonald, 1991). The gist of their memo was that students classified as having ADHD may qualify for special education services in one of three ways. First, a child with both ADHD and another "disability" (e.g., learning disability) could qualify for special education services under one of the existing disability categories defined in Part B of the Individuals with Disabilities Education Act (IDEA) of 1990 (i.e., reauthorization of the Education of the Handicapped Act). This was the only way a child with ADHD could qualify for special education prior to the issuance of this memo.

A second possibility for special education eligibility was identified under the "Other Health Impaired" category of Part B. The memo defined this eligibility as follows:

> The term "other health impaired" includes chronic or acute impairments that result in limited alertness, which adversely affects educational performance. Thus, children with ADD should be classified as eligible for services under the "other health impaired" category in instances where the ADD is a chronic or acute health problem that results in limited alertness, which adversely affects educational performance. *In other words, children with ADD, where the ADD is a chronic or acute health problem resulting in limited alertness, may be considered disabled under Part B solely on the basis of this disorder within the "other health impaired" category in situations where special education and related services are needed because of the ADD.* (Davila et al., 1991, p. 3, emphasis added)

The inclusion of ADHD an "other health impairment" (OHI) has been reaffirmed with the 1997 reauthorization of IDEA (hereafter referred to as "IDEA-1997"). Furthermore, the OHI provision has been the most commonly applied criterion to judge a student's eligibility for special education services on the basis of having ADHD: there has been a 280% increase in the number of students identified with OHI over the past decade (U.S. Department of Education, 1999). This provision clearly states that if the child's alertness is limited by chronic ADHD to the extent that his or her educational performance suffers, then the child may require special education services. The previous sentence describes most, if not all, children diagnosed with ADHD, as, by definition, it is a chronic disorder wherein they exhibit limited alertness and their academic performance is deleteriously affected. The difficult decision, therefore, is whether the child actually *needs* special education programming (i.e., the second criterion for determining special education eligibility, the first being the presence of a disability) to address these difficulties and/or academic competencies or whether interventions in the general education classroom will be sufficient.

A final criterion that could be used to determine a child's eligibility for instructional modifications on the basis of having ADHD is contained in Section 504 of the federal Rehabilitation Act of 1973. Such modifications may or may not require the provision of special education services. This is a civil rights law that states that schools must address the needs of children considered to be "handicapped" as competently as the needs of nonhandicapped students are met. A *handicapped person* is defined as "any person who has a physical or mental impairment which substantially limits a major life activity" (Davila et al., 1991, p. 6). Certainly, learning as related to academic performance and school functioning can be considered a "major life activity." Thus, even children with ADHD who are not eligible for special services under Part B could be considered in need of individualized intervention on the basis of being "handicapped" in accordance with Section 504.

If the above regulations are interpreted loosely, one could make a case that most children with ADHD are eligible to receive some degree of special education services. Given the high percentage of children already receiving such services and the limited database supporting the overall efficacy of special education, however, this may not be a prudent course of action. Rather, as is the case for children with other behavior disorders, one of the main criteria for receipt of special education services should be the child's response to interventions in the general education classroom (Gresham, 1991). Thus, the diagnosis of ADHD does not necessarily warrant the receipt of special education services, unless the child's behavior has not changed as a function of regular classroom interventions (National Association of School Psychologists, 1998; Silver, 1990).

From the standpoint of practice, a child diagnosed with ADHD who also is experiencing learning and/or achievement problems would likely be evaluated for special education eligibility purposes following a lack of responsiveness to interventions delivered within general education settings (see Telzrow & Tankersley, 2000). If that child is found eligible for special education services, a team of professionals would then design, implement, and evaluate an individualized educational program. If that child is found not eligible for special education services, school personnel would remain responsible for "removing barriers" to learning in the general education classroom/instruction. This removal of barriers has been referred to commonly as creating a "504 accommodation plan" (see Zirkel & Aleman, 2000, for a thorough treatment of Section 504 and students with disabilities).

In designing accommodations, educators should consider both the potential accommodation itself and the "barrier" to learning that is being removed. For example, in providing a student with task modifications in the form of allowing a choice of assignments, the barrier to learning of having one and only one assignment to work on is being removed. Similarly, allowing a student with ADHD to complete fewer items on an independent seatwork task (at the same level of accuracy expected of peers) is removing aspects of the assigned tasks known to exacerbate ADHD-related problems in the classroom—namely, repetitive work items. Finally, the use of peer tutoring and/or computer-assisted instruction as accommodations removes the barriers to learning of delayed feedback and large-group instruction, both known to be potential hindrances to the learning of students with ADHD (see Chapter 5 for a discussion of school-based interventions).

Zirkel (1992) has designed a checklist for determining the legal eligibility for special education services in accordance with the regulations enumerated above (see Appendix 3.1). Figure 3.3 presents a decision-making flow chart that has been adapted from Zirkel's checklist. Using this checklist and flow chart as guides, the following steps should be followed in determining whether a specific child will require special education services for ADHD:

1. Conduct an evaluation of ADHD and related difficulties, as discussed in Chapter 2. If the child is found to meet the criteria for ADHD, then, by definition, he or she has a chronic condition that significantly limits alertness, thus satisfying two components of the eligibility criteria for special education services under the "other health impaired" category of Part B, as discussed above.

2. If the child is found to exhibit behaviors related to one of the existing classification categories of IDEA-1997 (e.g., learning disability), then special education services may be warranted.

3. If the child does not qualify for special education services under one of the existing categories, then two more determinations must be made. First, does the child's ADHD-related behavior in the classroom significantly limit his or her educational performance? This can be determined using academic performance data, as discussed in Chapter 2. Usually, some aspect of a child's academic achievement is deleteriously affected by his or her ADHD symptomatology. Thus, some form of intervention will be necessary given that Section 504 stipulates such action given that the "handicap" substantially impairs a major life activity (i.e., education). The typical initial step is to design and implement an intervention program in the general education classroom (see Chapter 5). Such programs will include modifications to the child's instructional program based on behavioral principles. The child also may be referred to his or her physician for consideration of a trial of stimulant medication, as discussed in Chapter 6.

4. The last, and most critical, criterion for special education eligibility is whether the child *needs* such services because of his or her ADHD. This criterion could be interpreted in a variety of ambiguous

FIGURE 3.3. Flow chart for making special education eligibility decisions for students with ADHD. From Zirkel (1992). Copyright 1992 by LRP Publications. Reprinted by permission.

ways. Therefore, the most objective way to reach a decision regarding this criterion is through evaluating the efficacy of regular classroom interventions (Gresham, 1991). Baseline data should be collected on a number of target behaviors prior to implementing a specific intervention (including medication). After implementing the recommended treatment(s), data are collected again on the same variables to assess behavioral change. If the child does not exhibit significant improvement following a trial of general education classroom intervention(s), one of three possible courses of action is followed. First, changes could be made to the intervention program in the general education classroom. Second, the child could receive some form of special education programming. Third, changes could be made in general education interventions and special education programming could be provided.

5. Whether special education services are provided or not, interventions addressing the child's ADHD will be necessary. The efficacy of both general and special education interventions should be evaluated on a continuous basis to determine when changes in programming and/or placement are necessary.

SUMMARY

Most children with ADHD will exhibit significant problems with academic performance, such as slow work completion, inconsistent accuracy on seatwork and homework, and poor study skills. Furthermore, about 25% of these children will display academic skills that are significantly below average, and therefore will be characterized as having a learning disability. The fact that academic problems are consistently associated with ADHD has direct implications for the assessment and treatment of these students. The evaluation of ADHD must not only be directed toward behavior control difficulties, but should include measures of academic performance as well. Furthermore, such children should routinely be screened for academic skills deficits, with additional assessment of academic functioning conducted as necessary. In similar fashion, intervention programs designed to treat ADHD must include target behaviors related to academic performance. In the case of children who have both ADHD and academic skills deficits, treatment must be directed toward ameliorating both conditions simultaneously. Finally, federal guidelines allow for the provision of special education services to children with ADHD when they meet the criteria for learning disabilities, emotional disturbance, or other health impairment limiting their educational performance. Special education eligibility decisions should be made on the basis of a reliable assessment of ADHD, the degree to which the child's ADHD impacts academic and social functioning, and the success of general education classroom interventions in ameliorating academic and behavioral difficulties related to ADHD.

◆

Zirkel's Checklist for Determining Legal Eligibility of ADD/ADHD Students

PART I

1. Does the student evidence, to a preponderant extent, all the qualifications of "other health impaired" under the IDEA:

   - a chronic or acute health problem?   YES   NO
   - if YES, does this problem result in limited strength, vitality, or alertness?   YES   NO
   - if YES, does the limited strength, vitality, or alertness adversely affect the child's educational performance to the extent of necessitating special education?   YES   NO

2. Does the student evidence, to a preponderant extent, all the qualifications for "specific learning disability" under the IDEA:

   - a basic psychological processing disorder in understanding or using language that is manifested in a severe discrepancy between achievement and intellectual ability in (a) oral comprehension, (b) listening comprehension, (c) written expression, (d) basic reading skill, (e) comprehension, (f) mathematics calculation, or (g) mathematics reasoning?   YES   NO
   - if YES, is the severe discrepancy not correctable without special education and related services?   YES   NO
   - if YES, is the problem only secondarily or not at all attributable to (a) environmental, cultural, or economic disadvantage; (b) visual, hearing, or motor disabilities; (c) mental retardation; or (d) emotional disturbance?

Note. From Zirkel (1992). Copyright 1992 by LRP Publications. Reprinted by permission.

3. Does the student evidence, to a preponderant extent, all the qualifications for any other disability under the IDEA:

• severe emotional disturbance?	YES	NO
• mental retardation?	YES	NO
• autism or traumatic brain injury?	YES	NO

PART II

4. If the student does not qualify under *Part I*, does the child's ADD/ADHD condition meet all the qualifications under Section 504:

• is the condition mental or physical?	YES	NO
• if YES, does it impair a major life activity, such as learning?	YES	NO
• if YES, is the degree of this impairment substantial?	YES	NO

PART III

5. If the student does not qualify under *Part I* or *Part II*, is the child eligible under a state law that supplements the IDEA or Section 504?   YES   NO

CHAPTER 4

♦ ♦ ♦

Early Screening, Identification, and Intervention

♦

By definition, ADHD is a disorder of early onset with behavioral symptoms exhibited prior to or concurrent with early elementary school (American Psychiatric Association, 2000). Children usually are not diagnosed with ADHD until the onset of formal schooling (i.e., kindergarten and first grade). In recent years, however, more children are entering daycare and/or nursery school settings as early as infancy. Although preschool educational programs are typically play-oriented and offer more free-choice activities than later schooling, the preacademic tasks, social activities, and art projects comprising schooling during these years require sustained attention and compliance with rules for short periods of time. Thus, children with ADHD-related behaviors could significantly disrupt structured activities, transitions from one activity to another, and group interactions (e.g., circle times). Furthermore, preschoolers who are motorically overactive and more impulsive than their peers may have difficulties sharing, waiting turns, and controlling frustration even during less-structured activities such as free play. Thus, given the potential for early onset of ADHD symptoms, it is important for school personnel, particularly those working with young children, to be aware of (1) how this disorder manifests in early childhood, (2) how to identify young children at risk for ADHD, and (3) how to design programs for reducing symptoms and enhancing academic, social, and family functioning.

ADHD IN YOUNG CHILDREN

Despite the myriad difficulties associated with ADHD symptoms in young children, the vast majority of research studies on this disorder have been conducted with elementary school-age children (see Barkley, 1998). Available epidemiological data indicate that approximately 2% of children in this age group have ADHD (Lavigne et al., 1996). Keenan, Shaw, Walsh, Deliquadri, and Giovanelli (1997) found that 5.7% of 5-year-olds in a low-income sample met diagnostic criteria for ADHD. Furthermore, given that ADHD tends to be chronic, at least 50% of pre-school-age children with this disorder will continue to exhibit significant ADHD symptoms during elementary school (Campbell, 2002). Those children exhibiting high levels of hyperactive and impulsive behaviors (i.e., combined or predominantly hyperactive–impulsive types of ADHD) will be at higher than average risk for developing other disruptive behavior disorders (i.e., oppositional defiant disorder and conduct disorder) along with academic and social deficits (Campbell & Ewing, 1990). Young children exhibiting ADHD symptoms have significantly poorer social skills than their normal counterparts and exhibit significantly higher levels of verbal and physical aggression in preschool classrooms and when interacting with their parents (DuPaul et al., 2001). Of further concern, 59–67% of those children with ADHD whose difficulties are persistent at school entry will continue to show significant symptoms of disruptive behavior disorder during middle childhood and early adolescence (Pierce, Ewing, & Campbell, 1999). Thus, significant ADHD symptoms are associated with chronic behavioral/academic impairment for a large percentage of affected youngsters.

Aberrant mother–child interactions as well as disruptive and aggressive social behaviors are related to ADHD at a young age. Mothers of young children with ADHD issue significantly more commands, criticism, and punishment than mothers of nondiagnosed children (Barkley, 1988). In addition, mothers of preschool-age children with ADHD report greater levels of parenting stress than do mothers of similar-age normal children or even parents of older children with ADHD (DuPaul et al., 2001; Fischer, 1990). As a result, parents of young children with this disorder cope with behavior difficulties in a less adaptive fashion than do parents of young children without ADHD (DuPaul et al., 2001). In preschool/daycare settings, children with ADHD exhibit high levels of disruptive, noncompliant, and possibly physically aggressive behaviors (Campbell, Endman, & Bernfield, 1977; DuPaul et al., 2001). These behaviors not only affect interactions with adult caregivers but also could negatively impact peer relationships. In fact, peer rejection is strongly associated with aggression, as rated by peers and teachers, among preschool-age children (Milich, Landau, Kilby, & Whitten, 1982). This finding is not surprising given that children with ADHD who also are aggressive disrupt the play activities of other children and are excessively demanding and noisy during peer interactions (Campbell et al., 1977; Campbell, Schliefer, & Weiss, 1978). In some cases, ADHD-related behaviors are severe enough to warrant removal from preschool or daycare classrooms, thus reducing the opportunities for children to develop age-appropriate social interaction and preacademic skills (Blackman, Westervelt, Stevenson, & Welch, 1991).

Young children with ADHD may be more likely to utilize medical services relative to their normal counterparts for at least two reasons. First, young children with ADHD appear to be at greater than average risk for physical injuries and accidental poisonings, presumably due to high rates of impulsive and overactive behavior (e.g., Lahey et al., 1998). Furthermore, injured children with ADHD are more likely to sustain severe injuries (including loss of consciousness) than are injured children without ADHD (DiScala, Lescohier, Barthel, & Li, 1998; Lahey, 2000). The relationship between ADHD and accidental injuries appears to be strongest for children with the hyperactive–impulsive subtype (Lahey et al., 1998) and is exacerbated by aggressiveness (Bijur, Golding, Haslum, & Kurzon, 1988; Davidson, Hughes, & O'Connor, 1988). Second, as is the case for older children with ADHD, some preschool-age children with ADHD receive psychotropic medication (e.g., methylphenidate) to reduce symptoms of the disorder. In fact, approximately 1.2–2% of 2- to 4-year-olds are prescribed stimulant medication, presumably for treatment of ADHD (Zito et al., 2000).

Upon school entry, young children with ADHD are likely to be behind their nondisabled peers in basic math concepts, prereading skills, and fine motor abilities (Lahey et al., 1998; Mariani & Barkley, 1997; Shelton et al., 1998). For example, DuPaul and colleagues (2001) found that a sample of 58 preschool-age children with ADHD scored on average approximately 1 standard deviation below a sample of 36 normal peers on a test of cognitive development and preacademic skills. This is particularly concerning given the strong relationship between early skills and later achievement (e.g., Kameenui, 1993). The presence of academic (and other) risk factors in children with ADHD is supported by data indicating that young children with ADHD may be at higher than average risk to be placed in special education programs during the early elementary school years (Lahey et al., 1998) and that students with ADHD are less likely to complete high school than their nondisabled counterparts (e.g., Barkley, Fischer, et al., 1990).

The results of a recent investigation (O'Reilly, 2002) highlight the extent to which young children with ADHD enter elementary school trailing their peers in important areas of academic functioning. O'Reilly examined the trajectory of prereading and reading skills in a small sample of kindergartners and first graders exhibiting ADHD symptoms as well as in a matched sample of normal comparison children. The Dynamic Indicators of Basic Early Literacy Skills (DIBELS; Kaminski & Good, 1996) was used to assess acquisition of skills over three time points (fall, winter, and spring) in the school year. Results indicated that kindergartners with ADHD differed from the comparison sample by approximately 0.5 standard deviation in early literacy skills at all three assessment points. Similar group differences in terms of oral reading fluency were found for first graders. Furthermore, the first graders with ADHD showed a slower growth rate in oral reading fluency relative to the comparison group and the 50th percentile using local district DIBELS norms (see Figure 4.1). Thus, young children with ADHD *enter* elementary school behind their peers in critical academic skills and this deficit continues through the early elementary grades.

In sum, the behavioral, medical, social, and academic difficulties associated with ADHD typically begin at an early age and are usually unremitting (Pierce et al., 1999). Thus, the best opportunity to prevent significant behavioral, academic, and social deficits; to reduce the need for medical intervention; and to boost academic functioning of children with ADHD during the early elementary grades (i.e., kindergarten and first grade) involves early identification and intensive intervention.

FIGURE 4.1. Mean onset recognition fluency (OnRF) scores for kindergarten at-risk and comparison peer groups as compared to 50th percentile on district norms for fall and winter benchmarks. From O'Reilly (2002). Copyright by the author. Reprinted by permission.

SCREENING AND DIAGNOSTIC PROCEDURES

In order to identify young children who are at risk for ADHD, one must use reliable and valid methods to (1) screen for those youngsters who require further assessment and (2) assess behaviors related to ADHD and other disruptive behavior disorders. Although psychometrically sound assessment methods are available, evaluating preschool-age children for ADHD is fraught with difficulties. Chief among these is the fact that typical children in this age range often engage in inattentive, impulsive, and highly active behaviors. In many cases, these behaviors may simply be a manifestation of being a young child. A related concern is the ephemeral nature of behavior difficulties exhibited by young children. Although about 50% of young children exhibiting ADHD symptoms will show chronic difficulties in this area, the corollary is that these symptoms will remit in about 50% of affected children (Campbell, 1990). Furthermore, behavior in young children can be highly inconsistent across time and settings. Finally, differentiating behaviors that are a manifestation of ADHD versus other disorders (e.g., autism) is particularly challenging in young children given the natural variability in skill and ability development in this age group. Thus, screening and diagnosis of ADHD in young children must be conducted in a conservative manner while remaining cognizant of developmental considerations.

Screening

There are two approaches to screening for at-risk children: classroom-based and individual screening. Classroom-based screening is a proactive procedure designed to identify those children at risk for ADHD or related disruptive behavior disorders *before* a teacher or parent referral is made. Stated differently, given the prevalence of ADHD in the general population, it is assumed that one or two children in every classroom may have this disorder. Rather than waiting for concerns to be voiced regarding these children, methods can be used to identify them at the earliest point possible. For example, the Early Screening Project (Feil, Walker, & Severson, 1995) employs a multiple gating procedure to identify young children at risk for behavior disorders. Initially, the preschool teacher is asked to rank all children in terms of severity and frequency of externalizing behaviors. The top three children are then passed to the next "gate," wherein the teacher provides behavior ratings on a psychometrically sound questionnaire. Those children who receive teacher ratings that exceed normative criteria (e.g., 1.5 standard deviations above the mean) are then passed to the next gate where systematic behavioral observations and parent ratings are collected. If the latter measures result in scores that exceed normative criteria, then a classroom intervention is designed and implemented and/or the child is referred for a more comprehensive evaluation.

In contrast, individual screening is a reactive procedure wherein assessment takes place *after* a teacher or parent referral. This process is very similar to that described for Stage I of our assessment model (see Chapter 2). Thus, whenever a preschool teacher or parent states concerns about a young child's attention, impulse control, activity level, or behavior control, screening for possible ADHD is warranted. Furthermore, given the strong association between symptoms of this disorder and difficulties attaining early reading and math skills, screening for ADHD should take place when teachers or parents indicate concerns regarding a child's learning letters or numbers. As is the case for older children, the primary assessment methods used here are teacher or parent ratings of ADHD behaviors and/or a brief parent or teacher interview. To aid in this process, McGoey and colleagues (2002) have devised a preschool version of the ADHD Rating Scale–IV. The latter contains the 18 symptoms of ADHD that have been adapted for use with preschoolers. Specifically, behavioral items include examples of how symptoms might be manifested by young children (e.g., difficulties following instructions manifested by having problems making the transition from one activity to another). If a significant number of symptoms are reported to occur often or very often, then further assessment of ADHD may be necessary.

As part of the screening process, the following questions should be considered:

1. How much of the child's disruptive behavior is due to "immaturity"? Is the child immature in many areas of development in addition to attention span and distractibility? Have the child's behaviors improved over time and with careful attention to their amelioration? If not, a referral for an ADHD evaluation may be warranted.

2. Are the classroom expectations age-appropriate? For example, are children expected to sit still for too long? The curriculum may be too focused on academics and/or may be requiring skills beyond the child's instructional levels. Are the disruptive behaviors a function of frustration?

3. Are the classroom rules clear? Have these rules been taught to the children? Is the teacher's discipline style clear and consistent? Is the child oppositional and defiant toward the classroom rules?

4. Parents and professionals often are reluctant to "label" a child at a young age. They and the child's teacher may be more comfortable waiting until kindergarten or first grade to see if the child "grows

out of it" (i.e., behavior becomes less difficult to manage). Alternatively, if a child exhibiting ADHD-related behaviors receives no intervention during the preschool years, the "wait-and-see" approach may result in increased frustration in school activities, the development of poor peer relationships, and diminished self-esteem relative to school success. Thus, one must ask whether the benefits of identification and intervention at this age outweigh the costs.

When screening data warrant further assessment, then a multimethod protocol should be used as described Stage II of our assessment model (see Chapter 2). Although the questions guiding the process and the process itself is the same as with older children, there are several important differences. First, different assessment measures must be used with preschoolers than with older children. Specifically, one must use rating scales and other instruments that have been developed for use with preschoolers. At a minimum, assessment methods must include an adequate and representative normative sample of 3- to 5-year-olds. Some measures that meet this criterion are delineated below. Second, given the variable nature of preschooler's behavior, observations and ratings need to sample behavior over a wider range of time and settings than with older children. For example, teachers should be asked about behavior over the entire school year and parents should rate behaviors over a 6-month period. Observations need to be conducted during both structured (e.g., circle time) and unstructured (e.g., free play) activities. Finally, primary emphasis should be given to parent report of ADHD symptoms because parents typically spend the most time with young children. When additional adults (e.g., daycare personnel) spend considerable time with a child, then interview and/or rating scale data should be collected from these individuals.

A number of interviews and behavior rating scales have been developed for assessing the disruptive behavior of young children. Preschool versions of structured diagnostic interviews such as the Diagnostic Interview for Children and Adolescents (Reich, 2000) and the Diagnostic Interview Schedule for Children (DISC; Columbia University DISC Development Group, 2000) are now available. Although these interviews are somewhat lengthy (30–60 minutes), they provide a comprehensive and reliable way to assess symptomatic behaviors of various disorders that might affect preschoolers. Rating scales that contain items specifically addressing the behavior of young children also are available for completion by parents (or other caretakers) as well as by preschool teachers. Broad-band parent scales include the Preschool and Kindergarten Behavior Scale (PKBS; Merrell, 1994), the Conners Parent Rating Scale (Conners, 1997), the Early Childhood Inventory–4 (ECI-4; Gadow &

Sprafkin, 1997) and a young child version of the Child Behavior Check-list (Achenbach & Rescorla, 2000). Similar rating scales are available for teachers, including the PKBS, Conners Teacher Rating Scale, and the ECI-4. A narrow-band scale that can be used to obtain parent and teacher report of ADHD symptoms is the Preschool ADHD Rating Scale–IV (McGoey et al., 2002). As is the case with older children, rating scales can be used to assess developmental deviance in key areas that might be impaired in association with ADHD symptoms including preacademic and social skills. The SSRS (Gresham & Elliott, 1990) includes parent and teacher versions that are appropriate for assessing the social skills of young children. The Preschool Learning Behaviors Scale (McDermott, Leigh, & Perry, 2002) can be completed by teachers to indicate the degree to which children exhibit problems with learning-related behaviors and motivation.

Another critical component of the multimethod assessment of ADHD symptoms in young children is direct observation of child behavior in classroom and/or home settings. For example, DuPaul and colleagues (2001) used an adaptation of the Early Screening Project social behavior coding system (Feil et al., 1995) to obtain information regarding the behavior of young children at risk for ADHD in structured (e.g., listening to teacher reading) and unstructured (e.g., free play) situations in their preschool classrooms. This system uses a combination partial interval (15-second) system for negative behaviors, a whole interval system for positive behaviors, and a momentary interval system to record activity changes. The category of negative social behavior includes negative social engagement, disobeying established rules, off-task behaviors, and tantrumming. Positive social behavior includes positive social engagement, parallel play, and following established rules. Activity change is measured independently of negative and positive social behavior and is defined as a child engaging in an activity other than the activity engaged in at the start of the previous observation interval. DuPaul and colleagues found that young children with ADHD exhibited significantly higher rates of negative social behavior in structured situations than did typically developing peers.

Observations of parent–child interactions across a variety of situations may be helpful not only in determining the developmental deviance of a young child's behavior but also to provide information that could be helpful in designing behavioral interventions for the home. DuPaul and colleagues (2001) observed parent–child interactions in a clinic playroom setting across four different controlled situations, each of which was 10 minutes in duration, in the following order. The first situation consisted of a parent allowing his or her child to play with toys in a free play situation (FPS). The second situation consisted of a parent providing minimal attention to his or her child in a low adult attention situation (LAAS). The third situation involved a parent supervising his or her child's activity (e.g., puzzle making and drawing) in a parent-supervised situation (PSS). The final observation situation required each child to complete tasks (e.g., cleaning up playroom) in a parent-directed task situation (PDTS). Parent behaviors that were coded included alpha (i.e., direct) commands, beta (i.e., indirect and vague) commands, positive behavior, negative behavior, questions, and reinforcement of child compliance. Child behaviors included activity, compliance, noncompliance, inappropriate behavior, and on-task behavior. For all but the activity category, the percentage of observation intervals was calculated. The activity score represented the number of intervals when activity changes occurred.

This parent–child interaction coding system was found to discriminate between young children with ADHD and normal peers (DuPaul et al., 2001). Children with ADHD exhibited more than twice the level of noncompliance and greater than five times the level of inappropriate behavior displayed by controls when asked to complete activities and tasks by their parents. Furthermore, parents of children with ADHD exhibited negative behavior toward their children three times more frequently than parents of controls, particularly when asking their children to complete activities and tasks. Interestingly, minimal group differences in interactions were found during the LAAS, suggesting that for many young children with ADHD escape from parent-directed tasks is a prime motivation for noncompliant behavior (as opposed to displaying negative behavior to gain parental attention). Thus, this system can be helpful in suggesting directions for functional assessment.

Along these lines, it is imperative that functional assessment data be collected. The components of a functional behavioral assessment for young children are no different than those for older children (see Chapter 2) and include parent and teacher interviews as well as behavior observations. In most cases, assessment data will be descriptive such that antecedent and consequent events will be delineated as they naturally occur in home or school environments. When possible, experimental analysis procedures as described by Boyajian, DuPaul, Wartel Handler, Eckert, and McGoey (2001) can be used to more definitively identify the function(s) of a specific target behavior. More details regarding functional assessment with young children are provided later in this chapter (see "Project ACHIEVE Model" section).

The multimethod assessment protocol must include measures that go beyond simply assessing behavioral concerns. Specifically, evaluation of the young child's early literacy and numeracy skills should be conducted, given that children with ADHD are at higher than average risk for deficits in reading and math achievement. Optimally, the assessment of early literacy skills should not only assess relevant content but also should meet criteria regarding practicality, technical characteristics, and decision-making utility (see Good, Gruba, & Kaminski, 2002). Given these criteria, the most comprehensive method for assessing prereading skills is the Dynamic Indicators of Basic Early Literacy Skills (DIBELS; Kaminski & Good, 1996). The DIBELS is comprised of four measures, including onset recognition fluency, phoneme segmentation fluency, nonsense word fluency, and letter naming fluency. There is a fifth measure, Curriculum-Based Measurement (CBM) of oral reading fluency, that can be used for children who are beginning readers. Each of these measures is brief and can be repeated over time to assess progress. Furthermore, the reliability and criterion-related validity of the DIBELS are strong (for a review, see Good et al., 2002). Unfortunately, a similar set of measures is not available for assessing early numeracy skills, although Sokol (2002) has developed an assessment protocol as part of the Project ACHIEVE treatment protocol, described below. Clearly, assessment of numbers and quantity-related concepts is an important area in need of development for young children in general.

Once assessment data are collected, the results must be interpreted in a similar fashion to the interpretation process described Stage III of our assessment model (see Chapter 2). Diagnostic decisions must be made in the context of the degree to which assessment data are consistent with DSM-IV (American Psychiatric Association, 2000) criteria for one of the three subtypes of ADHD. Several caveats are important to consider here. First, a diagnosis of ADHD is made less confidently in young children because of the inherent variability of behavior in this age group as well as possible diminishment of symptoms over time. In fact, in our work with preschoolers, we use the term "at risk for ADHD" to describe young children who meet DSM-IV criteria for this disorder. This terminology acknowledges the severity of the symptoms while allowing for the possibility that these symptoms are merely precursors of the disorder and may remit with maturation. Also, we have found that qualifying the diagnosis with the term "at risk" is more acceptable to parents and teachers of young children who are concerned about the potential long-term stigma attached to a diagnostic label applied at an early age.

Another consideration at the interpretation stage is the degree to which apparent ADHD symptoms may have other causes. Although all of the alternative hypotheses enumerated in Chapter 2 for older children also are relevant for the evaluation of younger children, the need to differentiate ADHD from autism and other developmental disabilities is paramount in this age group. Autism and related pervasive developmental disorders are most likely to be identified in the preschool years (American Psychiatric Association, 2000). Furthermore, inattention, impulsivity, and high levels of gross motor activity may be exhibited by children who have developmental disabilities. Particularly when parent and teacher concerns are voiced regarding a child's language and social skills, the practitioner should include measures to screen for symptoms of autism. For example, the Autism Diagnostic Interview—Revised (Lord, Rutter, & LeCouteur, 1994) can be used to get parent and/or teacher report of autism symptoms in the context of a structured diagnostic interview. In addition, observations of child behavior, such as the Childhood Autism Rating Scale (Schopler, Reichler, & Renner, 1988), may be helpful in screening for behaviors related to autism.

As is the case for older children with ADHD, intervention strategies should be designed, evaluated, and modified based on assessment data (see Stages IV and V of our assessment model in Chapter 2). As part of the treatment plan, it is prudent to recommend periodic reevaluation of a child's ADHD diagnostic status to accurately ascertain whether the disorder is chronic. For example, a subsample of measures could be readministered once per year through early elementary school. Given that symptoms of this disorder can remit over time in some young children, one should track the trajectory of ADHD-related behaviors to aid in short- and long-term treatment planning.

EARLY INTERVENTION AND PREVENTION STRATEGIES

The most effective interventions for ADHD have been psychostimulant medication (e.g., methylphenidate) and behavior modification applied across home and school settings (MTA Cooperative Group, 1999; Pelham et al., 1998). Although most efficacy studies have been conducted with elementary school-age children (i.e., 6–10 year olds), empirical investigations with young children with ADHD also have provided support for these treatments (for a review, see McGoey, Eckert, & DuPaul, 2002). More specifically, stimulant medication and parent training applied in isolation have led to positive effects on behavior relative to control conditions. Parent behavior training programs appear to be an effective strategy for young children with conduct problems because this treatment can disrupt the coercive parent–child interactions that often are the source of problematic behaviors (Wierson & Forehand, 1994). Of particular note is the parent training program developed by Webster-Stratton (1996) that incorporates a videotape-based discussion model versus the more traditional didactic model of parent training. This program has extensive empirical support for its effectiveness in the treatment of young children with conduct problems (Webster-Stratton, 1998; Webster-Stratton, Hollinsworth, & Kolpacoff, 1989) and has been identified as one of two empirically supported treatments for conduct disorder (Brestan & Eyberg, 1998).

McGoey and colleagues (2002) conducted a comprehensive review of the literature examining interventions for young children with ADHD. A total of 28 studies published between 1967 and 2000 were identified wherein three primary treatment approaches were investigated, including psychotropic medication ($N = 14$), school-based behavior modification ($N = 9$), and parent education programs ($N = 4$). In addition, one study of a multicomponent treatment approach was found. These empirical studies provide support for the use of each of these treatments for ameliorating ADHD symptoms and related behaviors in young children. To illustrate what is known regarding the treatment of early childhood ADHD, examples of each treatment approach and supporting evidence are provided below.

Psychotropic Medication

The most widely studied treatment for ADHD in preschoolers has been psychotropic medication, specifically psychostimulant compounds. The vast majority of investigations have examined the effects of methylphenidate, although dextroamphetamine and lithium carbonate also have been studied. Most studies have focused on the extent to which medication reduces ADHD symptoms and related problem behaviors. For example, Barkley (1988) studied the behavioral effects of two dosages (0.15 mg/kg, 0.5 mg/kg) of methylphenidate in 27 children with ADHD between the ages of 2.5 and 4 years old. Observations of mother–child interactions in a clinic playroom were conducted wherein both dosages led to significant reductions in off-task and noncompliant behaviors. Conversely, children were more compliant with maternal commands during task situations. Similar reductions in inattentive noncompliant behavior have been obtained across various dosages and settings (home, clinic playroom, and preschool) in a number of related investigations. At the group level of analysis, higher dosages (e.g., 1.0 mg/kg) evince more ubiquitous effects across measures and settings, although these same dosages also are more likely to lead to side effects (e.g., decreased social interaction, loss of appetite, and dysphoric mood). Dextroamphetamine (also a psychostimulant) results in similar behavioral effects, while lithium does not appear efficacious for treating this disorder in young children.

McGoey and colleagues (2002) noted a number of limitations to medication studies with this population, including (1) absence of measures assessing adherence with medication protocols, (2) minimal study of behavioral effects in real-world preschool classrooms, and (3) short-term (e.g., several weeks) study of effects. In addition, several earlier studies of medication effects did not include placebo controls or double-blind methodology, which is critical for ruling out threats to internal validity. Furthermore, several investigators have reported that parents took their children off medication following completion of the study. Therefore, it appears that at least some parents did not perceive medication to lead to clinically meaningful changes in their children's behavior and/or were concerned about side effects. Thus, the most prudent conclusion is that methylphenidate and other stimulants are effective in reducing ADHD symptoms and related problem behaviors in young children; however, the extent to which pharmacotherapy is necessary in this age group beyond alternative interventions remains to be determined. A large-scale investigation (the Preschool Attention Treatment Study [PATS]; Greenhill, 2000) is currently being conducted that should shed further light on the role of psychostimulants in the management of ADHD symptoms in young children.

Preschool-Based Behavioral Intervention

In contrast to pharmacotherapy, relatively few studies have investigated the effects of behavioral and/or educational interventions in preschool classrooms. This is both surprising and sobering given the short- and long-term implications of disruptive behavior in preschool and elementary school settings. Furthermore, many of the "classroom" interventions studied thus far have been examined in laboratory rather than preschool settings, thus limiting the generalizability of obtained results. As an example of a classroom-based investigation, McGoey and DuPaul (2000) evaluated the effects of a behavioral intervention combining positive reinforcement and response cost on the disruptive behavior of four preschool-age children with ADHD. The children's teachers were asked to reinforce appropriate behaviors and to discourage inappropriate behaviors by the contingent awarding or removal of token reinforcers (i.e., buttons), respectively. Daily rewards were earned by children depending on the number of buttons they had earned during the school day. Direct observations of behavior indicated decreases in disruptive behavior during intervention relative to baseline conditions. The teachers and students reported this intervention to be acceptable and effective.

In general, it appears that as is the case for older children with ADHD, classroom interventions based on behavioral principles are effective in reducing disruptive behaviors in preschool settings. This conclusion is tempered by several limitations of the literature, including small sample sizes and a lack of treatment integrity, long-term follow-up, and generalizability data (McGoey et al., 2002). In addition, interventions have been applied following a "one-size-fits-all" approach with the underlying assumption that all young children with ADHD will respond to a particular intervention. More work is necessary along the lines of Boyajian and colleagues (2001), who designed preschool interventions using functional assessment data. The latter allow for individualizing behavioral interventions in an attempt to optimize outcomes.

Parent Education in the Use of Behavioral Interventions

A number of investigations have provided evidence that parent-mediated behavioral interventions can enhance compliance and reduce inappropriate behavior in young children with ADHD and similar disruptive disorders. Positive effects on child behavior appear to result from changes in the way the parents issue commands and respond to their children when the latter are cooperative. One of the most ambitious studies of parent training in this population was conducted by Strayhorn and Weidman (1989) who were able to obtain a sample of 98 parents of preschool-age children with ADHD. Parents were randomly assigned to a control or an experimental group; those in the latter group were taught to implement positive reinforcement for compliant behavior in the context of parent–child interaction training. The experimental group demonstrated statistically significant improvements on parent ratings of child behavior as well as in direct observations of parent–child interactions in the clinic setting. Parents also reported a high degree of satisfaction with training outcomes. These same investigators found that group differences were maintained a full year after treatment, attesting to the maintenance of treatment-induced behavioral change (Strayhorn & Weidman, 1991).

As is the case for preschool-based behavioral interventions, parent education in behavior management appears to be an efficacious treatment for young children with ADHD. However, this conclusion should be tempered by similar limitations, including a lack of treatment integrity assessment, reliance on indirect outcome measures (e.g., parent behavior ratings), and lack of data regarding generalization across settings (McGoey et al., 2002). Furthermore, most parent education training studies taught parents to implement multiple behavioral interventions (e.g., positive reinforcement, response cost, and time-out from positive reinforcement). Thus, it is difficult to discern which specific intervention strategies are effective and whether a comprehensive treatment package is necessary to obtain behavior change. Finally, most studies have included primarily white, middle-class samples, thus limiting the degree to which results can be generalized to diverse populations. Given that the parent training literature consistently has documented the limited effects of this treatment approach for single mothers from low socioeconomic backgrounds (Nixon, 2002), further work with more diverse samples is critically important.

COMMUNITY-BASED PREVENTION AND INTERVENTION

Despite empirical evidence that psychosocial interventions may help reduce the family and school difficulties of preschoolers with ADHD, it appears that these interventions are not implemented frequently in community or nonresearch settings. In short, there is a gap between what is needed by these children, what is known to work to address these needs, and what is actually provided in the real world. Eckert, DuPaul, McGoey, and Volpe (2002) surveyed parents of young children at risk for ADHD (N = 101), community-based service providers (e.g., early childhood educators, pediatricians, and school psychologists; N = 137), and national experts and researchers in the field of ADHD (N= 25) regarding the needs of preschoolers with this disorder. There was general agreement among the three samples that parents and preschool teachers required information and ongoing support relevant to behavioral and educational interventions. Although parents perceived that they were getting helpful information from their child's physician and teacher, they reported less satisfaction with parent support groups and other community sources. Service providers reported ongoing needs for early intervention services, parent education, and educational consultation. Experts reported a gap between research and practice, as well as a general need for more research on effective interventions with this age group.

The gap between research and practice does not appear to be due to a lack of acceptance or comfort with possible interventions on the part of parents and preschool teachers. Quite the contrary: Parents not only perceive the need for education in structured parenting strategies, surveys indicate that they find effective behavioral interventions, especially those incorporating positive reinforcement, to be highly acceptable and preferable to medication treatment (Wilson & Jennings, 1996). In similar fashion, Stormont and Stebbins (2001) found that preschool teachers rated various behavioral and educational interventions to be important in the management of young children with ADHD, and importance ratings were highly correlated with their comfort level with these strategies. Teacher ratings of importance and comfort level were not correlated with years of experience, education level, or other demographic factors.

Thus, parents and preschool teachers are in critical need of information and support in understanding and treating young children with ADHD. Although the empirical literature supports a number of treatments, there is a clear gap between research and community-based practice. In the following section, we advocate for greater involvement of school psychologists in early intervention with this population and articulate a prevention/intervention model that can be implemented by mental health, educational, and health professionals.

Prevention of Difficulties Associated with ADHD

As stated earlier in this chapter, early-onset ADHD symptoms are associated with a number of chronic difficulties that compromise children's success in a number of critical arenas (see top of Figure 4.2). By far, the two most problematic outcomes are the subsequent development of oppositional defiant disorder and for conduct disorder symptoms and academic underachievement. Over 50% of children, especially boys, with ADHD will be diagnosable with oppositional defiant disorder or conduct disorder at some point in their childhood (Barkley, 1998). Social development is dependent, at least in part, on the interaction between behavioral dispositions of children (e.g., ADHD) and parents' behavior management skills (Tremblay et al., 1992). The greatest number of reinforcers are delivered by the people who have the most contact with children (i.e., parents); therefore, positive exchanges with primary caregivers make a significant contribution to children's social development (Patterson, Reid, & Dishion, 1992). A key tenet of Patterson's theory (Patterson et al., 1992) of the development of antisocial behavior is that the latter begins in the home during the toddler/preschool years. More specifically, children learn that their own aversive behavior (e.g., crying, defiance) turns off the aversive behavior of parents (e.g., commands). Over time and with repeated trials, coercive interactions train children to use aversive behaviors as a method to control unpleasant and chaotic situations (Dishion, Patterson, & Kavanagh, 1992). As children develop, these coercive exchanges intensify in frequency and severity, leading to aversive behavior that generalizes across settings, is persistent over time, and results in rejection by parents and peers (Reid & Eddy, 1997).

The major variable underlying this coercive process is parents' skill and effectiveness in setting limits and in monitoring children's behavior (Dishion et al., 1992). Symptoms of ADHD are significantly associated with disrupted family management practices and can increase the probability of coercive parent–child exchanges (Dishion & Patterson, 1997). The key to change is to alter parental disciplinary practices, including reducing the frequency of coercive exchanges (while concomitantly in-

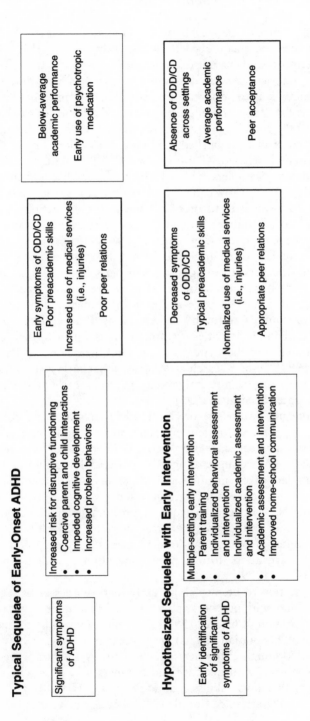

FIGURE 4.2. Typical and hypothesized sequelae of early-onset ADHD.

125

creasing positive exchanges) between parents and children. Furthermore, parents must be encouraged to consistently monitor their children to prevent antisocial behavior (e.g., physical aggression) and to prevent accidental injuries associated with impulsive behavior. Intervention is much more likely to be successful if conducted during what Patterson refers to as the "basic training" stage (i.e., preschool) rather than later in life when the coercive interaction style is well entrenched, antisocial behaviors are firmly established, and parent behavior is more distally related to child behavior (Patterson et al., 1992; Reid & Eddy, 1997). Given that preschoolers with ADHD are more likely than their nondisabled peers to show aggressive/defiant behavior in school settings, there is a pressing need to alter teacher–student interaction style as well.

The second common outcome associated with ADHD in early childhood is academic underachievement. As we stated earlier in this chapter, academic deficits often are evident from the very beginning of a child's schooling and persist throughout his or her school years. Numerous research studies have demonstrated that children's early experiences with literacy and numeracy have a significant influence on later academic skills. For example, research has demonstrated that children's experience with early literacy activities (i.e., phonemic awareness) makes a significant difference in their later language and literacy skills (e.g., Hart & Risley, 1995). Some research also suggests that early instruction in number activities may significantly reduce failure in early mathematics (e.g., Griffin, Case, & Siegler, 1994).

Phonemic awareness, or the insight that words are composed of sounds, is essential for reading acquisition. Children's knowledge in these areas at an early age is predictive of later literacy achievement (Adams, 1990). For example, at age 1–3 years, children should be exposed to vocabulary from interaction with adults and literature (Ninio & Bruner, 1978). Between the ages of 2 and 4 years old, with appropriate exposure, they will begin to acquire more complex linguistic knowledge, such as syntax and idiomatic expression (Snow & Goldfield, 1983). As children enter preschool and kindergarten, they should be prepared to begin to learn about formal print conventions and letter names and sounds (Clay, 1979).

In addition to literacy skills, early mathematics skills (i.e., fluidity and flexibility with numbers and a sense of what numbers mean) are important (Gersten & Chard, 1999). Early numeracy skills consist of identifying symbols (initially digits) and understanding linearity (i.e., bigger, smaller). Although still emerging, preliminary literature suggests that early experience with quantity and numbers may assist children in acquiring mathematical skills (e.g., addition, subtraction) once they enter kindergarten (Gersten & Chard, 1999). Because parents also are responsible for early cognitive and preacademic skill development, interventions to prevent later school failure must include enhancement of cognitive stimulation by parents (Hart & Risley, 1995).

Other than the investigation of individual treatment components (e.g., parent training and stimulant medication), there have been very few attempts to research the effects of comprehensive prevention/early intervention with this population. McGoey and colleagues (2002) conducted a pilot investigation of a community-based intervention program for young children with ADHD. A total of 57 children (3 and 4 years old) identified as having ADHD were referred by community service providers (e.g., pediatricians), preschool teachers, and parents. Children were randomly assigned to a combined intervention group or to a community treatment control group (wherein families obtained psychological, pediatric, educational, and/or psychiatric services available in the community). Complete results were available for 23 early intervention participants and 22 community control participants.

The combined intervention program included (1) weekly parent training sessions (using the program developed by Webster-Stratton [1996]) for 3 months followed by monthly parent training sessions for 9 months; (2) preschool-based behavioral interventions for 3 months followed by teacher consultation for the first 6 months of the following school year; and (3) open medication trials (methylphenidate or dextroamphetamine) for those children who did not respond to the psychosocial interventions.

Dependent measures were collected periodically over a 15-month period and included parent and teacher behavior ratings, observations of parent–child interactions and preschool behavior, documentation of injury rates and medical utilization, parent ratings of stress and family functioning, and a brief test of children's cognitive development. Furthermore, at two points in time, parents and teachers of children in the combined intervention group were asked to complete several consumer satisfaction ratings.

Results of this pilot investigation indicated that relative to community treatment controls, children who received the combined intervention showed statistically significant improvements in behavior control (at home and at school), their parents had reduced stress, and the family experienced more adaptive coping. The primary effect of the combined intervention was to alter the trajectory of child behavior over time relative to the community control participants. For example, the negative linear trend in teacher-rated antisocial/aggressive behavior (on the PKBS; Merrell, 1994) was significantly steeper for the combined intervention group (slope = –1.06) than for the community control group (slope = –0.2). In particular, the continued provision of teacher consultation seemed to help the combined intervention children to maintain a downward trend in antisocial behavior. Parents and teachers uniformly reported the combined intervention procedures to be highly acceptable and moderately effective. Although very few children who received early intervention were placed on psychotropic medication, statistically significant changes in medical utilization and cognitive development were not obtained in this pilot investigation.

At the individual level of analysis, the specific effects of preschool interventions based on functional assessment data were examined using single-subject designs employing more continuous data collection (Boyajian et al., 2001). Results indicated that determining the function of aggressive behavior (e.g., escape motivated vs. attention motivated) helped to develop classroom-based interventions that markedly reduced the frequency of aggressive behavior for three boys with ADHD relative to baseline conditions (see Figure 4.3).

Shelton, Woods, Williford, Dobbins, and Neale (2002) reported similar results with a comprehensive early intervention protocol for 184 young children at risk for ADHD. These preschoolers attended Head Start programs and were from diverse ethnic backgrounds. Behavioral interventions were implemented in home and preschool settings and were individualized using consultation procedures. After 1 year of intervention, children receiving early intervention showed reduced ADHD symptoms and aggression relative to an assessment-only control group. Although significant differences were not obtained regarding parenting competence, parenting stress, or family support, parents and teachers reported high satisfaction with the services they received.

Barkley and colleagues (2000) investigated the effect of a multicomponent prevention program for young children with disruptive behavior disorders. Although this program did not specifically target preschoolers with ADHD, their results are instructive regarding the promise and limitations of an early intervention approach with this population. A total of 158 children attending public school kindergarten who exhibited significant behaviors associated with ADHD and oppositional defiant disorder were randomly assigned to four experimental groups: parent training only, full-day treatment classroom only, combination of parent training and treatment classroom, and a no-treatment control. The parent training program developed by Barkley (1997b) was used on a weekly basis for 10 sessions followed by an additional five monthly booster sessions. Behavioral interventions were implemented in kindergarten classrooms using the model developed at the University of California–Irvine (see Pfiffner & Barkley, 1998). Classroom strategies included token reinforcement, response cost, group cognitive-behavioral

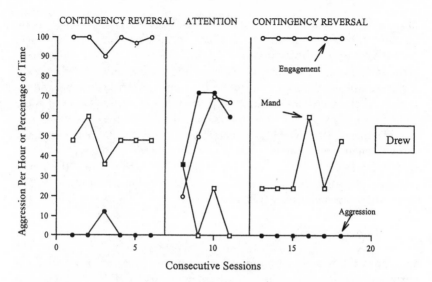

FIGURE 4.3. Level of aggression, requests (mands), and percentage of engagement in the contingency reversal (i.e., intervention) and baseline (attention) phases for Drew. From Boyajian, DuPaul, Handler, Eckert, and McGoey (2001). Copyright 2001 by the National Association of School Psychologists. Reprinted by permission.

self-control training, group social skills and anger control training, and a daily report card system.

Comprehensive data regarding child, family, and classroom functioning were collected at the beginning and end of the kindergarten year. The two groups who received the classroom treatment program showed significant improvements in adaptive behavior, social skills, and symptoms of ADHD and oppositional defiant disorder according to parent and teacher report as well as direct observations in the classroom. Unfortunately, no significant effects were found for the parent training component, perhaps because many parents did not attend these sessions on a consistent basis. Neither treatment component improved academic achievement or performance on clinic-based measures of attention and cognitive skills.

The results of these three promising investigations are consistent in indicating that psychosocial interventions primarily comprised of behavioral strategies can reduce ADHD and oppositional defiant disorder symptoms over the short term, particularly in classroom settings. Peer interactions and social skills also may be enhanced by early intervention

efforts. Unfortunately, more equivocal findings have been obtained regarding prevention efforts in the home setting. It appears that typical
parent education efforts may not be sufficient to produce even short-
term gains in parent and family functioning. A more intensive home intervention protocol incorporating both parent education sessions and individual behavioral consultation appears more effective. None of these
multicomponent programs were associated with improvements in academic achievement, which is a critical limitation. Furthermore, it is unknown whether short-term gains in behavioral functioning will maintain
over time. In fact, Shelton and colleagues (2000) found that the initial
gains in classroom functioning found by Barkley and colleagues (2000)
were not sustained after 2 years.

Project ACHIEVE Model

In light of the promise and limitations of prior efforts at prevention and
early intervention with young children at risk for ADHD, researchers at
Lehigh University and Lehigh Valley Hospital in eastern Pennsylvania
have developed a comprehensive, community-based early intervention
program called Project ACHIEVE. This intervention model is specifically designed to reduce and/or prevent the most problematic outcomes
associated with ADHD symptoms in early childhood (see bottom of Figure 4.2). Over the next several years, systematic data will be collected to
ascertain short- and long-term outcomes associated with implementation
of intensive school and home programming relative to a community
treatment control condition. Although this model program is only in the
beginning stages of evaluation, intervention components are described
briefly for illustrative purposes. We believe that school psychologists and
other educational personnel should be key participants in the design and
implementation of early intervention programs such as Project ACHIEVE
in their local settings.

The components of this intervention focus on three domains (behavior problems, academic readiness/skills, and child safety) across two
settings (home and school). Specific intervention components include
parent training, assessment-based behavioral intervention at home and
at school, preacademic readiness instruction at home and at school, and
home–school communication.

Parent Training

Parent training focuses on the domains of behavior problems, academic
readiness/skills, and child safety. Training typically is delivered to parents in groups of 10 who participate in 20 sessions over a 1-year period

led by a school psychologist or special educator. Of the 20 sessions, 12 consist of the original procedures outlined by Cunningham, Bremner, and Secord (1998) using the Community Parent Education (COPE) program. This program has been found effective in reducing noncompliance and aggression among at-risk children (for a review, see Cunningham, 1998). The remaining eight sessions include two introductory sessions (e.g., providing basic information about ADHD and related disorders), five sessions addressing functional assessment and promotion of academic readiness skills (described below), and one session devoted to injury prevention and home safety. Each parent training session lasts approximately 90–120 minutes.

The 12-session COPE program entails educating parents regarding effective behavioral procedures, such as positive reinforcement for compliance and use of problelm solving and mild punishment techniques to address problem behavior. Key behavioral concepts are delineated through videotaped vignettes of parent–child interactions followed by group discussion. In addition to the COPE program, parents are provided information and support regarding several related concepts and procedures. Philosophical components of the functional behavioral approach are a focus throughout parent training. Parents are introduced to the fundamental concepts concerning functions of behavior. For example, situations in which particular interventions are not likely to be effective (e.g., time-out in the context of escape-maintained problem behavior) are discussed. Using a consultative problem-solving process (Kratochwill & Bergan, 1990), parents are taught strategies for determining the function of challenging behaviors at home and then introduced to interventions that are matched to behavioral function. Instruction is provided in developing antecedent interventions (i.e., making changes in the environment to reduce the likelihood of problem behavior), skill building (teaching children alternative means to get their needs met), and providing consequences in a manner that is least likely to reinforce behavior.

Because a primary focus of Project ACHIEVE is to enhance academic and school readiness, two parent education sessions focus on this area of development. Four major topics are included in these sessions. The first is developing early literacy skills using the Ladders to Literacy curriculum (Notari-Syverson, O'Connor, & Vadasy, 1998). The second topic is "understanding your child's curriculum," wherein parents are helped to understand vocabulary they are likely to encounter as their child enters elementary school (e.g., phonics, readiness). The third topic that is covered is "reading to your child." Videotaped vignettes are used to illustrate reading at various developmental levels, including appropriate questions and expectations. The fourth major topic is "understanding your child's interests and attention span." This topic includes helping parents to select materials and learning opportunities that are likely to be motivational for their children.

Promotion of child safety is targeted in one session and is addressed in additional sessions throughout parent training. The primary method for accomplishing this is the use of The Injury Prevention Program (TIPP; American Academy of Pediatrics, 1999). Specifically, parents are provided with TIPP handout materials and group discussion of safety issues and strategies ensues. The implementation of safety promotion strategies also is imbedded into behavioral interventions designed as part of the parent training. Specifically, safety-related behaviors will serve as targets for intervention.

Assessment-Based Intervention: Home

Functional behavioral assessment and intervention is facilitated through a collaborative consultative model (e.g., Kratochwill & Bergan, 1990). Parents participate in a behavioral consultation procedure with a school psychologist or special educator once every month, as necessary, to facilitate the development and implementation of individualized intervention plans for each child. As part of this process, a functional behavioral assessment is conducted collaboratively wherein parents and the psychologist collect descriptive assessment data regarding possible antecedents and consequences surrounding challenging behavior. Hypotheses regarding the functions of behaviors are tested in the home using a brief functional analysis procedure (Northup et al., 1991). This assessment procedure requires approximately 90 minutes. Once hypotheses are developed regarding potential functions of problem behaviors, conditions are devised to confirm these functions. For example, if a parent request to complete a task is hypothesized to be associated with problem behavior, parents will be asked to provide multiple requests during a 5–10 minute observation period. To establish experimental control, this request session is alternated with a no-request session. If high rates of problem behavior are observed during the request session and low rates are observed during the no-request session, the function (escape) of problem behavior is experimentally supported. If differential rates of the problem behavior are not observed, alternative hypotheses are developed.

After the functional behavioral assessment has been completed and a behavioral function is identified, an individualized intervention is developed for each child/family. Interventions typically consist of three components, including antecedent strategies, skill building, and consequent approaches. Parents are trained to implement specific interventions through didactic instruction, modeling, practice, and feedback. Finally, a goal is established for the target behavior.

In subsequent months, parents are contacted periodically to discuss whether treatment goals are being met. Existing interventions are reviewed and problems with interventions assessed and remedied. Intervention decisions are made collaboratively by the parent(s) and psychologist based on data collected by the parents and parental report. Once a goal for a target behavior has been reached, maintenance is programmed and, if necessary, a new target behavior is selected, thus restarting the consultation process.

Assessment-Based Intervention: School

As in the home, functional behavioral assessment and intervention is facilitated through a collaborative consultative model in the preschool setting (see Table 4.1). Teachers receive behavioral consultation from the same psychologist or special educator who is working with the children's parents. Initially, a functional behavioral assessment is conducted in each child's preschool classroom consistent with guidelines developed by the Pennsylvania Department of Education (Bambara & Knoster, 1995). This functional behavioral assessment process includes the following five steps: (1) conduct a functional assessment, (2) develop hypothesis statements, (3) design an effective behavioral support plan, (4) evaluate effectiveness, and (5) modify support plan as needed. Preschool teachers are asked to collect data across 2 weeks regarding the antecedent and consequent events for a single problem behavior and to complete the Functional Analysis Screening Tool (FAST). Based on information from these two assessments, hypotheses are collaboratively formulated by the teacher and the psychologist. These hypotheses are tested by the psychologist using brief reversals (e.g., Kern, Childs, Dunlap, Clarke, & Falk, 1994). For example, if assessments identify escape from difficult work to be the function of behavior problems, work difficulty will be systematically manipulated across brief (e.g., 5–15 minutes) periods of time. If problem behavior systematically varies with work difficulty, hypotheses will be confirmed. Interventions then are individually developed based on the assessment information. These interventions typically consist of antecedent modifications, skill development, and consequent strategies. As was the case for parents, teachers are trained to implement specific interventions through didactic instruction, modeling, practice, and feedback. A treatment goal is selected collaboratively between the teachers and the psychologists, and teachers are asked to collect data on a target behavior to monitor progress toward achieving that goal.

In subsequent months, teachers are contacted to review progress toward intervention goals. Existing interventions are reviewed and problems with interventions are assessed and remedied. Once a goal for a tar-

TABLE 4.1. Steps to Functional Analysis and Intervention Evaluation

1. Consultant conducts Problem Identification Interview with teacher to determine problem behavior and possible environmental events (e.g., attention from teacher) maintaining behavior.
2. Consultant conducts Brief Functional Analysis with child in preschool classroom. This step involves:
   a. Analogue Assessment to get initial data on what environmental events might be following problem behavior.
   b. Replication of conditions that produced the highest and lowest rates of problem behavior to check on reliability of analogue assessment.
   c. Contingency Reversal to see if problem behavior will decrease and appropriate replacement behavior (e.g., verbal request) will increase if the latter is followed by the same environmental event (e.g., attention) that was found to follow problem behavior in the analogue assessment.
3. Consultant implements intervention based on results of contingency reversal. Each child's teacher gradually takes over implementation of the intervention after observing the consultant. Intervention effects are evaluated by looking at changes in problem behavior and appropriate, replacement behavior across baseline and intervention conditions.

Note. From Boyajian, DuPaul, Handler, Eckert, and McGoey (2001). Copyright 2001 by the National Association of School Psychologists. Reprinted by permission.

get behavior has been reached, maintenance is programmed and, if necessary, a new target behavior is selected.

Children with ADHD typically do not fully benefit from the preschool experience because they miss preacademic information due to inattention and may be excluded from playtime as punishment for disruptive behavior. Furthermore, the classroom ecology is changed by the presence of a child with ADHD because the classwide level of disruption may increase. Thus, the preschool teacher must evaluate the physical space, the daily schedule of activities, and her or his teaching techniques to help the child with ADHD to succeed and to manage the class as a whole. Classroom interventions for ADHD in preschool settings have not been studied in any detail to date. Thus, as part of the consultation process, preschool teachers are asked to consider possible accommodations, as delineated below.

1. Redesign the physical space. Tables where more formal activities, such as those designed to teach early academic skills, should be positioned away from indoor climbers, block areas, water tables, or other distractions (e.g., bright, three-dimensional bulletin boards). Use shelves or furniture as boundaries to play areas (e.g., book corner, dramatic play area) so that there are physical cues as to the type of play that is appropriate in a given area. These types of environmental arrange-

ments may help the child to focus on one activity at a time while minimizing the probability of becoming distracted by other classroom activities.

2. Adopt a step-by-step approach to activity setup. For example, rather than setting up an art activity by placing paper, crayons, scissors, and glue on a table all at once, the teacher would provide materials necessary for only the first step in the process (e.g., paper and crayons for coloring). As children complete each step of the activity, materials successively are added and then removed from the table when no longer needed. This reduces distractions and minimizes potential disruptions. During the presentation of activity directions, the child with ADHD should be seated as close as possible to the teacher with an uninterrupted view of the teacher's demonstrations. Finally, chairs should be spaced so that children are not seated too close together.

3. Evaluate and modify the daily schedule and activity transitions. The teacher should be encouraged to critically examine the content and timing of scheduled activities. Specific modifications will vary as a function of the classroom. Several questions could be considered. Is it preferable to schedule two short circle times versus one longer one? The former may be more adaptable to children with a short attention span. What time of the day does the child sit better for activities? Perhaps the schedule could be adjusted based on observations of the child's behavior. Must everyone actually form a line to go outside? Can transitions be shortened so that there is less waiting (e.g., to get everyone dressed to go outside, to serve snack to everyone)? Finally, it may be beneficial to "talk through" transition times. For example, impending transitions can be announced, as can the requirements for completing the present activity.

4. Vary the curriculum. To maximize interest level, the teacher should be encouraged to be creative in planning innovative and engaging activities (e.g., flannelboard stories, puppet shows) for the entire class and should include those of special appeal to the child with attention and behavior problems.

5. Give individual directions clearly. The teacher should not assume that the child will follow directions presented to the group on a consistent basis. While giving directions, the teacher should make eye contact and gently touch the child to encourage attention. Commands should be made in a straightforward, direct manner (e.g., "Johnny, please pick up these toys") rather than posed as a question or favor (e.g., "Johnny, could you do me a favor and pick up these toys?"). Multistep directions should be broken down into individual steps. Finally, the child should be asked to repeat directions to ensure attention and understanding.

6. Increase the ratio of adults to children. Recruit and use volunteers (e.g., grandparents, college students) to provide the child with ADHD more individualized attention during structured activities, circle times, and transitions. Also, having extra help can ensure greater consistency and follow-through on any interventions that might be implemented.

Assessment and Training of Preacademic Skills: Home

Ladders to Literacy: A Preschool Activity Book (Notari-Syverson et al., 1998) is used as a curriculum guide to create early literacy experiences. The program is readily individualized, offering choices, self-direction, and multiple opportunities for practice, thus making it appropriate for children at a variety of developmental levels. Activities and experiences contained in *Ladders to Literacy* fall into three broad areas that have been identified to influence children's literacy development. These are print/book awareness, metalinguistic awareness, and oral language.

Ladders to Literacy contains activities designed for "busy parents" that are simple and can be completed in the context of other activities (e.g., while washing the dishes, while driving the car). For example, one activity suggests that parents ask their child to predict what will happen next when reading a familiar story. Parents are provided activities on index cards for easy access. They are instructed to complete at least one activity daily, lasting approximately 15–20 minutes.

Parents also are exposed to several activities to assist their child with early numeracy skills. These activities are designed to reinforce number identification and linearity. For example, children are exposed to number lines and thermometers, which provide visual representations of the early numeracy concepts of bigger/smaller and going up/going down.

Assessment and Training of Preacademic Skills: School

Assessments based on children's preschool curricula occur on a monthly basis. In addition, phonemic segmentation fluency, letter-naming fluency, and picture-naming fluency are assessed using the Dynamic Indicators of Basic Early Literacy Skills (DIBELS; Kaminski & Good, 1996). A modified version of the DIBELS focusing on numeracy skills is used to allow for dynamic assessment of premath abilities. Specific skills assessed include numeric character naming, counting, character–set matching, set–set matching, and pattern matching. These data will help teachers to individualize instruction on an ongoing basis.

The *Ladders to Literacy* program is used as the instructional intervention because it contains an extensive curriculum for early childhood teachers. Each activity is used to teach or reinforce a specific skill (e.g., awareness of sounds). Activities are categorized into three levels of task demand, including "high demand/low support," "medium demand/medium support," and "low demand/high support." These correspond to the demand of the task on the child and the level of adult assistance needed to complete the activity. This system of categorization facilitates selection and scheduling of tasks depending on child characteristics and ongoing demands on the teacher. In addition, tasks contain multiple skills or goals along with adaptations for children with disabilities (e.g., hearing, motor, or visual impairments). Thus, they are suitable for children with diverse needs.

Home–School Communication

Preschool teachers are asked to send brief notes home to parents so that the latter can review the day's academic and behavior issues. In these notes, teachers provide parents with a brief description of the lesson plan for the day (e.g., "We reviewed words that begin with C today"). If a child is having difficulty, teachers are asked to provide parents with a simple exercise to improve the skill. Teachers also are asked to report any behavior problems that were exhibited by children that day, as well as examples of positive behaviors or areas of improvement in that regard. Parents are guided by the psychologist or special educator in providing positive consequences (e.g., praise and rewards) for appropriate school behavior and performance.

In sum, the purpose of the Project ACHIEVE protocol is to address the areas of greatest risk for young children exhibiting behaviors symptomatic of ADHD. Specifically, the objective is to prevent more serious antisocial behaviors from developing as well as to promote early literacy and numeracy skills. Although systematic evaluation of outcomes associated with this prevention program is in the beginning stages, we present this protocol as a contemporary model for early intervention with this population. It is hoped that this will stimulate further research and practice in this important area.

CONCLUSIONS

ADHD is a disorder that typically begins early in life, with most symptoms becoming evident prior to elementary school. Yet, until recently, minimal research has been conducted to aid practitioners in identifying and supporting young children at risk for this disorder. In this chapter, we have described methods for (1) screening preschool children to delineate those youngsters requiring further assessment and intervention, (2) adapting our multimethod assessment model for the evaluation of ADHD in young children, and (3) intervening early to reduce the frequency and severity of ADHD-related behaviors as well as to prevent the emergence of common outcomes (e.g., academic deficits and conduct problems) associated with this disorder. Given the chronicity of ADHD in many children, it is hoped that early identification and intervention may enhance the school, social, and family functioning of these children such that more expensive and intensive services are not necessary later in life. Although this assumption requires empirical verification, in keeping with recent calls for school psychologists to be preventionists (Power, 2002), we strongly believe that school practitioners should be engaged with these children and their families and teachers as early as possible.

CHAPTER 5

♦ ♦ ♦

School-Based
Intervention Strategies

♦

Children spend 6–8 hours per day, 5 days per week in classroom and other school settings throughout each school year. These environments require children to follow rules, interact appropriately with other children and adults, participate in adult-directed instructional activities, learn what is being taught, and refrain from disrupting or disturbing the learning and activities of others. For teachers, imparting the knowledge and skills comprising the curriculum and teaching children to behave in a manner consistent with organizational, social, and cultural expectations are demanding tasks. This work is even more demanding when it involves children diagnosed with ADHD, as the behaviors characteristic of these children frequently interfere with classroom learning and impede positive social interactions. The purpose of this chapter is to present and discuss school-based intervention and support strategies for promoting the learning and prosocial behavior of children diagnosed with ADHD, and for facilitating the smooth conduct of classroom teaching where these children are involved. We begin with a discussion of conceptual foundations for these interventions, and then discuss contingency management- and instructional strategy-based interventions.[1] We then

---

[1]Many of the intervention strategies described in this chapter are demonstrated on the videotape *Classroom Intervention for ADHD* (DuPaul & Stoner, 1999), available from Guilford Publications.

move to discussions of intervention strategies capable of delivery by a range of individuals and specific considerations for students with ADHD in secondary school settings. We end the chapter with a discussion of considerations for supporting teachers responsible for students with ADHD.

CONCEPTUAL UNDERPINNINGS
OF INTERVENTIONS FOR ATTENTION PROBLEMS

Given the challenging and chronic nature of ADHD, we recommend that involved professionals take a systematic and ongoing approach to designing, implementing and evaluating classroom-based accommodations that combines both preventive and remedial approaches to dealing with presenting problems, and that involves multiple intervention agents. To facilitate such an approach, the strategies presented are reviewed based on empirical support for them in the research literature of education and psychology as well as the National Association of School Psychologists (NASP; 1998) *Position Statement on Students with Attention Problems.* In addition, we review promising and newly investigated approaches to behavioral and instructional management with children with ADHD.

To begin, we examine our assumptions. The first is that ADHD should be considered a serious concern that will be enduring over time and will be associated with difficult-to-manage behavior in classroom settings (Barkley, 2002). Children diagnosed with ADHD likely will experience academic and social learning difficulties across many, but not all, classroom situations and throughout their school-age years (Teeter, 1998). To date, the vast majority of research in the area of interventions for children with ADHD has focused on issues and strategies pertaining to managing social behavior and deportment in the classroom, primarily via medication and contingency management. However, this focus on optimizing children's social behavior, behavioral maladjustment, and prevention of antisocial behavior represents only "one side of the coin" regarding ADHD. The other side is focused on optimizing the academic achievement and performance of identified children.

Social and academic problems can be seen as related. Viewing them as such leads to our second assumption. Specifically, we assume that the social and achievement problems of childhood can both be understood as instructional problems (Colvin & Sugai, 1988). That is, we as educators and psychologists have a critical role to play in arranging for and conducting instruction to promote both academic and social skill development such as to prevent and solve problems in these areas.

In a related fashion, then, our third assumption is that professionals involved with children with ADHD should take an educative approach to behavior problems (Evans & Meyer, 1985; Meyer & Evans, 1989). From this perspective, interventions for behavior problems have as their explicit goals to teach identified children the skills and knowledge necessary to replace problem behaviors with acceptable ones. An educative approach represents an alternative to interventions that are solely child-focused and primarily concerned with the elimination or reduction of problem behaviors.

Taking an educative approach to behavior problems leads us to our fourth assumption: dealing effectively and in an educative manner with behavior problems will require the development and implementation of programmatic behavior and teacher support plans (Horner, Albin, & O'Neill, 1991) Contemporary approaches to prevention of school-based problems, often referred to as "positive behavior support" programs, employ school- and classwide approaches to facilitate the learning and behavior of all students (see Sugai, Horner, & Gresham, 2002, for a thorough treatment of this topic). In doing so, such programs have the ability to "jump-start" individually focused intervention/support strategies.

Finally, it is assumed that persons responsible for supporting behavior of children with ADHD will have completed appropriate professional training (see Barnett et al., 2002; Jenson, Clark, Walker, & Kehle, 1991; McConnell & Hecht, 1991; and Power, 2002, for discussions of professional training needs in the area of interventions). Such training should include conceptual and practical preparation as regards intervention design, delivery, and outcome evaluation.

Given these assumptions, classroom-based intervention strategies for ADHD should be grounded in the guidelines for interventions presented in Table 5.1. First and foremost, the development and evaluation of interventions for ADHD are empirically based. Treatment strategies are chosen based, in part, on their demonstrated efficacy in the research literature. Furthermore, the relative success of an intervention program is assessed by using appropriate evaluation measures (see Chapter 2). For example, data regarding the possible reinforcement value, or functions, of problem behavior can be used to develop interventions that directly address the presumed function of problematic behavior (for a review, see DuPaul & Ervin, 1996). In a similar fashion, curriculum-based measurement data regarding a child's academic skills development can be used to set appropriate targets for and assess the benefit of academic interventions (Shinn, 1998).

School professionals also should consult the research literature regarding the most effective interventions for students with ADHD. There is clear evidence, for example, that manipulating environmental events

TABLE 5.1. Guidelines for the Design, Implementation, and Evaluation of Interventions for Learning and Behavior Problems

1. Intervention development, evaluation, and revision are *data-based* activities.

2. Intervention development, evaluation, and revision are driven by *child advocacy* and focused on attainment of clearly identified, socially valid *child outcomes*.

3. Intervention procedures must be thoroughly identified and defined, as well as implemented with integrity by persons with clearly delineated responsibilities.

4. Effective interventions produce or lead to increased rates of appropriate behavior and/or improved rates of learning, not solely decreases in undesirable or disturbing behavior.

5. Prior to its implementation, an intervention's effects on the behaviors of the identified child, the teacher, and on the classroom are unknown.

in the classroom leads to large changes in behavior among students with even the most severe symptoms of this disorder (see meta-analysis by DuPaul & Eckert, 1997).

Second, the child's needs are paramount in the selection of intervention strategies. Treatment goals are delineated relative to socially valid outcomes for the child with ADHD. Third, given that a team of professionals typically is involved in the treatment of students with ADHD, the responsibilities of each team member must be delineated clearly to ensure that intervention strategies are implemented with integrity. Fourth, the focus of treatment is primarily on *increasing* the frequency and/or duration of appropriate behaviors (e.g., academic productivity and accuracy) rather than primarily on *decreasing* disruptive classroom behavior. Finally, each child's response to intervention is presumed to be unique, and therefore the effects and side effects of a particular treatment are unknown prior to its implementation. This perspective implies the need for ongoing and comprehensive evaluation of all intervention strategies.

In addition to our assumptions about students with ADHD, and the noted intervention guidelines, we rely on several other conceptual and practical foundations in designing interventions for students with attention problems and ADHD-related difficulties. First, school professionals often rely on reactive and punitive procedures in attempting to change the behaviors of inattentive students. In fact, the most common classroom intervention for disruptive behavior is a verbal reprimand from the teacher and/or removal from the classroom (White, 1975). Such procedures are likely to be successful only when they are used sparingly, with minimal affect, and in the context of a positively reinforcing environment. Alternatively, an approach more likely to be successful is a balanced approach wherein both *proactive and reactive* strategies are employed. Specifically, antecedent events that typically precede inattentive and disruptive behaviors should be manipulated to prevent problematic interactions from arising. In addition, reactive strategies should not be confined to punitive approaches, but should be heavily weighted toward providing positive reinforcement when attentive and appropriate behaviors occur.

Another conceptual principle useful in designing effective interventions for students with attention problems is to intervene at the point of performance (Goldstein & Goldstein, 1998). Stated differently, to be optimally effective, strategies must be implemented in close proximity (i.e., in time and place) to the target behavior. For example, if the behavior of concern is attention to and completion of math work, then the most effective intervention strategies will be those used in math class at the time when students are expected to complete math work. Interventions further removed in time and place from the behavior of interest are likely to be less effective. This guiding principle is based on growing evidence that impulsivity is the primary deficit underlying the attention difficulties and other symptoms of ADHD (Barkley, 1997). Changing or preventing impulsive behavior typically requires that interventions be implemented when and where the problem behaviors occur..

In addition to intervening at the point of performance, intervention design for students with attention problems needs to be individualized. That is, we need to avoid a "one-size-fits-all" approach, based on the notion that all children sharing the ADHD diagnosis or behavior profile have the same support needs (DuPaul, Eckert, & McGoey, 1997). This process of individualizing intervention plans should take into account (1) the child's current level of academic skills; (2) the topography and possible environmental functions of a child's inattentive/problem behavior; (3) the target behaviors and/or outcomes of greatest concern to the teacher, parents, and/or student; and (4) elements of a teacher's approaches to classroom management and instruction that might limit the effectiveness of some interventions. Individualized interventions should be developed through a consultative problem-solving process using assessment data and collaborative interactions among teachers, parents, and other school professionals (Bergan & Kratochwill, 1990; Sheridan, Kratochwill, & Bergan, 1996).

Finally, recognition that interventions for students with ADHD can and should be mediated by a number of individuals is another important contemporary intervention design issue. Specifically, effective strategies can be implemented by teachers, parents, peers, and the identified students themselves (Teeter, 1998). When available, computers also can be used to improve task engagement and/or work completion, especially with drill-and-practice types of activities. The guiding principle here is that the classroom teacher should not be expected to be solely responsible for addressing all difficulties related to a student with ADHD. Other important resources (e.g., peers) in the classroom and home environments (e.g., parents) can be used to support and deliver interventions, thus creating a more comprehensive and perhaps cost-effective intervention strategy. Table 5.2 contains a matrix of some of the most effective intervention strategies in the context of both academic settings (i.e., elementary vs. secondary level) and mediating agent. These specific strategies are described later in this chapter, after the following sections addressing more general considerations in treatment design for students with ADHD.

BASIC COMPONENTS OF
CLASSROOM-BASED INTERVENTIONS

As already noted, there is a tendency to focus on the manipulation of consequences when designing classroom interventions for children identified with ADHD (for reviews, see DuPaul & Eckert, 1997; Pfiffner & O'Leary, 1993; Rapport, 1987a). Here, intervention research has emphasized the use of positive reinforcement and positive reinforcement coupled with mild forms of punishment (e.g., response cost and time-out from positive reinforcement). In the field of applied behavior analysis in general, research in the last decade has emphasized the prevention and

TABLE 5.2. Possible Mediators for School-Based Interventions

Intervention type	Elementary	Secondary
Teacher-mediated	Instructional strategies Token reinforcement systems	Study skills instruction Contingency contracting
Parent-mediated	Goal setting Contingency contracting Home-based reinforcement Parent tutoring	Negotiating Contingency contracting Home-based reinforcement
Peer-mediated	Peer tutoring	Peer coaching Peer mediation
Computer-assisted	Instruction Drill and practice	Instruction Word processing
Self-directed	Self-monitoring	Self-monitoring Self-evaluation

Note. From DuPaul and Power (2000). Copyright 2000 by the American Psychiatric Association. Adapted by permission.

management of behavior and achievement problems through antecedent manipulations and environmental arrangements (Sugai, Horner, & Gresham, 2002; Sulzer-Azaroff & Mayer, 1991). Similar emphases are warranted in the area of classroom-based management of children with ADHD.

Intervention procedures based on principles of human behavior have a long and well-documented history of effectiveness in ameliorating children's learning and behavior problems in school settings, including children with ADHD (Sulzer-Azaroff & Mayer, 1991). For example, these behavior change strategies have been successful in reducing the disruptive, off-task behavior of children identified with ADHD and increasing their academic productivity (e.g., Rapport, Murphy, & Bailey, 1980, 1982). Given the difficulties hypothesized to underlie the problems exhibited by children with ADHD (e.g., problems with impulsivity, self-control, and delayed responding), this finding is not surprising. It may be that behavioral interventions increase the overall level of appropriate classroom behavior through provision of external cues and prompts (e.g., rules, directions, contingencies) that supplement those "privately" operating for the target student. In designing behaviorally based interventions for classroom problems related to ADHD, the following issues warrant consideration:

1. A thorough assessment of the specific presenting problems, including a functional assessment, should be conducted to guide the design and selection of intervention components (e.g., target behaviors and their function(s), instructional strategy, motivational program).

2. Children diagnosed with ADHD typically require more frequent and specific feedback than their classmates to optimize their performance. As such, initial phases of interventions aimed at ADHD-related problems should incorporate contingencies that can be delivered in a relatively continuous manner. Leaner schedules of reinforcement should be introduced gradually, as some laboratory-based evidence indicates that children with ADHD have more difficulty maintaining their behavior under intermittent reinforcement schedules than do their peers (Douglas, 1984). Related to the issue of timing of reinforcement, in one study (Rapport, Stoner, DuPaul, Birmingham, & Tucker, 1985) children with ADHD tended to choose smaller, more immediate rewards over larger, delayed rewards contingent upon completion of academic work. These results serve to emphasize the need to attend to the general notion that to be effective, contingencies need to be in place at the "point of performance."

3. Contingent positive reinforcement should be the primary component of a behaviorally based intervention program for problems re-

lated to ADHD. But some evidence exists to suggest that exclusive reliance on reinforcement may distract the child from the task at hand. Alternatively, this concern may be ameliorated by the use of positive reinforcement coupled with the use of mild negative consequences (e.g., prudent reprimands; Abramowitz, O'Leary, & Rosen, 1987; Rosen, O'Leary, Joyce, Conway, & Pfiffner, 1984) and redirection of the child toward appropriate task behavior. The effectiveness of verbal reprimands and redirections can be enhanced through *specificity* of communication regarding the teacher's concerns and through *consistent delivery immediately* following the occurrence of problem behavior(s) (Pfiffner & O'Leary, 1993). Furthermore, treating children with dignity and respect requires that reprimands and redirection statements be made in a *brief, calm, and quiet* manner. As much as possible, reprimands should be delivered *privately* while making eye contact with the child.

4. When student behavior during independent work periods is targeted for change, initial task instructions should involve no more than a few steps. The child then should be asked to repeat directions back to the teacher to demonstrate understanding. Similarly, student homework and related tasks/projects should be assigned one at a time, with more complex tasks broken into smaller units. In some cases, the overall amount of assigned work would be reduced for the child with ADHD. The length and complexity of the workload would be increased gradually as the child demonstrates successful independent completion of increasingly larger units. Repetitive material (e.g., reassigning erroneously completed worksheets) should be avoided. Alternatively, an assignment focused on the same skill or concept area could be substituted to avoid boredom and potential exacerbation of attention problems.

5. Academic products and performance (e.g., work completion and accuracy) are preferred as targets of intervention as compared with specific task-related behaviors (e.g., attention to task or staying in one's seat) for several reasons. First, this preference promotes teacher monitoring of important student outcomes. Second, this preference promotes attention to the organizational and academic skills (e.g., working with the appropriate materials for an assignment, soliciting formative feedback on initial task performance) necessary for independent learning and for completing academic assignments. Third, a focus on active academic responding does not violate the "dead man test for behavior" (i.e., desired behavior) articulated by Lindsley (1991). This "rule" stated that "if a dead boy could do it, it wasn't behavior" (Lindsley, 1991, p. 457). Employing treatment targets like "sitting still" and "not calling out" violate the dead man test. Finally, this preference for academic responding as a treatment target promotes a focus on behavior that is incompatible with inattentive and disruptive behavior, and as such may lead to multi-

ple desired outcomes, including a reduction in disruptive behavior (Pfiffner & O'Leary, 1993).

6. Preferred activities (e.g., free-choice activity time, access to a classroom computer) should be used as reinforcers rather than tangible rewards (e.g., stickers and consumable items) whenever possible. Such contingencies may include making access to a preferred classroom activity contingent upon completion of an assignment in a less-preferred subject area (e.g., completion of a math worksheet leads to access to reading activities). Also in this vein, the specific rewards or reinforcers employed should be varied or rotated as needed to prevent disinterest with them, and thus with the program (i.e., reinforcer satiation). Finally, rather than assuming that specific activities will be motivating for the child, reward "menus" should be developed through direct questioning of the child as to what she or he wants to earn or by observing her or his preferred activities.

7. To enhance the positive incentive value of classroom privileges, employ a "priming" procedure with the child prior to academic assignment periods (Rapport, 1987b). "Priming" involves the teacher and student in reviewing a list of possible classroom privileges *prior* to beginning an academic work period wherein the student chooses which activity he or she would like to participate in following the work period.

8. The integrity or fidelity with which an intervention program is implemented must be monitored and evaluated (Gresham, 1989). Such monitoring can serve as the basis for making changes in program components, justifying additional resource needs, and/or developing and providing additional training materials or coaching with those carrying out the procedures. An intervention integrity checklist (Gresham, 1989) is provided in Figure 5.1, as an example of one method for monitoring program integrity. Gresham (1989) employed this checklist to assess the accuracy of implementation of a classroom response-cost lottery system. An independent observer evaluated the degree to which the classroom teacher completed the 11 main steps of this intervention on a daily basis. Thus, intervention integrity could be evaluated by component across days or vice versa. Such information is invaluable in determining the need for additional teacher training and support in implementing classroom interventions. This type of checklist, of course, would be altered to reflect the specific components of a particular intervention procedure.

CONTINGENCY MANAGEMENT PROCEDURES

Positive reinforcement of appropriate academic and social behavior should be viewed as the cornerstone of classroom-based behavior man-

Components	Monday	Tuesday	Wednesday	Thursday	Friday	% Component Integrity
1. Describes system	XI	XI	XI	XI	XI	100%
2. Displays/Describes reinforcers	XI	IO	IO	XI	XI	60%
3. 3 × 5 card placed on desks	XI	XI	XI	XI	XI	100%
4. Card taped on 3 sides	XI	XI	XI	XI	XI	100%
5. 4 slips of colored paper placed in cards	XI	XI	XI	XI	XI	100%
6. Lottery in effect ½ hour	XI	IO	IO	IO	XI	40%
7. Slips removed contingent on rule violation	XI	IO	XI	IO	IO	40%
8. Restates rule contingently	IO	IO	IO	XI	XI	20%
9. Tickets placed in box	XI	XI	XI	XI	XI	100%
10. Drawing on Friday	NA I	NA I	NA I	NA I	XI	100%
11. Winner selects reinforcer	NA I	NA I	NA I	NA I	XI	100%
Daily Integrity =	91%	64%	73%	82%	82%	

X = Occurrence
O = Nonoccurrence

$\bar{X}$ Integrity = 78%

FIGURE 5.1. Direct observation form for recording treatment integrity of the response-cost lottery. From Gresham (1989). Copyright 1989 by the National Association of School Psychologists. Reprinted by permission.

agement strategies. By definition, a *positive reinforcer* is an event, condition, or stimulus that increases the future likelihood of an action or behavior that it immediately follows (Sulzer-Azaroff & Mayer, 1991). For children with ADHD, the research literature indicates that several different behavior management strategies based on positive reinforcement can favorably enhance classroom behavior. In fact, the meta-analysis conducted by DuPaul and Eckert (1997) indicated that manipulation of antecedent and consequent events in the classroom was associated, on average, with a moderate-to-large effect size with respect to behavior change. Contingency management interventions have had less pronounced effects on academic achievement in this population.

A representative range of such strategies includes the use of contingency contracting, the use of positive reinforcement coupled with penalties or redirection contingent on problematic behavior, and the use of home-based contingencies to influence in-school behavior. Although most of these procedures involve contingent social praise from the teacher (e.g., O'Leary, Pelham, Rosenbaum, & Price, 1976), research indicates that children with ADHD may not exhibit consistent behavioral change in the absence of more powerful contingencies (Barkley, 1998). Thus, formal classroom behavior change programs are likely to require one or more of the following components: token reinforcement, contingency contracting, response cost, and time-out from positive reinforcement. Each of these techniques is described below, along with additional discussion of factors to consider when preparing for their use in classrooms.

Token Reinforcement Programs

Contingent social praise and attention can be effective in producing positive behavioral change with many children. Typically, however, praise alone is insufficient to bring about consistent improvement in the classroom behavior and academic performance of children with ADHD (Pfiffner & Barkley, 1990). Behavioral strategies that incorporate secondary generalized reinforcers (e.g., token economies) can provide the reward immediacy, specificity, and potency that often are required for children diagnosed with ADHD. Behavior management systems incorporating these components have been shown to be highly successful in enhancing the academic productivity and appropriate behavior of inattentive children (e.g., Ayllon, Layman, & Kandel, 1975; Robinson, Newby, & Ganzell, 1981).

Designing a school-based token reinforcement system involves the following steps:

1. One or more problematic classroom situations are targeted for intervention. These situations may be determined through a teacher interview and/or use of an objective rating scale such as the School Situations Questionnaire—Revised (DuPaul & Barkley, 1992). Direct observations in the classroom should be used to validate the selection of these problematic situations and behaviors (see Chapter 2). Typically, classroom work periods requiring independent completion of tasks present the greatest difficulty in terms of behavior control for children with ADHD.

2. Target behaviors are selected. They typically include academic products (e.g., number of math problems completed in a given amount of time) or specific actions (e.g., appropriate interactions with peers during recess). In general, products are preferred due to the relative ease of their collection and monitoring. In addition, academic productivity typically involves behaviors that are incompatible with inattentive and disruptive behavior (see Robinson et al., 1981).

3. Types of secondary reinforcers (i.e., tokens) to be used are identified; these may include multicolored poker chips, check marks or stickers on a card, or points on a card stand. Younger children (e.g., up to 9 years old) generally prefer tangible rewards (e.g., poker chips), while older children and adolescents respond more positively to points or check marks. Token economy systems typically are considered too complicated for children under 5 years of age. With preschool-age children, the use of primary reinforcers (e.g., parental or teacher praise, hugs, or other social attention) contingent upon the occurrence of appropriate behavior is recommended.

4. The values of target or goal behaviors must be determined. That is, the number of tokens earned by completing each target behavior or its subcomponents should be determined by task difficulty, with completion of more difficult or time-consuming tasks worth more tokens than less involved assignments. More complex behaviors are broken down into their component parts (e.g., "successful work completion" can be defined as completing a certain number of items within a specified time period, attaining a certain level of accuracy, and reviewing the work before requesting the teacher's feedback) to allow children to earn tokens for partial completion of a task or reaching a certain performance criterion. In these instances, a task analysis may be necessary to explicitly delineate the components of expected behaviors.

5. The teacher and the student should jointly develop a list of privileges or activities within the classroom and/or school for which tokens may be exchanged. The list should include low-, medium-, and high-"cost" items. It can be beneficial to ask parents to collaborate on the development of this list and, in addition, to make privileges available at home in exchange for tokens. The amount of tokens or points necessary to "purchase" each privilege can be determined collaboratively among those individuals involved in the program. As a rough guide, estimate the maximum number of tokens that could be earned on a daily basis and divide this sum evenly among available reinforcers, then add or delete tokens to the cost of each item in accordance with the "value" of the privilege or activity to the child.

6. The value of the tokens should be taught or demonstrated to involved children (i.e., via token-backup reinforcer exchanges accompanied by discussion), and initial criteria for earning tokens should be set to ensure early success. Take, for example, a child for whom the percentage of assigned math problems completed is chosen as a target behavior. The child typically completes somewhere between 50–60% of math problems. An initial completion rate of 50% might be the criterion selected for the first few days of the program.

7. Tokens are exchanged for classroom privileges on at least a

daily basis. However, as a rule, shorter delays between receiving tokens and exchanging them for backup reinforcers will result in a more effective program. Although tokens can serve as immediate rewards of an interim nature, they may lose their value as reinforcers if they cannot be "cashed in" until after a long period of time has elapsed.

8. The effectiveness of the intervention program should be evaluated in an ongoing fashion, using multiple outcome measures. Based on the results of this ongoing evaluation, new behavioral targets may be added, old ones deleted or modified, and privileges rotated or varied. Also, the delivery of tokens and the timing of token exchanges may be altered. Response cost procedures (as discussed below) also may be incorporated into the system when some improvement in appropriate behavior has been achieved, yet disruptive or inattentive behaviors remain problematic.

9. Following initial implementation and behavioral improvement, several additional procedures may be necessary to ensure the generalization of obtained effects across time and settings. First, any additional problematic situations must be identified and targeted for change by implementing the above strategies (i.e., steps 2–8). It is erroneous to assume that one need only obtain performance in one situation for such behavior to spontaneously generalize to other settings (Stokes & Baer, 1977). Second, the use of tokens and backup reinforcers should be faded in a gradual fashion. For example, rather than continuing to provide tokens following successful completion of each step in an academic task, reinforcement would be provided contingent upon completion of several steps first, and then following completion of the entire assignment. Eventually, the system would evolve into a contingency contract as discussed below. Numerous other strategies are available in the professional literature for enhancing both generalization and maintenance of treatment gains (see Horner, Dunlap, & Koegel, 1988; Stokes & Osnes, 1989).

Contingency Contracting

Contingency contracting is a behavior management technique that involves the negotiation of a contractual agreement between a student and a teacher (DeRisi & Butz, 1975). Typically, the contract stipulates the desired classroom behaviors and consequences available contingent upon their performance. As with a token economy program, specific academic and behavioral goals are identified for the child to meet in order to gain access to preferred activities or other rewards. Contracting typically involves a direct connection between target behaviors and primary contingencies rather than the use of secondary reinforcers such as tokens. As such, there may be a longer time delay between behavior completion and reinforcement than with a token economy program. A sample contract appears in Figure 5.2.

Although contingency contracting is a relatively straightforward procedure, a number of factors may directly influence its efficacy with the ADHD population. First, the age of the child is an important consideration. Contracting procedures typically are unsuccessful with children under the age of 6, perhaps due to a lack of sufficiently developed rule-following skills and an inability to delay reinforcement for longer time

---

I, _____, agree to do the following:
[insert student's name]

1. Complete all of my written math and language arts assignments, with at least 80% accuracy, before lunch time.
2. Give [insert teacher's name] my full attention when he or she is speaking to the class or to my reading group.
3. Remain quiet, and follow directions when lining up for recess, lunch, and music class.
4. Follow all playground rules (e.g., no fighting) during recess.

Each day that I do these things, I will be allowed to choose **one** of the following:

1. 15 minutes' time at the end of the school day to play a game with a classmate.
2. Use the classroom computer for work or play for 15 minutes.
3. Assist my teacher by completing some errands (take attendance forms to the office) or in-class jobs (collect student math assignments).

If I have a successful week, I will have earned one of the special weekend activities with my parents, such as: [e.g., a trip to the park, a bicycle ride, having a friend visit for lunch or dinner]. If I do not complete these classroom responsibilities, then I will lose the opportunity to participate in daily free-time activities.

I agree to fulfill this contract to the best of my abilities.

Signed,

_____   _____
      Student's signature   *Teacher's signature*

Date _____

FIGURE 5.2. A sample classroom behavior contract for a student with ADHD. From *ADHD in the Schools* (2nd ed.) by George J. DuPaul and Gary Stoner. Copyright 2003 by The Guilford Press. Permission to photocopy this figure is granted to purchasers of this book for personal use only. See copyright page for details.

periods on the part of young children. A second consideration is the length of the time delay between the required behavior and reinforcement. For example, a procedure requiring an 8-year-old child with ADHD to accurately complete math problems at a rate of 80% of assigned problems each day for a 1-week time period before earning a reward is doomed to failure. Timing of reinforcement is a crucial issue in implementing behavior management programs with children, especially those with ADHD. To increase the probability of improved outcomes in the example given, access to preferred activities should be provided at the conclusion of the successful work period or school day.

The choice of target behaviors and the manner of incorporating them into an intervention program are important determinants of a behavioral contract's success. For example, during the *initial* stages of a contracting procedure care should be exercised to avoid large numbers of goals, extremely high standards of quality, and completion of complex (e.g., multistep) tasks. For the child with ADHD, these types of initial requirements likely will lead to failure. A preferable approach would be to target a few simple behaviors or products so that the child can achieve success right from the start. More difficult or complex goals could be incorporated gradually into later iterations of the contract such that terminal objectives are reached with minimal failure along the way.

A final consideration of importance in designing a behavioral contract is the identification of appropriate reinforcers. All too often identified reinforcers take the form of activities or items that are assumed by school personnel to be motivating for children. Assumptions about the reinforcer preferences of the children we work with are a good starting point for designing contracts and contingency management procedures. However, reinforcer preferences can be very idiosyncratic, and as such it is suggested that individual reward menus be derived. Two alternatives for doing so are suggested. First, it is advisable, especially with older children, to negotiate directly with the student regarding possible privileges. Direct negotiation not only assures identification of potent reinforcers, but also enlists the student's cooperation and investment in the contractual process. Second, naturalistic observations can be conducted to identify a child's preferred activities for use as reinforcers. Such observations might include identifying those off-task behaviors (e.g., drawing, playing with objects at seat) that the child frequently engages in while assigned to do independent work. This strategy would be helpful especially when a child is unable to provide suggestions for rewards.

Response Cost

Contingency management strategies consisting solely of positive reinforcement procedures are rarely effective in maintaining appropriate levels of academic and social behavior among children with ADHD (Pfiffner & O'Leary, 1993). In fact, several studies have documented the effectiveness of levying mild penalties following inappropriate (i.e., off-task) behavior in promoting consistent behavioral change (Pfiffner & O'Leary, 1987; Pfiffner, O'Leary, Rosen, & Sanderson, 1985; Rosen et al., 1984). For example, in addition to prudent reprimands and verbal redirection, penalties involving the loss or removal of privileges, points, or tokens (i.e., response cost) contingent upon inattentive, disruptive behavior has proven beneficial when used in combination with reinforcement-based procedures.

The concurrent use of token reinforcement and response cost has been demonstrated to increase the levels of on-task behavior, seatwork productivity, and academic accuracy of children with ADHD (DuPaul, Guevremont, & Barkley, 1992; Rapport et al., 1980, 1982). In several cases, obtained classroom improvement was equivalent to that obtained with stimulant medication (Rapport et al., 1982). For example, Rapport (1987a, 1987b) describes a token delivery system that incorporates response cost. The student and teacher are each supplied with a card stand or electronic apparatus serving to display point totals earned by the child.[2] Points are earned for in-seat, academically engaged behavior on a fixed-interval schedule and are deducted following incidents of off-task behavior. Points are awarded or deducted by the teacher changing the card displayed on his or her card stand (or by pressing a button on a remote control device). With this system, students change their own cards to match the teacher's or receive/lose points on the electronic apparatus via the remote mechanism controlled by the teacher. Thus, "token" delivery and deduction are accomplished on a remote basis by the teacher, allowing for simultaneously teaching and/or involvement in activities with other students. As with other token systems, at the conclusion of an academic work period a child's accumulated points are traded for various backup reinforcers (e.g., a choice activity).

The efficacy of response-cost programming can be illustrated by examining Figures 5.3 and 5.4 from Rapport (1987a). These data represent the response of an 8-year-old boy with ADHD to varying doses of methylphenidate (Ritalin) and to a response-cost system implemented in his regular classroom. Figure 5.3 shows treatment-related changes in this boy's on-task behavior and teacher ratings of classroom deportment over the course of the school year. Response-cost procedures were imple-

---

[2]An electronic response-costs system based on the prototypes used in this research is the Attention Training System, or ATS. The ATS is available from Gordon Diagnostic Systems, Inc., of DeWitt, New York (*www.gsi-add.com*).

FIGURE 5.3. The mean percentage of intervals of daily on-task behavior across academic areas (closed circles = math; open circles = phonics) and experimental conditions. The right-hand ordinate represents teacher-rated social behavior (open triangle = Abbreviated Conners Teacher Rating Scale) whereby the numbers become smaller as the child improves. From Rapport (1987a). Copyright 1987 by John Wiley & Sons. Reprinted by permission.

mented in a staggered fashion (i.e., using a multiple baseline design) across math and phonics class periods. During baseline conditions, this boy was observed to attend to task materials during an average of 40–50% of observation intervals. The implementation of response-cost procedures led to an increase in the frequency of on-task behavior to approximately 90% of observation intervals. This improvement in attentiveness was similar to or, in the case of some doses, superior to that obtained with methylphenidate. Response cost also enhanced this boy's completion of academic problems relative to baseline conditions (see Figure 5.4). In fact, improvements in academic productivity were superior to that obtained with methylphenidate. Thus, response-cost procedures can be used to improve both task-related attention and academic performance.

Several issues should be considered in the use of response-cost procedures. For example, response cost is a form of punishment, and its use could result in the child taking a negative view of the entire token system. Thus, in introducing the program and its components to the student and the teacher, emphasis should be placed on the program's positive as-

FIGURE 5.4. The mean percentage of daily problems completed across academic areas (closed circles = math; open circles = phonics) and experimental conditions. The right-hand ordinate represents teacher-rated social behavior (open triangle = Abbreviated Conners Teacher Rating Scale) whereby the numbers become smaller as the child improves. From Rapport (1987a). Copyright 1987 by John Wiley & Sons. Reprinted by permission.

pects (e.g., emphasize that the student will have a chance to earn points and rewards for completing work accurately). In addition, initial and ongoing efforts should be made to adjust and arrange contingencies such that the child is earning more points than he or she is losing. For example, students may initially test the system by deliberately engaging in off-task behavior to see if they will lose points. To prevent teachers from being caught up in a "point reduction game" of this sort, it is recommended that point reductions not occur more than once per minute regardless of the frequency of off-task behavior. Also, the teacher should be instructed to look away from the child immediately following point reductions (Rapport, 1987b). Finally, a child's point total should never fall below 0; when a point total is 0, all disruptive, off-task behavior should be ignored. If 0 point totals are a common occurrence, the contingencies may need to be revised so that point reductions do not occur for minor infractions. Once the child begins to experience success and is invested in the system, the criteria for point reductions can become more stringent in efforts to further improve classroom behavior and performance.

Time-Out from Positive Reinforcement

Another type of mild punishment strategy that may be appropriate for classroom use consists of various forms of time-out from positive reinforcement. Time-out from positive reinforcement, as its name implies, involves restricting the child's access to positive reinforcement (e.g., teacher and peer attention). An adaptation of Barkley's (1987) procedures designed for use within the home may be most applicable. To be effective, time-out procedures should be: (1) implemented only when there is a reinforcing environment to be removed from, (2) implemented when the function of the child's disruptive behavior is to gain teacher or peer attention, (3) implemented swiftly following a rule infraction, (4) applied with consistency, and (5) employed for the smallest amount of time (e.g., 1–5 minutes) that proves effective. Lack of available reinforcement is the most salient feature determining the effectiveness of this procedure, *not* the amount of time spent in actual time-out. If the child is to be moved to a time-out area, this area should be located in a relatively dull location within the classroom (*not* a separate room, closet, cloakroom, or hallway) to allow for monitoring of the child's activities. Criteria for terminating the time-out period should include (1) a time-out period sufficiently long enough to be effective (i.e., 1 minute for every 2 years of age of the child); (2) a short period of calm, nondisruptive behavior required prior to its termination; and (3) the child's expressed willingness to correct, amend, or compensate for the misbehavior that led to the time-out contingency. Finally, children who leave the time-out area without permission should have their time interval lengthened by a fixed amount for each violation, or lose points or tokens if a token economy system is also being used.

As with response cost, it is imperative that restrictive procedures such as time-out be employed only in the context of ongoing positive reinforcement programming. Furthermore, time-out contingencies should be an intervention of last resort following implementation of a hierarchy of both positive and less restrictive behavior management procedures. For example, inappropriate behavior would lead initially to brief, prudent reprimands, followed by response cost, followed by time-out with head down at desk, followed by time-out in a corner of the room. More severe disruptive behaviors (e.g., physical aggression) should lead to immediate application of the more restrictive time-out procedures or to other procedures consistent with classroom or school rules. When used, time-out procedures need to be monitored very carefully, as they are not considered viable ongoing management strategies. They are best viewed as short-term behavior reduction techniques.

Home-Based Contingencies

Home-based contingency management procedures, based on the child's behavior and/or academic performance at school, can be used as an effective supplement to classroom-based behavior change systems. These procedures have several beneficial features. First, on a daily basis the child receives direct feedback from his or her teachers as to performance in several areas of classroom functioning. Second, parents receive daily information about the child's classroom performance, thus providing an ongoing forum for teacher–parent communication. For children experiencing classroom difficulties, this schedule of communication is preferable to waiting for a parent–teacher conference or an end-of-the-term report card. Finally, the system circumvents some of the practical limitations (e.g., restricted range of possible reinforcing activities) of classroom-based contingency management systems because it involves the parents in providing reinforcement for in-school behavior.

An example of a home-based reinforcement program for a student with ADHD has been proposed (DuPaul, Guevremont, & Barkley, 1991) that employs a daily report card similar to the one displayed in Figure 5.5. For each child, several behavioral goals are identified, such as paying attention to class activities, completion of assigned work, accuracy of work, and following rules. The specific goals should vary with respect to the presenting problems of the individual student (e.g., interactions with classmates may be targeted if the child is prone to arguing and fighting with peers). The columns of the card can be used to convey information across different subject areas or periods of the school day. Thus, if the child has more than one teacher, they all may participate. The teacher enters ratings (on a 5-point scale from "excellent" to "terrible") of the child's performance in the appropriate area of the card, initials the card, and provides comments where necessary. Ratings and comments are made in ink to prevent their alteration by the child. The student is responsible for giving the card to each teacher and bringing it home on a daily basis.

Given the use of quantitative ratings, school–home notes can be used within a token economy system based at home. For example, the teacher provides quantitative ratings of performance in each goal area, as discussed above. When the card is brought home, the parent(s) briefly discusses the positive and negative ratings with the child. Then, specified point values are assigned to the numbers on the card and summed to yield the net total points earned for the day. For example, each teacher rating of "1" could be converted to 25 points, each "2" to 15 points, each "3" to 5 points. Ratings of "4" or "5" would result in the deduction of 15 and 25 points, respectively. To produce positive behavior

```
┌─────────────────────────────────────────────────────────┐
│                                                          │
│           DAILY STUDENT RATING CARD                      │
│   NAME _____ DATE _____              │
│     Please rate this child in each of the areas listed below │
│     as to how he performed in school today using ratings of  │
│     1 to 5.  1=excellent, 2=good, 3=fair, 4=poor, 5=terrible │
│     or did not work.                                         │
│                         CLASS PERIODS / SUBJECTS          │
│     AREA              1   2   3   4   5   6               │
│   ┌──────────────────┬───┬───┬───┬───┬───┬───┐           │
│   │ participation    │   │   │   │   │   │   │           │
│   ├──────────────────┼───┼───┼───┼───┼───┼───┤           │
│   │ class work       │   │   │   │   │   │   │           │
│   ├──────────────────┼───┼───┼───┼───┼───┼───┤           │
│   │ handed in homework│  │   │   │   │   │   │           │
│   ├──────────────────┼───┼───┼───┼───┼───┼───┤           │
│   │ interaction      │   │   │   │   │   │   │           │
│   │ with other children│ │   │   │   │   │   │           │
│   ├──────────────────┼───┼───┼───┼───┼───┼───┤           │
│   │ teacher's initials│  │   │   │   │   │   │           │
│   └──────────────────┴───┴───┴───┴───┴───┴───┘           │
│                                                          │
│     Place comments on back if needed:                    │
│                                                          │
└─────────────────────────────────────────────────────────┘
```

FIGURE 5.5. Daily report card for use in a home-based reinforcement program for ADHD. From Barkley (1990). Copyright 1990 by The Guilford Press. Reprinted with permission.

change, a home token reinforcement program must be arranged such that these points can lead to the "purchase" of backup reinforcers (e.g., household privileges, television time, spending a night at a friend's home). As with other token programs, this system's effectiveness is dependent upon its motivational value and the availability of a variety of backup reinforcers.

Kelley (1990) has written a text that provides thorough coverage of this topic, focused on developing and using what she calls "school–home notes" as a means of communication among parents, teachers, and children. A variety of school–home notes are presented in her text, all of which could be adapted for use with students who are exhibiting ADHD-related behaviors. For example, a school–home note that could be used in treating a student with ADHD at the secondary school level is displayed in Figure 5.6. There is an increased emphasis on homework completion and test grades at this level. The teacher is able to alert parents about upcoming homework assignments on a regular basis, as well. At the secondary level, teachers typically prefer to complete school–home notes on a weekly rather than a daily basis.

Several factors may limit the effectiveness of home-based reinforce-

SCHOOL–HOME NOTE

Name __Richard_____   Date ___10/20_____

SUBJECT___Math_____

Was prepared for class	(Yes) No NA		Homework assignment:
Used class time well	(Yes) No NA		Test Friday on
Handed in homework	(Yes) No NA		Chapter 3

Homework/Test Grade   F D (C) B A NA   Teacher's Initials _WJ_

Comments: Seems to be paying attention better and using his time well.

SUBJECT___Social Studies_____

Was prepared for class	Yes (No) NA	Homework assignment:
Used class time well	(Yes) No NA	Answer questions
Handed in homework	Yes (No) NA	1–10, page 113

(Homework) Test Grade   F (D) C B A NA   Teacher's Initials _MS_

Comments: Did not bring notebook; he talked a good bit during class.

SUBJECT___English_____

Was prepared for class	(Yes) No NA	Homework assignment:
Used class time well	(Yes) No NA	None
Handed in homework	Yes No (NA)	

Homework (Test) Grade   F D (C) B A NA   Teacher's Initials _JL_

Comments: Participated nicely in class.

Parent Comments: ___Ms. Sessions, Richard says he handed in his___

___homework. Would you mind checking with him?___

FIGURE 5.6. Abbreviated school–home note used with middle and high school students. (This note was completed by Richard, his teachers, and his parents.) From Kelley (1990). Copyright 1990 by The Guilford Press. Reprinted with permission.

ment programs (Rapport, 1987a). One primary drawback of such a system is that, by definition, it involves a delay in the provision of reinforcement. Given that children with ADHD have difficulty delaying reinforcement (Barkley, 1998), home-based reinforcers may be less powerful relative to classroom-based contingencies that are more immediately linked to the behaviors of interest. This issue is particularly important in working with children younger than the age of 6. Second, school personnel have limited means for assessing parental implementation of the procedures. Finally, when home-based reinforcers are used, parents should be discouraged from relying solely on material rewards, which can lose some of their potency over long periods of time. Instead, parents should be provided with assistance in developing an array of potential reinforcers of an activity, social, or material nature. These reinforcers should be salient to the child, readily available in the home or community, inexpensive if they involve a monetary cost, and rotated on a regular basis to prevent boredom with the "same old rewards." It is particularly important to use reinforcers that are viewed as "necessities" by the child (e.g., watching television, playing video games, riding bicycle) rather than an exclusive reliance on "luxury" items that the child could live without (e.g., going to a favorite restaurant, a trip to the amusement park).

In view of the limitations to home–school communication systems enumerated above, it is worthwhile to delineate the factors that will enhance the efficacy of home-based contingencies. These factors are listed in Table 5.3. First, daily and weekly goals are specified in a positive manner. As noted earlier, to pass the "dead man test," target behaviors involve the active performance of classroom responsibilities (e.g., work completion) rather than an absence of inappropriate behavior. Second, both academic and behavioral goals are included. In an effort to increase the chances of initial success, one or two goals should be readily attainable by the child. This will serve to "hook" the child into cooperating with the system before increasing standards or expectations for performance. Third, it is important to employ only a few goals at a time so that the student and teacher are not overwhelmed by the system. Fourth,

TABLE 5.3. Components of Effective Home–School Communication Programs

1. Daily and/or weekly goals are stated in a positive manner.
2. Both academic and behavioral goals are included.
3. A small number of goals are targeted at a time.
4. The teacher provides quantitative feedback about student performance.
5. Feedback is provided by subject or class periods.
6. Communication is made on a regular basis (either daily or weekly).
7. Home-based contingencies are tied to school performance. Both short- and long-term consequences are employed.
8. Parental cooperation and involvement are solicited prior to implementation.
9. Student input into goals and contingencies is solicited, particularly with older children and adolescents.
10. Goals and procedures are modified, as necessary.

teacher feedback about the child's performance should be quantitative. Although qualitative statements can be informative, they are often vague and nonspecific (e.g., "Johnny had a good day today"). Fifth, feedback is provided by subject or class period. This provides the student with specific information about performance, allows for more frequent feedback, and circumvents a loss of motivation if the child experiences difficulties in the early part of the day. In the latter situation, if ratings on the daily report card were based on the entire day's performance, it is likely that the child would still obtain low ratings even if his or her behavior improved over the course of the day. Sixth, home–school communication occurs on a daily or weekly basis to facilitate the provision of frequent reinforcement. Seventh, a hierarchy of short- and long-term privileges at home are tied directly to teacher ratings on the daily report card. It is unlikely that a child with ADHD will exhibit improvement in the absence of external reinforcement. Eighth, parents should be involved in planning the home–school communication program from the onset to ensure their understanding of and cooperation with the procedures. Older children and adolescents should be included in planning the program for the same reasons. Ninth, goals and procedures are modified on an ongoing basis in accordance with student progress or lack thereof.

Another possible parent-mediated intervention is for parents to provide academic support to their children. For example, Hook and DuPaul (1999) evaluated the effects of a *parent tutoring* intervention for four second- and third-grade students with ADHD who exhibited reading difficulties. Parents were trained to monitor their children's reading using passages provided by the children's teachers. Tutoring was implemented over a 4- to 8-week period using a multiple baseline across participants experimental design. Reading achievement was assessed at home and at school using brief curriculum-based reading probes that were administered two times per week across experimental phases. All four children showed gains in reading on home-based probes, with more variable improvements evident on school-based reading probes. The results indicated that parent tutoring may be a promising intervention for enhancing reading achievement for some children with ADHD, particularly those whose parents are invested in their child's education.

In summary, parent-mediated strategies, particularly home-based contingency systems, can be effective in enhancing school performance, especially when used to supplement classroom-based behavior change procedures (e.g., cover periods of the school day when the latter procedures are not in effect). Students who display ADHD-related behaviors that are considered milder in severity should be particularly responsive to home–school programming. As with other contingency management strategies, attention to the details of identifying target behaviors and reinforcers, linking the two, and monitoring and managing the system to ensure its integrity will be critical to successful outcomes.

Functional Behavior Assessment

The contingency management strategies discussed above focus on altering target behaviors primarily through the manipulation of consequences following the occurrence of targeted problem and appropriate behaviors. From a technical standpoint, these procedures focus on what behavior looks like, or its topography, rather than what function a behavior serves for an individual student. Recent technical advances in classroom-based behavior management, however, make prominent the notion of linking intervention to an assessment of behavioral function.

Functional assessment strategies include interviews, observations, and environmental manipulations (e.g., changing a seating arrangement) intended to identify environmental variables that reliably precede or reliably follow problem behaviors of concern. Such variables are then hypothesized, in a behavior analytic formulation, to prompt or promote the occurrence of problem behavior, in the case of preceding variables. And in the case of variables reliably following problem behavior, these are hypothesized to reinforce or maintain problem behavior (see Nelson et al., 1998; O'Neill, Horner, Albin, Storey, & Sprague, 1997).

Understanding the factors that maintain problem behaviors, along with the situations that appear to cue or prompt those behaviors, is an essential first step in individualizing interventions (DuPaul et al., 1997). For example, consider the disruptive classroom behavior (e.g., verbal disruptions, speaking out of turn) of an identified student. Assume that we know the behavior is reliably occasioned by the teacher's instructional presentation of new math material. It is highly probable in such circumstances that the child's disruptive behavior is motivated by the desire to avoid and/or escape from math instruction. Here, then, one potential intervention could involve provision of teacher assistance at the beginning of that activity to ensure that rules and expectations are understood, that the student has all materials needed to participate in the instruction, and that the student is able to clearly see and hear the teacher's presentation. This would constitute a preventive or proactive strategy.

Alternatively, consider the same student and behavior but a different formulation of the problem. Suppose, for example, the student's disruptive behavior reliably results in teacher attention (e.g., "William, please stop disrupting the lesson. Don't you remember the class rules?"). These circumstances might lead to a hypothesis that William's disruptive behavior is being reinforced through teacher-delivered social attention. At least one component of a "functional" approach to intervention would include behavior management strategies intended to strengthen an alternative behavior that would produce the same type of reinforcement—in this case, teacher attention. For example, the teacher might use a strategy that included providing attention contingent upon William responding appropriately to a question posed by the teacher and/or otherwise maintaining appropriate attention to the lesson, and withholding attention when disruptive behavior occurs.

Once the function of a child's behavior is determined, then an intervention is designed that leads to functionally equivalent behavior. Functionally equivalent interventions provide access to desired consequences contingent upon appropriate behavior rather than the problematic behavior. Connections between behavioral functions and possible functionally equivalent interventions are displayed in Figure 5.7. For example, if a child is engaging in disruptive behavior in a classroom to gain teacher attention, then the intervention should arrange for teacher attention to be contingent only upon the display of appropriate behavior, while disruptive behavior is ignored (i.e., differential reinforcement of incompatible behavior). It is assumed that function-based interventions will be more effective than strategies implemented based on broader diagnostic data and/or a trial-and-error approach. Furthermore, because function-based interventions provide access to desired consequences, it is presumed that these strategies will result in outcomes that are maintained over time.

Based on a formulation of this type, Ervin, DuPaul, Kern, and Friman (1998) used functional assessment strategies to guide the development of classroom-based interventions for four adolescents diagnosed with ADHD. For two of these students, the interventions used were linked to problems hypothesized to serve the functions of escape from written tasks and access to peer attention, respectively. The former student was allowed to complete written assignments using a computer rather than writing by hand—the problem behavior was hypothesized to be escape-motivated. The latter student was provided with peer attention contingent on the display of on-task behavior—the problem behavior was hypothesized to be maintained by peer attention. Results of this work suggested that the classroom interventions based on functional assessment strategies resulted in significant improvements in the task-related behavior of both students

SELF-MANAGEMENT STRATEGIES

A primary goal of treatment for ADHD is to enable a student to develop adequate levels of self-control. The latter term implies that a child will

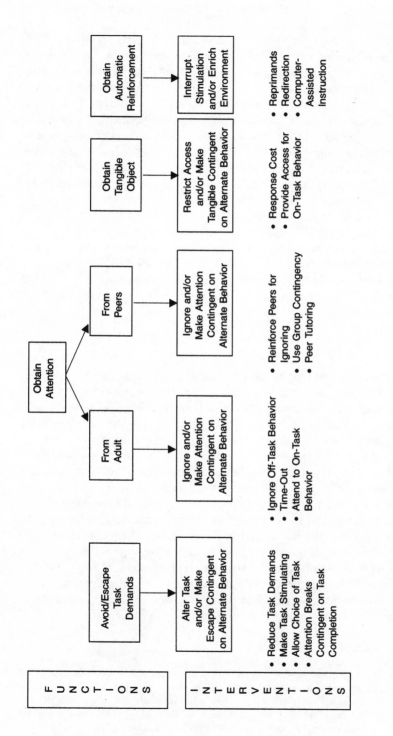

FIGURE 5.7. Possible functions for child behavior and associated interventions. From DuPaul and Ervin (1996). Copyright 1996 by the Association for Advancement of Behavior Therapy. Reprinted by permission.

exhibit age-appropriate social and academic behaviors on an independent basis (i.e., with a minimum of accommodation on the part of the environment). Although this is a desirable treatment goal, it is quite difficult to obtain in practice given the chronic and multifaceted nature of ADHD. Self-managed interventions for ADHD are comprised of strategies incorporating self-monitoring, self-reinforcement, and/or self-instruction (Barkley, 1989). These strategies, especially those incorporating self-instruction, sometimes have been referred to as *cognitive-behavioral interventions* given their emphasis on changing children's thinking, behavior, and their interaction. In recent years, self-management interventions have become increasingly popular as treatments for a variety of classroom difficulties, including ADHD (see Shapiro & Cole, 1994). In general, despite their apparent potential in ameliorating ADHD symptoms, these interventions, particularly self-instruction training, have not been uniformly successful (Abikoff, 1985). Nevertheless, we will review findings relevant to self-monitoring and self-reinforcement approaches enumerated above while highlighting procedures that of relevance for practitioners.

Self-Monitoring

Children can be taught to observe and record the occurrence of their own behaviors. For instance, a child with ADHD might be taught to recognize and record instances of on-task behavior during academic work. Typically, an auditory or visual stimulus (e.g., beep from a tape recorder, hand signal from the teacher) is used periodically throughout a specific time period to signal the child to observe his or her current behavior.[3] The child then records whether he or she was on-task on a grid or chart taped to his or her desk. This type of self-monitoring can be used alone or, more typically, in combination with other self-management procedures. Although this intervention has not been studied extensively with children diagnosed with ADHD, attention-related behaviors have been found to increase as a function of self-monitoring, especially when combined with self-reinforcement or external reinforcement (e.g., Barkley, Copeland, & Sivage, 1980). Also, some research indicates that it may be more effective to have the child monitor task completion and/or accuracy than to simply monitor attentive behavior (e.g., Lam, Cole, Shapiro, & Bambara, 1994).

---

[3]A less intrusive method for signaling self-monitoring is available through the use of a vibrating device attached to the child's clothing. This device, called the MotivAider, can be programmed to signal the child at various intervals. The MotivAider is available through Behavioral Dynamics, Inc., P.O. Box 66, Thief River Falls, MN 56701. You can also get product information on the Internet at www.habitchange.com/index.html.

Self-monitoring may be a particularly viable intervention for adolescents with ADHD, especially when organizational skills are a concern. For example, Gureasko-Moore, DuPaul, and White (in press) evaluated the use of a self-monitoring strategy for three seventh-grade students with ADHD. All of these participants were reported by their teachers to have significant problems being prepared and organized for class (e.g., coming to class with correct textbook, pencils, and notebook). A checklist of preparatory behaviors was constructed for each student by his teacher. This checklist was used to determine the percentage of preparatory steps completed across experimental phases in the context of a multiple-baseline, across-participants design. Following a baseline phase, a school psychologist provided brief training in self-monitoring to each participant. All three students showed substantial gains in the percentage of steps completed as a function of self-monitoring (see Figure 5.8). In fact, several weeks later, students were observed to complete nearly 100% of required preparatory behaviors on a consistent basis, even without external prompting and reinforcement.

Self-Reinforcement

The most promising self-management intervention for ADHD requires students not only to monitor their behavior but also to evaluate and reinforce their own performance (Barkley, 1989). In fact, the combination of self-monitoring and self-reinforcement has been found effective in improving on-task behavior, academic accuracy, and peer interactions for students with ADHD (Barkley et al., 1980; Hinshaw, Henker, & Whalen, 1984). These effects are enhanced further when stimulant medication is used in combination with these procedures (Barkley, 1989).

Self-reinforcement strategies may be particularly helpful for addressing ADHD-related problems in two situations. First, a student can be taught to monitor and reinforce his or her own behavior while fading the use of an externally based, contingency management program (Barkley, 1989). The premise is that positive behavioral change will be maintained despite the reduction in teacher feedback or other forms of reinforcement. Of course, backup reinforcers (e.g., classroom or home privileges) *must* be used as teacher monitoring and feedback are faded. The fading of backup reinforcement must take place over an extended time period. A second situation where self-reinforcement is an appropriate treatment for ADHD is at the secondary level where teachers and students are reluctant to employ contingency management procedures. Thus, self-management may be a more acceptable intervention at the secondary level, and therefore presumably more likely to be implemented on a consistent basis.

An example of self-monitoring and self-reinforcement procedures

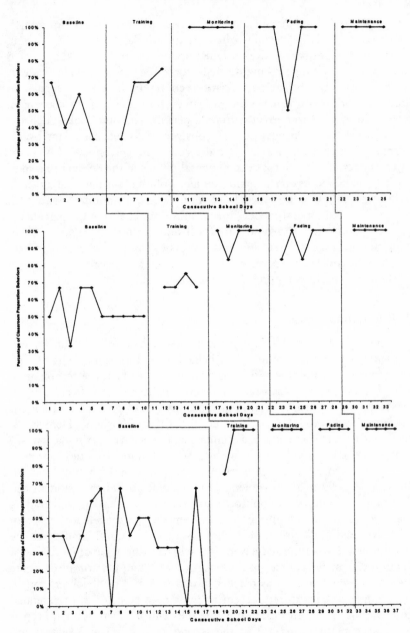

FIGURE 5.8. Percentage of classroom preparation behaviors for three adolescents with ADHD receiving self-monitoring training. From Gureasko-Moore, DuPaul, and White (in press). Copyright by Sage Publications, Inc. Reprinted by permission.

useful for ameliorating ADHD symptoms is based on the work of Rhode, Morgan, and Young (1983). These researchers used these strategies to facilitate the mainstreaming of six elementary students with "behavioral handicaps." The initial stages of the program involve the use of a token reinforcement program and verbal feedback from the teacher based on teacher ratings of student behavior during specific intervals in the classroom. Ratings are provided using a 6-point criterion hierarchy as displayed in Table 5.4. Separate evaluations of behavioral and academic performance can be made using this system. Teacher-provided points are exchanged for backup reinforcers in school or at home as in a standard token economy.

Once behavioral and/or academic gains are exhibited by the student, he or she is trained in evaluating his or her own behavior using the criteria displayed in Table 5.3. At this stage, the teacher's ratings continue to be used to determine how many points the student has earned. In addition, the student can earn one bonus point for matching teacher ratings exactly. If the student's ratings deviate by more than one point from the teacher ratings, the student does not earn any points for that interval. Thus, contingencies are associated with both behavioral improvement *and* rating one's performance in a manner similar to the teacher.

Over the course of time, the teacher ratings are gradually faded such that the student ratings are the primary arbiter for earning backup reinforcement. This is facilitated by (1) the use of random "matching challenges" that occur on a periodic basis; and (2) the gradual reduction in frequency of these matching challenges. For example, the initial cutback in teacher ratings may involve a matching challenge that occurs every other day, on the average. Then the teacher matches are faded to every third day, once weekly, and once biweekly, on the average. If, at any point in time, the student's performance deteriorates and/or the teacher suspects inflation of student ratings, then matching challenges are conducted more frequently.

In the program described by Rhode and colleagues (1983), the students eventually employed self-ratings only, with no backup reinforcers. This led to maintenance of significant behavioral improvements across resource and regular classroom settings. This self-reinforcement system has been extended to children with ADHD and related disruptive disorders in elementary (Hoff & DuPaul, 1998), middle (Shapiro, DuPaul, & Bradley, 1998) and high (Smith, Young, Nelson, & West, 1992) school settings. Thus, it would seem that the use of variations of this program could have applicability for the treatment of ADHD-related behaviors across a wide age span. Nevertheless, it is important to note that a key variable influencing the success of these procedures is the continued use of external reinforcers contingent on student ratings. It is unlikely that the effectiveness of this intervention would be maintained if backup reinforcement was reduced or eliminated earlier in the sequence of program steps.

Designers of self-management interventions need to keep in mind that children with ADHD often lack the skill to be accurate judges of their own behavior. Because they may have a tendency toward recalling their positive behaviors and not recognizing the problem behaviors that affect their ratings, a brief discussion or reminder of the behaviors that led to a lower rating may be useful (Hinshaw & Melnick, 1992). Designing a self-management system in a classroom for a child with ADHD would involve teaching the child to use the system, providing clear descriptions of the expected behaviors, and drawing up a list of privileges the student would like to earn. The goal of such a system is to eventually train the child to monitor his or her own behavior in the classroom, without constant feedback from the teacher.

EFFECTIVE INSTRUCTIONAL STRATEGIES

In addition to the documented benefits of contingency management strategies, students identified with ADHD are likely to benefit from prevention-oriented behavior-management and classroom-management strategies. Furthermore, children with this disorder may require remedial or supplemental instruction aimed at improving basic academic skills, learning, and study. In general, ameliorating the classroom difficulties experienced by target students should involve multiple prevention and intervention approaches including (1) active and ongoing teaching of classroom rules, routines, and expectations for appropriate classroom behavior; (2) grading practices and contingencies to support the rules, routines, and expectations; (3) changes in instructional routines and curricula to improve rates of learning; (4) ongoing monitoring of progress in basic skill areas (i.e., reading, writing, math, and spelling); and (5) teaching students to be competent at organizing and studying academic materials.

In considering the classroom learning and performance of children with ADHD, a number of variables will need to be analyzed, ranging from the child's basic academic skills to the observable classroom behaviors that are potentially interfering with the child's classroom performance. A nonexhaustive list of such variables is provided in Table 5.5. For many children experiencing achievement and/or behavior problems in the classroom, a first step in pursuing problem resolution is to determine whether the problem is a skills or a conditions problem so that an appropriate intervention might be designed. One of the difficulties facing professionals serving children with ADHD, however, is that classroom difficulties are likely to be a combination of *both* skills and conditions

TABLE 5.5. Skills and Conditions to Consider in Evaluating and Treating Classroom-Based Problems Associated with ADHD

Skills	Conditions
Reading skills	Severity of ADHD symptomatology
Writing skills	Classroom management and motivational strategies
Spelling skills	Instructional routines
Math skills	Curricula
Study skills, organizational skills, and self-management skills	Home–school communication
Social and interpersonal skills	Community-based interventions (e.g., medication)

problems. Because of this likely interaction, multiple interventions typically will be implemented across settings and intervention agents.

The strategies discussed in this section are those with empirical support for their effectiveness in ameliorating some of the difficulties listed in Table 5.5. However, it must be noted that these routines, strategies, and approaches to teaching have only recently begun to be researched specifically with respect to their effects on the learning and behavior of children with ADHD. Researchers at Lehigh University are developing and testing a consultation model (Promoting Academic Success for Students [PASS]) for designing academic interventions for students with ADHD. This data-based decision-making model includes elements of consultative problem solving (Bergan & Kratochwill, 1990), curriculum-based measurement (Shinn, 1998), and functional assessment of academic behavior (Witt, Daly, & Noell, 2000). Over the next several years, academic outcome data will be collected to determine the cost-effectiveness of instructional interventions based on this model relative to more typical "trial-and-error" approaches to intervention design. Many of the strategies discussed in this section will be evaluated in the context of this research project. We begin our discussion with a focus on proactive teacher behaviors (i.e., proactive strategies occurring prior to the display of problem behaviors).

Teaching Classroom Rules and Expectations (Prevention)

Teacher-provided cues, prompts (including performance feedback), or signals to do or not do something can be quite effective in managing problem behaviors and promoting active engagement in academic work, task completion, and performance accuracy (Paine, Radicchi, Rosellini, Deutchman, & Darch, 1983; Sulzer-Azaroff & Mayer, 1991). Simply put, if one person wants something to be done by another, the easiest way to promote its occurrence is by communicating those expectations in an unambiguous fashion. This is not to suggest or imply that teachers have been remiss in what they have asked or required of children with ADHD. The point is, however, that at times all of us forget to do the "simple things" in carrying out our educational responsibilities. At other times, we firmly believe that we already have communicated our expectations clearly, and no further explanation is necessary.

Take, for example, the issue of classroom rules. It seems safe to assume that all children, including those identified with ADHD, who understand and follow classroom rules will experience greater success in school than children who do not understand and follow these rules (Madsen, Becker, & Thomas, 1968; Paine et al., 1983). However, the clarity with which classroom rules are taught and understood by students, in general, is not fully understood. In one pilot study investigating children's understanding of classroom rules, Stoner and Green (1992a) found that fewer than 10% of first-, second-, and third-grade students interviewed could accurately state or identify the rules pertaining to their own classrooms. Of further interest and importance here is that each of the involved teachers firmly believed that her or his classroom rules had been taught clearly and unequivocally. In a follow-up investigation with older students, Johnson, Stoner, and Green (1996) found that the active teaching of classroom rules to an entire classroom of seventh-grade math students resulted in significant behavioral improvement, including improvement on the part of initially identified individual students. Further studies of this type are needed to help us better understand the roles and uses of rules in preventing and remediating problem behavior in the classroom.

Initial directions for variables to include in such work have been identified by educational researchers such as Martens and Kelly (1993), Ysseldyke and Christenson (1987, 1988), and others (e.g., Elliott, Witt, & Kratochwill, & Stoiber, 2002; Paine et al., 1983; Paine & Paine, 2002; Sprick, Borgmeier, & Nolet, 2002). These professionals have suggested that the following proactive teacher behaviors can be effective in promoting appropriate classroom behavior:

1. Teachers remind students of the classroom rules, and actively teach these rules by discussion and by pointing out examples of students following them (i.e., "catch" students following the rules).

2. Teachers maintain eye contact with students as appropriate to the particular lesson or activity in progress.

3. Teachers remind students about expected behaviors that are critical to an activity *before* the start of the activity.

4. Teachers circulate throughout the classroom while monitoring student behavior and providing feedback in an unobtrusive fashion.

5. Teachers use nonverbal cues and signals to redirect a student while teaching others.

6. The pace of instructional lessons is brisk and directed by the teacher.

7. Teachers ensure that academic and nonacademic activities and routines are understood by students (e.g., when a project is considered complete, what expectations and activities are involved in today's math class). Teachers manage transitions from one activity to another in a brief and well-organized manner (e.g., state the expectations and activities involved in a transition from math period to recess).

8. Teachers frequently communicate their expectations about the use of class time in a clear manner. For example, Sprick and colleagues (2002) suggest posting (e.g., written on the blackboard) class schedules broken down into blocks of time with clear expectations for student behavior noted for each time block. In addition, they recommend providing students with "challenge problems" at the beginning of a given class period. These challenges provide students with an activity related to the lesson to get them involved in the subject matter while the transition is completed and to pique their interest in and attention to the lesson.

Incorporating these strategies into daily classroom routines can be useful in preventing and managing challenging classroom behavior. In addition, many of these procedures are correlated with improvements in student achievement (Martens & Kelly, 1993).

In addition to careful consideration of classroom and instructional routines, in working with children identified with ADHD, teachers should consider environmental arrangement strategies that will allow for more careful monitoring of the activities of identified students. For example, placing the child's desk near the teacher's may promote monitoring of student behavior as well as decrease the likelihood of misunderstanding of directions for an assignment. Teachers also should consider arrangements that will ensure student participation in class activities and not restrict opportunities to learn and benefit from instruction, while limiting proximity to potential distractions inherent in any given classroom. For example, a child identified with ADHD probably will not do well when seated beside a frequently used classroom activity center.

Instructional Management and Remediation in Basic Skill Areas

Classroom-based research efforts involving children with ADHD have tended to focus on the issues of behavior management as discussed in the previous sections of this chapter. In contrast, relatively little research has been conducted regarding instructional, curricular, or classroom environment manipulations aimed at enhancing the learning and academic performance of these children. Our speculation is that this phenomenon is a result of a combination of two variables. First, disruptive behaviors frequently are paramount concerns to teachers, and lead them to refer children to specialists. Second, historically, research knowledge and practices regarding ADHD and related problems have emerged from within the domains of medical and clinical professionals rather than from the educational arena. However, this set of circumstances has begun to change as educational researchers have now investigated intervention approaches including peer tutoring, computer-assisted instruction, task and instructional modifications, and strategy training on the learning and achievement of students with ADHD. These strategies are described below following a brief discussion of some basic issues in instruction, as well as strategies for remediation in basic skill areas such as reading, writing, and spelling.

A complete treatment of the topic of instruction is well beyond our scope, and numerous books are available on the topic (see Berliner & Rosenshine, 1987, for a thorough, readable treatment of critical issues in classroom teaching; see Shinn et al., 2002, for thorough coverage of interventions for academic and behavior problems). However, it is our hope that this presentation will spark the further development of needed classroom-based research and practices linking ADHD and instructional strategies.

Basic Instructional Processes

As reviewed and discussed by Rosenshine (1987), effective teaching involves the sequential arrangement of six primary instructional functions: review, presentation, guided practice, corrections and feedback, independent practice, and weekly/monthly reviews. For example, *review* involves checking for prerequisite skills and knowledge, and discussion of previously taught material and information relevant to the current lesson. Next, *new information or material* (i.e., facts, discriminations, basic concepts and relations) is presented in manageable steps or units, using clear positive and negative examples. Once the new material and examples have been presented, students are provided with numerous opportunities for *guided practice* with high rates of success. Then, based on student performance during the practice exercises, teachers provide students with *feedback and corrections*, and reteaching of material as needed to strengthen the new learning. When students are able to respond correctly a high percentage of the time to questions and problems involving the new material, they are ready for independent practice. *Independent practice* is intended to build fluency and autonomy with newly learned material, so that students can apply the new learning to various problems and understand it within a variety of contexts. Finally, *weekly and monthly reviews* are provided, again in the interest of building fluency and independent application of the learned material.

In a discussion of what he calls "simple views of effective teaching," Berliner (1987, p. 93) suggests that these teaching functions promote student learning for two primary reasons. First, the strategies ensure that students are provided with the opportunities to learn what they are supposed to learn. Second, working through cycles of review, practice, feedback, corrections, and more practice, teachers ensure that students are performing accurately and becoming more fluent. Doing so helps to avoid situations in which students repeatedly practice or perform their schoolwork inaccurately, thereby strengthening "mis-rules" (e.g., add when I see a "–" sign and subtract when I see a "+" sign). Furthermore, these factors can be manipulated and individualized with respect to difficult-to-teach material or students. For example, more opportunities to practice and a greater frequency of feedback might be provided around material broken down into smaller units when teaching a student who is experiencing difficulty in a particular subject area.

The instructional support and remediation strategies discussed below incorporate factors that have been associated with improved performance among children with ADHD. These include opportunities to learn via active responses to teacher directions and instruction, coupled with opportunities for the provision of frequent feedback and corrections. These strategies are presented only briefly here, with the intent of providing the interested reader with direction for further reading or study.

Reading Skills

Research findings suggest that success in reading in the early school years is related to later school achievement and adjustment (Chall, 1983). As such, skill in reading is a critical building block for a child's successful school experience (Anderson, Hiebert, Scott, & Wilkinson, 1985). Children with ADHD appear to be at greater risk for reading problems than their typically developing peers (O'Reilly, 2002). Reading instruction and remediation can be construed broadly as divisible into the two related areas of *decoding* and *comprehension*.

Gaining meaning from written information involves the decoding of text. The importance of children learning to decode text is such that the National Research Council (1998) and the National Reading Panel

(2000) have discussed the importance of *all children* receiving instruction in phonics as part of early reading instruction. Similarly, other leading researchers in the field of reading instruction (Adams, 1990; Carnine, Kameenui, & Silbert, 1990; Simmons et al., 2002) suggest that systematic phonics-based training should be a part of a student's first 2 years of reading instruction. Grossen and Carnine (1991) discuss four primary components of such instruction: (1) teaching letter–sound correspondence in isolation; (2) teaching the blending of sounds; (3) providing immediate feedback and corrections on oral reading errors; and (4) providing for extensive practice using sounds in isolation, word lists, and words in the context of reading passages. Students who develop fluent decoding skills are well prepared to become skilled readers who obtain meaning from text, as decoding skills are complemented with other forms of reading instruction.

Comprehensive reading instruction includes a great deal more than teaching phonics skills. For example, Sindelar, Lane, Pullen, and Hudson (2002) have suggested that students experiencing difficulty with reading may benefit from a variety of other strategies within three primary areas: (1) building fluency in reading/decoding, (2) building vocabulary, and (3) strengthening comprehension skills. A few of these strategies are noted here. Instruction for building reading and decoding fluency includes such strategies as repeated readings wherein passages are read several times (O'Shea, Sindelar, & O'Shea, 1987; Samuels, 1979) and previewing new readings (Rose & Sherry, 1984). Both interventions have been shown to enhance the reading fluency and comprehension of students with learning disabilities. Baker, Gersten, and Grossen (2002) also suggest that systematic instruction in vocabulary is warranted as part of comprehensive reading instruction. Sindelar and Stoddard (1991) note several research studies documenting the effectiveness of vocabulary-building strategies such as teaching synonyms via matching of printed words (Pany, Jenkins, & Shreck, 1982), teaching sets of words that belong within categories (Beck, Perfetti, & McKeown, 1982), and preteaching vocabulary words contained in a new reading assignment (Wixon, 1986).

Last, but certainly not least, we identify some instructional strategies to promote reading comprehension. First, as noted by Grossen and Carnine (1991), reading for comprehension assumes skill in decoding. Given fluent decoding skills, a number of instructional activities can be utilized to enhance reading comprehension (for reviews, see Baker et al., 2001; Simmons et al., 2002; Sindelar et al., 2002). For example, prereading discussions of the assignment can help to put the reading into a context that the student can understand and relate to. Background knowledge or information related to the reading can be checked for and supplemented, as can necessary vocabulary. In addition to these prereading activities, several strategies to enhance comprehension can be used either during reading or following the completion of a passage. Students can be taught to understand readings and their structure by learning to ask a series of questions, known as "story grammar" or "story patterns" (Carnine & Kinder, 1985). Students also can be taught to draw diagrams or maps of the text that they are reading to help support their comprehension of material (Grossen & Carnine, 1991). Reading comprehension also can be facilitated by the development of writing and spelling skills (Anderson et al., 1985).

In addition to instruction in reading, language arts instruction typically focuses on the development of writing and spelling skills. Skills in both these areas are critical to the development of functional communication abilities. Stated differently, writing and spelling skills allow writers to have their intended effect on their reader(s). The treatment of this topic is beyond our scope here, and we direct readers to excellent work of Graham and Harris (2002) on writing/spelling and interventions to improve these skills among low-performing students.

Clearly, this discussion of academic skills and instructional strategies is far from comprehensive. However, teachers and school psychologists with thorough knowledge of these and other procedures can utilize instructional interventions to build comprehensive and effective educational programs for students with ADHD who exhibit academic skills deficits.

Study and Organizational Skills

Children diagnosed with ADHD often present with a variety of academic performance problems in the areas of work completion, organization of desks and other materials, following directions, and studying for tests (Barkley, 1998; Todd et al., 2002). Children experiencing such difficulties may benefit from direct instruction in study and organizational skills. An organized and thorough set of field-tested materials for teaching study and organizational skills to students in grades 3–6 has been published as *Skills for School Success* by Archer and Gleason (1989), with both elementary- and secondary-level materials. The goal of these authors was to prepare a curriculum to teach study skills for gaining, responding to, and organizing information. In this fashion, students would be encouraged to become more actively engaged in the classroom learning process. Similar work has been conducted at the University of Kansas, by Donald Deshler, Jean Schumaker, and their colleagues, with a focus on strategies for use by secondary-level students (Deshler & Schumaker, 1988; Ellis, Deshler, & Schumaker, 1989; Schumaker, Deshler, & McKnight, 2002).

As discussed by Gleason, Archer, and Colvin (2002), students can be taught several strategies related to gaining information from written materials. These strategies involve previewing readings to identify main ideas and topics, reading text and concomitantly answering prepared questions about the reading, and utilizing strategies for taking careful and complete notes about the reading. In gaining meaning from text, children also must learn to read and understand the maps, graphs, pictures, and other visual aides that frequently accompany text. A second study skills area involves utilizing information gleaned from texts to respond to questions or other assignments based on the material. In this domain, the *Skills for School Success* curriculum contains lessons on carefully reading and answering end-of-unit questions, organizing and preparing written summaries of material that has been read, and taking quizzes and tests. For example, in learning to take quizzes and tests, students are taught how to anticipate the content of a forthcoming test, how to study and prepare for tests, and how to respond to particular types of questions, such as multiple-choice items.

Finally, Archer and Gleason (1989) have developed lessons for elementary-age children on how to manage time and materials in school. Three main topics are covered, including the organization of a school materials notebook, preparation and use of an assignment calendar, and the setup and completion of a neat, well-organized paper. For example, in setting up assignment papers, students are taught what is referred to as the HOW strategy. Here, the components and organization of a paper *Heading* are learned, including name, date, and subject. Next, children are taught the components of a paper's *Organization*, including the use of margins and blank lines. Finally, instruction focuses on what it means to produce a paper that is *Written* neatly, including writing on lines and erasing neatly when necessary. Across each of these study skills areas, it is suggested that teachers first must provide appropriate models, then supply regular opportunities for the study and organizational skills to be practiced by students, and finally, give positive feedback and corrections as necessary. Few would disagree that these study and organizational skills are invaluable to all students, including those with ADHD. And it seems clear to us that the effects of direct instruction in these skills on children with ADHD needs to be investigated. Other instructional strategies that have the potential to directly address the academic difficulties experienced by students with this disorder include peer tutoring, computer-assisted instruction, task and instructional modifications, and strategy training.

PEER TUTORING

According to Greenwood, Delquadri, and Carta (2002), *peer tutoring* can be defined as any instructional strategy within which two students work together on an academic activity with one student providing assistance, instruction, and/or feedback to the other. A number of approaches to peer tutoring exist that share the characteristics of this definition exist, yet differ along the lines of instructional variables. For example, the range of models differs regarding instructional focus (e.g., skill acquisition vs. skill practice), tutoring structure (e.g., reciprocal vs. nonreciprocal tutoring), and procedural components (e.g., numbers of sessions per week, methods of pairing students, types of motivational systems used) (for reviews, see Fuchs, Fuchs, Phillips, Hamlett, & Karns, 1995; Greenwood et al., 2002). Despite these differences, all models of peer tutoring share instructional characteristics that are known to enhance the sustained attention of students with ADHD. These characteristics include instruction that involves (1) a one-to-one student–teacher ratio/arrangement; (2) self-paced instruction determined by learner; (3) continuous prompting of academic responding; and (4) frequent immediate feedback about quality of performance (Pfiffner & Barkley, 1998).

Several research investigations have employed ClassWide Peer Tutoring (CWPT; Greenwood et al., 1988, 2002) in general education classrooms that included students with ADHD. CWPT has been found to enhance the mathematics, reading, and spelling skills of students of all achievement levels (for a review, see Greenwood et al., 2002). This form of peer tutoring includes the following components: (1) division of the class into two teams; (2) formation of tutoring pairs among classmates within each team; (3) students take turns tutoring each other; (4) tutors are provided with academic scripts (e.g., math problems with answers); (5) praise and points are delivered contingent on correct answers; (6) errors are corrected immediately along with an opportunity for practicing the correct answer; (7) the teacher monitors tutoring pairs and provides bonus points for pairs who are following prescribed procedures; and (8) points are tallied by each individual student at the conclusion of each session. Tutoring sessions typically last 20 minutes with an additional 5 minutes for recording of student progress and putting materials away. Interestingly, earned points typically are not exchanged for backup reinforcers. Rather, at the conclusion of each week, the team with the most points is applauded by the other team.

A controlled case study of CWPT conducted with a 7-year-old boy with ADHD in a second-grade general education classroom found promising results (DuPaul & Henningson,1993). The influence of CWPT, relative to baseline conditions, during instruction followed by independent seatwork was investigated, with a focus on on-task behavior, fidgeting, and math performance. CWPT was found to produce reliable increases in on-task behavior and similarly reliable reductions in fidgeting during math class relative to typical instructional conditions. Less consistent findings were obtained with respect to math performance, although the student did make measurable gains in this area.

In a replication and extension of this work with a larger group of students exhibiting significant ADHD-related behaviors, DuPaul, Ervin, Hook, and McGoey (1998) evaluated the effects of CWPT on the academic performance and behavioral control of 19 students (16 boys, 3 girls; median age = 7.5) with ADHD in first- through fifth-grade general education classrooms. Outcome measures included direct observations of ADHD-related behavior, teacher ratings, self-report ratings, and weekly pre- and posttests. CWPT was implemented for math, spelling, or reading depending on the academic area that each teacher identified as weakest for the student with ADHD.

The results of the DuPaul and colleagues (1998) study indicated that the active engagement of students with ADHD significantly increased from an average of 21.6% during baseline to an average of 82.3% when CWPT was implemented. Concomitant reductions in off-task behavior also were obtained. In addition, children's weekly posttest scores increased from an average of 55.2% during baseline to 73% for CWPT conditions, thus indicating that this intervention affected both attentional behavior and academic performance. Similar improvements in behavior and academic performance were exhibited by typically functioning classmates, thus attesting to the fact that peer tutoring can help *all* students, not just those with disabilities. Furthermore, the teachers and students in the DuPaul and colleagues study all reported CWPT to be effective and acceptable.

In general, these studies provide consistent evidence that peer tutoring is an intervention strategy that is able to improve the active engagement, academic performance, and, possibly, the social interactions of a wide variety of students, including those with ADHD. Given that students with ADHD have significant problems when asked to complete independent assignments, peer tutoring provides an alternative instructional mode providing for practice and refinement of academic skills.

COMPUTER-ASSISTED INSTRUCTION

The use of computer-assisted instruction (CAI) has been recommended for increasing the on-task and work production behaviors of students with ADHD. It has been suggested that the instructional features of CAI allow students with ADHD to focus their attention on academic stimuli (Lillie, Hannun, & Stuck, 1989; Torgesen & Young, 1983). That is, CAI has the potential to readily present specific instructional objectives, provide highlighting of essential material (e.g., with large print, color), use multiple sensory modalities, divide content material into smaller bits of information, and provide immediate feedback about response accuracy. In addition, CAI can readily limit the presentation of nonessential features that may be distracting (e.g., sound effects, animation). A few studies have shown positive effects of CAI with students diagnosed with ADHD.

As an example of a *computer-assisted academic intervention*, Ota and DuPaul (2002) examined the effects of using computer software with a game format (Math Blaster) to improve math achievement. The participants were three male, white, fourth- through sixth-grade students with ADHD. Following baseline (observation under normal classroom conditions), the math software was introduced sequentially in a multiple baseline fashion for each participant. Observational data were collected during the baseline and experimental conditions along with a set of instructional-level math probes, which were administered several times per week throughout the study. All three participants showed some improvement in their performance on curriculum-based math probes; however, the strength of these improvements varied across individuals (i.e., effects were particularly pronounced for two of the three participants). Furthermore, all three participants showed substantial reductions in off-task disruptive behavior as a function of interacting with the computer software.

The results of these studies provide preliminary evidence for school personnel that CAI may be an effective instructional alternative for at least some children with ADHD. Allowing students to receive CAI may result in improvements in work completion and attending behaviors. However, characteristics of the software packages may affect the attending behaviors of students with ADHD. Software packages that include game formats and animation may be more effective than drill and practice or tutorial programs. Clearly, there is a pressing need for continued research on CAI for students with this disorder.

TASK AND INSTRUCTIONAL MODIFICATIONS

Task Modifications

Another type of academic intervention that can improve the academic performance of students diagnosed with ADHD is task modification (TM). TM involves revising the curriculum or aspects of it in an attempt to reduce problem behaviors and increase appropriate classroom behaviors. In addition, TM is a proactive strategy, as changes are made before the curriculum is presented to the student. It has been argued that this type of positive academic modification is more responsive to the individual needs of the student (Meyer & Evans, 1989).

One type of TM, choice making, requires the student to choose activities from among two or more concurrently presented options. Previous studies examining the effects of choice making on students with developmental disabilities have demonstrated increases in social behavior and decreases in levels of disruptive behavior (Dyer, Dunlap, & Winterling, 1990; Koegel, Dyer, & Bell, 1987). The effects of classroom-based choice making were recently examined in a study conducted by Dunlap and colleagues (1994). In this study, the effects of choice making on the task engagement and disruptive behaviors of three students with emotional and behavioral disorders were examined. Of these three participants, one 12-year-old male was identified as having ADHD. This student was provided with a menu of academic tasks in English and Spelling from which to choose. The results of the study indicated that choice making led to reliable and consistent increases in task engagement with concomitant reductions in disruptive behavior. Therefore, choice making may be a valuable task modification for students with ADHD. Not only does allowing students to chose their assignments reduce disruptive behaviors and improve task engagement, but this strategy promotes student initiative and independence. However, it is not clear whether this type of TM is effective at improving academic performance.

Based on the premise that children with ADHD have a greater need for cognitive stimulation than their nondiagnosed peers, a few TM studies have investigated the effects of modifying intratask stimulation (Zentall, 1989; Zentall & Leib, 1985). In one study conducted in a classroom setting, Zentall and Leib (1985) investigated the effects of added structure on the activity levels and performance of children using a repeated-measures design. Eight participants identified as hyperactive were randomly assigned to one of two experimental art conditions in which the structure of the task requirement was manipulated (explicit instructions combined with task materials vs. nonspecific instructions without task materials). Results indicated significant decreases in activity level of the participants, and suggested that modifying task requirements may affect activity levels of children identified as hyperactive.

In another classroom-based study, Zentall (1989) examined whether adding color to relevant cues in a spelling task improved the performance of children diagnosed as hyperactive. Participants included 20 hyperactive and 26 comparison boys who were preassessed on spelling achievement and randomly assigned to one of two condition-order groups. Results of this study indicated the participants identified as hyperactive demonstrated better performance than the comparison participants when relevant color was added to spelling tasks. Interestingly, the addition of color to irrelevant aspects of the task resulted in decreases in spelling performance. The educational implications of these results suggest that adding color to relevant components of a task may increase attention to detail and improve the academic performance of children with ADHD. However, the highly controlled spelling task and limited measures of academic achievement reduces the degree to which these findings can be generalized to classroom settings.

In one of the first studies to utilize classroom-based functional assessment procedures, Ervin, DuPaul, Kern, and Friman (1996) examined the effect of TM on the academic performance of children with ADHD. Based on the results of descriptive analyses and hypothesis development, it was purported that the task engagement of two male students diagnosed with ADHD would improve if a task modification were conducted. Using a brief reversal design, the effects of an alternative writing method were examined with one male participant. This method included peer discussion, brainstorming of ideas, and the use of a computer for journal writing. Allowing the participant to modify his written assignments resulted in clinically significant decreases in off-task behavior. Specifically, the percentage of intervals in which off-task behavior was not observed was greater when the participant was able to use the computer ($M = 96.8\%$) than when the participant completed the written task by hand ($M = 64.8\%$). For the second male student diagnosed with ADHD, it was hypothesized that allowing him to take notes during a lecture would result in less frequent off-task behaviors than if he passively listened to the lecture. The results of a brief experimental manipulation indicated that the percentage of intervals without off-task behavior was consistently higher when the note-taking strategy was employed ($M = 97.8\%$) than when the participant did not use the strategy ($M = 54.5\%$). The results of this study are limited by the brief intervention period and the absence of academic performance data; however, they are intriguing and suggestive of future research directions.

Instructional Modifications

Similar to TM, specific instructional modifications (IM) can be implemented to improve the academic environments of students experiencing difficulties with inattention, impulsivity, or hyperactivity. As stated earlier, few studies have examined this form of intervention with students displaying ADHD-related behaviors.

For example, Skinner, Johnson, Larkin, Lessley, and Glowacki (1995) examined the influence of two taped-words interventions, fast-taped words (FTW) and slow-taped words (STW), on word reading list performance. One of the three participating students was identified as having ADHD. Outcome measurement focused on reading accuracy rates across baseline conditions and the FTW and STW procedures. Relatively higher rates of accurate reading were demonstrated in the STW condition. Results of this study suggest that taped-words interventions can be effective procedures for improving reading accuracy rates for students with ADHD.

Results from the available research literature suggest that task and instructional modifications can lead to decreased disruptive behavior, increased task engagement, and increased academic performance. Furthermore, these types of modifications can occur within the context of the daily classroom routine, requiring minimal teacher preparation. However, it should be noted the results have been limited to immediate, short-term intervention effects. Again, this is an area in need of further investigation.

STRATEGY TRAINING

Finally, one other type of academic intervention involves teaching students to use specific classroom strategies while completing academic work. Strategy training (ST) involves teaching students to use a set of procedures or strategies that specifically address the demands of an academic situation. This type of intervention is promising for students diagnosed with ADHD because it can facilitate students becoming more responsible for their own academic behavior. Again, however, very few empirical investigations have examined the use of ST in this population.

Strategy training seems particularly applicable to adolescents with ADHD, though again few studies have been conducted in this area. At the secondary school level, students with ADHD may exhibit poor organization and study skills, which contributes to their elevated risk for poor scholastic achievement (Shapiro, DuPaul, Bradley, & Bailey, 1996). For example, students with this disorder may have difficulty attending to classroom instruction and taking organized notes for later review. Perhaps improving the note-taking strategies of adolescents with ADHD may enhance their academic and behavioral performance in the classroom. One such note-taking strategy is the Directed Notetaking Activity (DNA; Spires & Stone, 1989). Here, students learn the strategy through teacher-directed lectures and prompts in attempts to increase students' on-task behavior, improve comprehension of classroom materials, and reduce the frequency of disruptive behaviors. Specifically, the teacher instructs the students on the note-taking process by illustrating how to outline notes based on main ideas and details. The number of teacher prompts is slowly faded until students are able to independently produce an outline based on the presented lecture material.

Evans, Pelham, and Grudberg (1995) examined the effects of DNA with adolescents diagnosed with ADHD. In the first experiment, 16 adolescents with ADHD (13 males, 3 females) attending a summer treatment program received DNA instruction during their classroom period. The summer treatment program included both academic and recreational activities. Each week of the intervention, the amount of teacher instruction and prompts provided in note taking were reduced from a teacher-provided outline of lecture material to a blank page for taking notes. Results showed that the participants achieved significant improvements in the quality of notes over time. In addition, significant increases in the recording of details were observed. These results suggested that adolescents with ADHD may improve their note-taking skills with the DNA instruction procedure.

In the same study, Evans and colleagues (1995) examined the efficacy of the DNA procedure on the process and products of note taking. Here, 14 adolescents participating in a summer treatment program received DNA instruction for 3 weeks. The participants' proficiency in using the note-taking strategy was assessed across four experimental conditions, with results indicating the note-taking intervention significantly improved the on-task behavior and daily assignment performance of the participants. It should be noted, however, that this intervention did not significantly improve quiz scores or reduce disruptive behaviors. Overall results of this study indicate that note-taking strategies can enhance the on-task behavior and academic performance of adolescents with ADHD in the classroom. In addition, the greater the quality and organization of the notes, the fewer disruptive behaviors are displayed.

CONSIDERATIONS WITH SECONDARY-LEVEL STUDENTS

Research on effective academic intervention strategies for adolescents is sparse. In fact, in their meta-analytic review of school-based interventions for students with ADHD, DuPaul and Eckert (1997) were able to locate only two studies that specifically targeted the performance of students with ADHD over the age of 13 years old. Given the problems that secondary students with ADHD encounter with respect to academic achievement, organization, study skills, test taking, and adjustment in general, this is yet another important area for future investigation in the field of ADHD.

Strategies discussed thus far that warrant consideration with secondary students include contingency contracting, self-monitoring and self-reinforcement, computer-assisted instruction, and instruction in study and organizational skills. Additionally, a recent book by Robin (1998) provides excellent guidelines and directions for professionals and families working with adolescents with ADHD across both home and school settings. This group of students represents a significant challenge to us, as a result of the interaction of the chronic nature of ADHD and the more general characteristics of adolescence. These include demands and expectations for increasing academic, social, and behavioral independence, judgment, and self-regulation. Furthermore, these expectations take place in the increasingly complex contexts of completing high school and planning for postsecondary work and/or education; negotiating within-family responsibilities surrounding automobile use, social engagements and activities, substance use, and romantic and sexual interests/activities; and, ultimately, independent living.

Support for adolescents with ADHD in these endeavors is likely to take many forms. For example, academically students are likely to need assistance and direct instruction in study and organizational skills including note taking, preparing for and taking tests, and completing long-term assignments (see Robin, 1998, for a thorough discussion of possible accommodations). In addition, these students may need greater then typical amounts of support in planning for their educational and employment futures. For example, many colleges and universities have excellent support programs for students with disabilities; learning to explore such options is likely to be important for these students. Becoming an effective self-advocate also will be important, including understanding one's rights, one's disability, and one's skills/weaknesses. Such understanding will likely be critical to postsecondary academic success—as will availing oneself of available supports and resources.

One promising avenue for the support of adolescents with ADHD is that of being "coached" in a one-to-one relationship intended to support the adolescent in achieving her or his self-selected goals. In this regard, Dawson and Guare (1998) have developed a *Coaching the ADHD Student* resource workbook that provides guidelines organized into three brief chapters on the foundations, mechanics, and applications of coaching students with ADHD, as well as appendices with materials for use within coaching activities. Briefly, Dawson and Guare describe the following steps to coaching: do a needs assessment, obtain commitment from participants, select a coach, arrange an initial meeting between the student and the coach, and initiate regular coaching sessions (daily is recommended). Further suggestions are offered as to the focus of the coaching relationship on goal setting, developing plans for attaining goals, identifying and overcoming obstacles to goal attainment, and evaluation of progress.

This coaching model is based on correspondence training research (Paniagua, 1992; Risley & Hart, 1968) with its focus on promoting a match between what a person says he or she will do and what he or she actually does. The model and methods make good conceptual sense; however, empirical investigations are needed to further validate this approach to intervention.

In the context of the family, adolescents with ADHD and their parents are likely to benefit from some form of counseling support (Robin, 1998; also see Chapter 8 for further discussion). Such support may range from understanding ADHD and its influence on the family's interaction patterns, to supporting and planning the education of an adolescent with ADHD, to negotiating privileges and responsibilities in the context of the family. As with previous examples, individualizing the nature and type of academic, family, and individual support will be one of the keys to successful outcomes.

PROVIDING TEACHER SUPPORT

Given evidence that a student is not meeting the expectations of his or her current classroom, reasonable interventions and accommodations should be made in attempts to allow the student to meet those expectations and achieve academic success. Such accommodations might include matching instructional materials with current academic skills, providing more frequent positive and corrective feedback, enhancing motivation to engage in academic work, and increasing opportunities to learn and practice newly acquired skills. It also must be recognized, however, that teachers who are expected to make such accommodations should themselves be able to expect systematic assistance in the way of consultation and support services for the design, implementation, and evaluation of classroom-based interventions.

"Teacher support systems" have been identified by Horner and colleagues (1991) as being critical to the successful education of students with challenging behaviors. These researchers have noted that teacher support systems rely on instructional and behavioral programs that are grounded in three important commitments. These commitments are to (1) teaching students in those classrooms or schools in which they would be educated were they not exhibiting challenging behaviors, (2) providing support in an ongoing fashion, and (3) producing positive and broad lifestyle outcomes, including preparing the student to participate successfully in the community and society.

Given these commitments, teacher support systems for providing services to students identified with ADHD should consist of the following components, as identified by and adapted from Horner and colleagues (1991):

1. A systematic screening and identification process to ensure identification of all students in need of the behavioral or instructional support. For example, the Systematic Screening for Behavior Disorders (Walker & Severson, 1988) and Early Screening Project (Feil et al., 1995) approaches are a viable choices for this purpose.

2. Comprehensive procedures linking assessment and program development to address achievement and behavior problems. For example, the use of functional behavioral assessment and curriculum-based measurement procedures would fulfill this need.

3. Procedures to ensure the design, implementation, and evaluation of interventions and accommodations to support student learning and behavior.

4. Procedures to ensure the transfer of responsibility for intervention program continuance to regular classroom staff.

5. Provision of ongoing supervision and monitoring across classrooms and other school settings, with a focus on structuring educational environments that are purposeful, organized, and supportive, while producing positive student outcomes.

6. Provision for evaluations of and revisions to the support system.

Mechanisms for providing teacher support are considered necessary components in the treatment of children with ADHD. Given the frequency and severity of disruptive behaviors that these students exhibit, it is not uncommon for teachers to express feelings of frustration and helplessness when attempting to manage their classrooms. These feelings should be expected and validated by professionals and parents who are interacting with classroom teachers. Furthermore, efforts should be made to help teachers deal with these feelings in a productive fashion (e.g., by providing instructional materials related to stress management). A second, related factor to consider is that making teaching accommodations often requires time, patience, resources, and training beyond that which is currently available to the teacher. For instance, the implementation of an individualized token reinforcement program in the context of a classroom of 25–30 children often is a prohibitive enterprise for the teacher. Thus, the selection of treatment strategies should be made in view of constraints placed on the teacher. The characteristics of the teacher support system enumerated above are designed to address these practical issues in a proactive fashion rather than waiting for teacher complaints to occur.

Implementation of teacher support systems will require professionals with assessment and program development expertise, educators with supervisory or administrative rank and responsibilities for monitoring ongoing educational programs, and personnel to provide intervention assistance as needed in support of regular classroom staff. Ideally, this type of commitment to teacher support would be coupled with staff who are knowledgeable and skillful in the areas of instructional and behavioral support. In schools where such circumstances exist, it would not seem unreasonable for parents and teachers to expect higher rates of academic, behavioral, and social success for students with ADHD.

CONCLUSION

Children with ADHD frequently experience difficulty in the areas of classroom behavior, academic performance, and scholastic achievement. Maximizing each child's likelihood for school success will require a variety of behavioral, instructional, and learning strategies aimed at the prevention and management of problems in these areas. This chapter has provided a review of effective behavior management interventions and instructional strategies, as well as review of promising instructional and self-management strategies. The need for systematic teacher support was also noted. In addition to further research on promising intervention approaches, the challenge before us is one of integrating the various strategies into treatment programs that are based on individual student needs such that all students with ADHD experience success in school.

CHAPTER 6

♦ ♦ ♦

Medication Therapy

♦

The prescription of psychotropic medication is the most common treatment for ADHD. For example, approximately 1.5 million children (or greater than 4% of the school-age population) are treated with psychostimulant medications (e.g., methylphenidate) in the United States (Safer & Zito, 2000). Psychostimulant medication use has grown steadily throughout the last two decades, particularly among preschool and secondary school populations (Olfson, Marcus, Weissman, & Jensen, 2002; Safer & Zito, 2000). The average duration of medication use is between 2 and 7 years, depending upon the age of the child (Safer & Zito, 2000). Furthermore, more research has been conducted on the effects of stimulant medications on the functioning of children with ADHD than any other treatment modality for any childhood disorder (DuPaul, Barkley, & Connor, 1998).

Numerous studies have consistently demonstrated short-term enhancement of the behavioral, academic, and social functioning of the majority of children being treated with stimulant compounds (see DuPaul et al., 1998, for a review). Alternatively, the limitations of pharmacotherapy (e.g., possible side effects, lack of evidence of long-term efficacy) have led to the adoption of multimodal treatment approaches for ADHD (Barkley, 1998). Stimulants appear to exert greater effects on problems associated with ADHD symptoms (e.g., academic underachievement) when combined with other effective treatment approaches, such as behavior modification (MTA Cooperative Group, 1999). But given the demonstrated efficacy and widespread use of psychotropic medications in treating ADHD, it is important for school-based personnel to become familiar with (1) the types of medications used to treat ADHD; (2) possible behavioral and side effects associated with these medications; (3) factors to consider in recommending medication trials for individual children; (4) methods to assess treatment response within school settings; (5) how to communicate assessment data to physicians and other medical professionals; and (6) the limitations of pharmacotherapy.

TYPES OF PSYCHOTROPIC MEDICATIONS EMPLOYED

Central Nervous System Stimulants

Psychostimulant medications are so named because of their demonstrated ability to increase the arousal or "alertness" of the central nervous system (CNS). Their effects on children with ADHD are not "paradoxical," as they exert similar physiological and behavioral effects with the normal population (Rapoport et al., 1980). Given the structural similarity of psychostimulants to certain brain neurotransmitters (e.g., dopamine), they are considered sympathomimetic compounds (Donnelly & Rapoport, 1985). The most commonly employed CNS stimulants are methylphenidate (Ritalin, Concerta, Metadate), dextroamphetamine (Dexedrine), and mixed amphetamine (Adderall). Of the three medications, methylphenidate is the most widely employed: it is used in over 80% of children treated with stimulants (Safer & Zito, 2000). Pemoline (Cylert) has been used in the past to treat ADHD; however, its use has diminished significantly in recent years due to serious concerns about hepatoxicity. Other types of stimulants (e.g., caffeine) are not discussed here because they have not been found to be as effective as the above medications nor are they typically used clinically.

Dose Ranges

The CNS stimulants, their available tablet sizes, and typical dose ranges are displayed in Table 6.1. Fixed dose ranges, as opposed to those based on body weight (i.e., mg/kg), are given to reflect typical prescribing practice. Also, research indicates that neither gross body weight nor body area is a significant predictor of dose–response to methylphenidate in the pediatric age range (Rapport & Denney, 1997). Once a child's "optimal" dose is established, as discussed below, medication is usually dispensed once per day (in the case of sustained-release preparations) or twice per day (at breakfast and lunch for standard preparations).

Given the relatively short behavioral half-lives of these compounds,

TABLE 6.1. Stimulant Medications, Tablet Sizes, and Dose Ranges

Brand name[a]	Tablet sizes	Dosage regimen	Dose range[b]
Ritalin	5–20 mg	Twice daily	2.5–25 mg
(methylphenidate)	SR, 20 mg	Once daily	20–40 mg
Concerta		Once daily	
(methylphenidate)			
Metadate		Once daily	
(methylphenidate)			
Dexedrine	5-mg spansule		2.5–25 mg
(d-amphetamine)	10-mg spansule		
	15-mg spansule	Once daily	
	5-mg tablet		
	5 mg/5 ml (elixir)	Twice daily	2.5–25 mg
Adderall	5–20 mg	Once daily	5–20 mg
(mixed amphetamine)			

[a]Generic name in parentheses.
[b]Dose range for each administration is provided.

school personnel have a greater opportunity to observe the child with ADHD when medicated than do parents and therefore must be included in the assessment of treatment response.

Both methylphenidate (MPH) and dextroamphetamine are available in short-acting and sustained-release forms. Because the behavioral effects of the latter compounds purportedly last longer (i.e., 8 hours postingestion) than the short-acting derivatives, they (along with Adderall, which is also a long-acting preparation) have several advantages, including the preclusion of noontime medication administration at school and greater confidentiality of treatment (DuPaul, Barkley, & Connor, 1998). Thus, at present, sustained-release medications are preferred over short-acting preparations for treating most children.

Tricyclic Antidepressant Medications

Antidepressants, such as desipramine (Norpramine) and imipramine (Tofranil), are slower acting medications that have been shown to produce behavioral effects similar to those of the stimulants with children with ADHD (Spencer, Biederman, & Wilens, 1998). For instance, both antidepressant medications have been found to result in improved teacher ratings of inattention, hyperactivity, and aggression in up to 70% of treated children. Furthermore, these medications may be particularly helpful for children who are nonresponders to stimulants (e.g., Biederman, Baldessarini, Wright, Knee, & Harmatz, 1989). Desipramine has been found to enhance performance on laboratory-based measures of short-term memory and visual problem solving, but does not affect learning of higher order relationships unless combined with MPH (Rapport, Carlson, Kelly, & Pataki, 1993).

Potential side effects of antidepressant medications include increases in blood pressure and heart rate, as well as possible slowing of intracardiac conduction (Spencer et al., 1998). Thus, a child's response to these medications requires more intense monitoring (e.g., frequent electrocardiograms) than is necessary with the stimulants. Desipramine also has been associated with growth deficits, although these are not as pronounced as found with the stimulant medications (Spencer, Biederman, Wright, & Danon, 1992).

Other Antidepressant Medications

Monoamine oxidase inhibitors (MAOIs) have been found to be clinically effective for problems related to ADHD (Rapoport, 1986; Zametkin, Rapoport, Murphy, Linnoila, & Iamond, 1985). Unfortunately, certain dietary and multidrug restrictions must be followed when MAOIs are administered, thus rendering the use of MAOIs problematic given the impulse control problems of children with ADHD (Hunt, Lau, & Ryu, 1991). Nortriptyline has been found to be helpful in reducing tics associated with Tourette's disorder and symptoms of ADHD in a majority of children with both ADHD and Tourette's (Spencer, Biederman, Wilens, Steingard, & Geist, 1993). Bupropion (Wellbutrin) has been found to be mildly effective, at best, in reducing ADHD symptomatology (Casat, Pleasants, Schroeder, & Parler, 1989; Simeon, Ferguson, & Van Wyck Fleet, 1986). There is a possibility that bupropion may exert both antiaggressive and antihyperactive effects in some children with ADHD (Hunt et al., 1991). The results of an open trial of bupropion indicated positive behavioral effects for a sample of adolescents with ADHD, conduct disorder, and substance use disorder (Riggs, Leon, Mikulich, & Pottle, 1998). Effects on academic performance are more variable and require further exploration (Nebrig & DuPaul, 2001).

Antihypertensive Medications

Clonidine, an antihypertensive agent, is moderately effective in reducing ADHD symptoms (for a meta-analysis, see Connor, Fletcher, & Swanson, 1999). For example, Hunt, Mindera, and Cohen (1985) obtained clonidine-induced enhancement of teacher and parent ratings of hyperactivity and conduct problems in 70% of children treated. But it should be noted that when the effects of clonidine are directly compared to those of MPH, the latter is found to be superior (Connor et al., 1999).

Alternatively, clonidine may be preferred in certain situations due to continued effects in the evening and an absence of the sleep or appetite disturbance that is sometimes found with MPH. In fact, the combination of clonidine and MPH may be helpful in those cases where MPH alone has led to side effects such as insomnia (Connor, Barkley, & Davis, 2000; Hunt et al., 1991). The most frequent side effects of clonidine are sedation, irritability, and a drop in blood pressure (Connor et al., 1999). Guanfacine (Tenex) is another antihypertensive agent that has been found to lead to similar behavioral effects as clonidine in several open trials. Side effects appear to be less frequent and severe than those found with clonidine (Connor, 1998). But given the lack of controlled trials on this compound, use of gaunfacine in the clinical treatment of ADHD appears premature. Given its modest efficacy and association with side effects, it appears that clonidine is a viable second-tier treatment for ADHD, with effects equivalent to tricyclic antidepressants (Connor et al., 1999).

Atomoxetine

Atomoxetine (Strattera) is a nonstimulant compound that affects norepinepherine in a similar manner to stimulants. Although this drug has not been extensively studied, the results of an initial controlled trial are promising (Michelson et al., 2002). Specifically, a large sample of children and adolescents with ADHD were treated with several dosages of atomoxetine over an 8-week time period. Results indicated a majority of participants showed a positive behavioral response, including children with the inattentive subtype. Although further investigation of this medication is necessary, atomoxetine may play an increasingly important role in the treatment of children who do not respond to the stimulants.

Summary

Although these and other initial results are promising, most of the available research with medications other than stimulants has been conducted with small samples employing only teacher and parent ratings as outcome measures. Furthermore, some initial studies did not employ double-blind methodology, a crucial control in pharmacological research. Effects on academic performance and cognitive functioning must be studied prior to these compounds being considered viable alternatives to stimulant medications. In addition, the magnitude of treatment effects associated with alternative drugs and stimulants need to be compared directly within large samples of children with ADHD. Pending the results of such investigations, stimulants remain the medication of choice for the treatment of ADHD. For this reason, the remainder of this chapter will focus on CNS stimulants, primarily MPH.

BEHAVIORAL EFFECTS OF STIMULANTS

Based on the empirical literature, approximately 75% of elementary school-age children with ADHD treated with stimulant medications respond positively to one or more doses (see Rapport & Denney, 2000). Remaining children either exhibit no change or their ADHD symptoms worsen with treatment, thus implicating the need for alternative medications or treatment approaches. Thus, it is not guaranteed that a given child with ADHD will respond to a particular stimulant nor should medication response be used as a confirmation of diagnosis (i.e., a positive response does not confirm an ADHD diagnosis, nor does a negative medication response indicate that a child does not have ADHD). Furthermore, a lack of response or adverse effects associated with one of the stimulants does not rule out the possibility of a positive response to one of the remaining medications in this class (Elia & Rapoport, 1991). At the present time, MPH is by far the most commonly employed stimulant; it is prescribed in greater than 80% of children receiving such medications (Safer & Zito, 2000). Several investigations have delineated that the behavioral effects of MPH, dextroamphetamine, and mixed amphetamine compounds are quite similar (e.g., James et al., 2001).

The effects of stimulant medications upon nearly every area of behavioral, emotional, and physical functioning of children with ADHD have been investigated (for reviews, see DuPaul, Barkley, & Connor, 1998; Spencer et al., 1996). The areas of greatest potential concern to school professionals will be reviewed briefly below.

Effects on Behavioral Control and Attention

Stimulant medications have been found to have positive effects on the ability of children with ADHD to sustain attention to effortful tasks (Barkley, DuPaul, & McMurray, 1991; Douglas, Barr, O'Neill, & Britton, 1986; Rapport et al., 1987) and to inhibit impulsive responding (Brown & Sleator, 1979; Rapport et al., 1988). In many cases, attention to assigned classwork is improved to the extent that the child's behavior appears similar to his or her "normal" classmates (Abikoff & Gittelman, 1985; DuPaul & Rapport, 1993). Furthermore, these medications significantly reduce disruptive motor activity, especially task-irrelevant movements during work situations (e.g., Cunningham & Barkley, 1979). Problems with aggression (Hinshaw, 1991; Klorman et al., 1988), classroom disruptive behavior (Barkley, 1979), persistence with frustrating tasks (Milich, Carlson, Pelham, & Licht, 1991), and noncompliance with authority figure commands (Barkley, Karlsson, Strzelecki, & Murphy, 1984) also have been shown to improve with these medications. A meta-analysis conducted by Connor, Glatt, Lopez, Jackson, and Melloni (2002) found moderate-to-high effect sizes for stimulant-induced improvements in overt and covert aggression. In fact, effects on aggressive behavior were equivalent to effect sizes obtained for ADHD symptoms. In general, improvements in behavior control and sustained attention are strongest at the higher doses and are ubiquitous across home, clinic, analog classroom, and school settings. Similar behavioral effects have been obtained for adolescents with ADHD; however, the percentage of positive responders is lower (i.e., 50–70%) than among elementary school children (Evans & Pelham, 1991; Pelham, Vodde-Hamilton, Murphy, Greenstein, & Vallano, 1991).

Behavioral effects of stimulants are, in part, moderated by environmental factors. Northup and colleagues have conducted several studies explicating the relationship between environmental contingencies and MPH response (e.g., Northup et al., 1997, 1999). These investigations demonstrated that MPH effects vary across situations as a function of contingencies operating in the environment. For example, in a laboratory situation where children were asked to complete tasks under differing conditions, MPH effects on disruptive behavior were strongest when an adult was present in the room and weakest when the child was alone (Northup et al., 1999). Although MPH operates directly on biological factors (i.e., brain functioning), the effects of this and similar drugs are dependent on prevailing contingencies and the rates of behavior that the latter elicit (Murray & Kollins, 2000; Rapport, DuPaul, & Smith, 1985). Thus, Northup and Gulley (2001) have recommended that school psychologists evaluate medication effects in the context of functional behavioral assessments, wherein MPH dosage and environmental factors are systematically manipulated to find optimal combinations of each treatment approach. The applicability of this laboratory paradigm to school settings awaits investigation; however, it is clear that the behavioral effects of stimulants do not occur in a vacuum and environmental factors must always be considered when evaluating medication response.

Effects on Cognitive and Academic Performance

Stimulant medication effects on the cognitive performance of children with ADHD traditionally have been studied using laboratory-based paradigms such as the Paired Associates Learning test (Swanson & Kinsbourne, 1975) and tests of short-term recall (Sprague & Sleator, 1977). Salutary effects of MPH on children's cognitive functioning have been found on tests of verbal retrieval (Barkley, DuPaul, & McMurray, 1991; Evans, Gualtieri, & Amara, 1986), paired associates learning (Rapport et al., 1985), stimulus equivalence learning (Vyse & Rapport, 1989), and short-term recall of visual stimuli (Sprague & Sleator, 1977). In general, the dose–response effects of MPH on cognitive performance have been found to be linear, with the greatest enhancement occurring at the highest doses (Rapport & Kelly, 1991; Solanto, 2000). It is important to note, however, that these dose–response effects have been delineated at the group level and there are substantial differences in dose responsivity across individual children, as will be explicated below.

Reviews of stimulant medication effects on the academic performance of children with ADHD have generally concluded that this area of functioning is not impacted significantly by pharmacotherapy over the *long term* (Barkley & Cunningham, 1978). Of course, the studies conducted through the late 1970s had primarily utilized traditional academic achievement tests (e.g., Wide Range Achievement Test) or intelligence batteries. Such measures may not be sensitive enough to detect short-term or more subtle changes in cognitive functioning associated with treatment. Several additional factors limit the utility of norm-referenced achievement tests for treatment evaluation purposes, including (1) a failure to adequately sample the curriculum in use; (2) the use of a limited number of items to sample various skills; (3) the use of response formats that do not require the student to perform the behavior (e.g., writing) of interest; and (4) an insensitivity to small changes in student performance (Marston, 1989; Shapiro, 1996).

Research studies conducted by several independent research teams have found acute MPH-induced improvements in academic productivity and accuracy among large samples of children (Douglas, Barr, O'Neill, & Britton, 1988; Pelham, Bender, Caddell, Booth, & Moorer, 1985; Rapport et al., 1987, 1988) and young adolescents with ADHD (Evans & Pelham, 1991; Evans et al., 2001; Pelham et al., 1991). Attention to teacher lectures, completion of study hall assignments, and quiz and test scores among junior high school students with ADHD also are enhanced by MPH (Pelham et al., 1991). As with other domains, these effects have been strongest in the higher dose range when analyzed at the group level. Rather than standardized achievement tests, these investigators employed written tasks assigned by each child's classroom teacher to assess academic performance. Although such measures may be more sensitive to treatment-related change and presumably possess greater ecological validity than do published, norm-referenced instruments, their reliability (i.e., stability over time) must be established prior to evaluating intervention effects. It remains to be seen whether short-term improvements in academic performance lead to greater scholastic success in the long run. However, these results would indicate a high probability of obtaining such findings if medication dosage is initially determined based on the enhancement of academic functioning rather than simply on behavioral control, as has been done in the past (Rapport & Kelly, 1991).

Several studies emanating from independent investigative teams have delineated MPH effects on the trajectory of academic skill acquisition. Specifically, dose–response effects are evident on curriculum-based measures of reading and math that parallel findings with other academic measures (Roberts & Landau, 1995; Stoner, Carey, Ikeda, & Shinn, 1994). However, findings typically show a wide range of individual responsivity to medication for this area of functioning. As discussed in Chapter 2, CBM probes are an efficient and sensitive means for evaluating intervention effects on academic skills. As such, greater use of these measures is strongly recommended for both clinical practice and research.

Effects on Social Relationships

MPH has been found to significantly improve the quality of social interactions between children with ADHD and their parents, teachers, and peers. For example, several studies have shown that stimulants increase children's compliance with parent or teacher commands and enhance their responsiveness to the interactions of others (for a review, see DuPaul, Barkley, & Connor, 1998). These same investigations found that negative and off-task behaviors are reduced in compliance situations, resulting in a decrease in the frequency of authority figure commands and an increase in positive adult attention to child behavior. In fact, the effects of stimulants on both overt and covert aggression are nearly of the same magnitude as medication effects on ADHD symptoms (Connor et al., 2002).

Similar results have been obtained for the peer relations of children with ADHD. When treated with MPH, children with ADHD are found to be less aggressive with others, behave more appropriately with other children, and to be accepted to a greater degree by their peers (Cunningham, Siegel, & Offord, 1985; Gadow, Nolan, Sverd, Sprafkin, & Paolicelli, 1990; Hinshaw, 1991; Pelham & Hoza, 1987; Whalen et al., 1989). In a similar fashion, the social behavior of adolescents with ADHD is improved with MPH, particularly at lower dosages (Smith et al., 1998). The effects of MPH on the prosocial behavior of children with ADHD remains unclear. Some studies have found no change in the frequency of initiating interactions with others (Hinshaw, Henker, Whalen, Erhardt, & Dunnington, 1989; Wallander, Schroeder, Michelli, & Gualtieri, 1987), while others have found a reduction in positive interactions with peers (Buhrmeister, Whalen, Henker, MacDonald, & Hinshaw, 1992). Beyond direct effects on social behavior, MPH has been found to enhance other areas of functioning that may indirectly impact social status. For example, a group of children with ADHD was found to pay attention better during softball games (e.g., greater recall of the game score) when receiving MPH versus a placebo (Pelham et al., 1990).

Dose–Response and Individual Responsivity

Beyond a delineation of specific behavioral effects, the results of empirical investigations of stimulants with children with ADHD have led to a number of important conclusions regarding the general properties of these drugs. First, MPH-induced changes in a specific behavioral realm vary across dose in a systematic fashion, at least at the group level of analysis (e.g., Barkley, Anastopoulos, Guevremont, & Fletcher, 1991; Pelham et al., 1985; Rapport & Denney, 2000; Rapport et al., 1985; Sprague & Sleator, 1977). For most areas of functioning (i.e., cognitive, social, behavior control), these dose–response effects have been linear, with higher doses leading to the greatest change. Second, at an individual level of analysis, separate classes of behavior may be affected differently by MPH even at the same dose (Rapport & Denney, 2000; Sprague & Sleator, 1977). For instance, a given child may show the greatest improvement in academic performance at a different dose than that level of medication that was "optimal" for impulse control or sustained attention. Finally, although linear dose–response effects are consistently found at the group level of analysis, individual children vary considerably with respect to behavior change across doses (Douglas et al., 1986; Pelham et al., 1985; Rapport & Denney, 2000). Even when children share similar characteristics (e.g., diagnosis, age, and body weight), there may be considerable variability in dose-responsivity presumably due to individual differences in CNS functioning (Rapport & Denney, 2000).

To illustrate the idiosyncratic nature of MPH effects, Figure 6.1 presents school-based, dose–response data for three individual children with ADHD who were participants in a study conducted by Rapport, DuPaul, and Kelley (1989). Behavioral changes for three measures are presented, including percentage of on-task behavior during independent work, percentage of academic work completed correctly (i.e., Academic Efficiency Score [AES]), and teacher ratings on the Abbreviated Conners Teacher Rating Scale (ACTRS; Werry, Sprague, & Cohen, 1975). A double-blind, placebo-controlled experimental design was employed wherein each child received four active MPH doses (i.e., 5 mg, 10 mg, 15

FIGURE 6.1. Dose–response curves of three dependent measures for three individual children of similar body weight ($M= 25$ kg). Percentage of on-task frequency and Academic Efficiency Score (AES) are plotted along the left-hand ordinate. Total score on the Abbreviated Conners Teacher Rating Scale (ACTRS) is plotted on the right-hand ordinate. Improvement for all three measures is indicated by an upward movement on the axis. From Rapport, DuPaul, and Kelly (1989). Copyright 1989 by M. D. Rapport. Reprinted by permission.

mg, 20 mg) and an inert placebo in a randomly determined sequence. The children were of similar age and body weight, but exhibited rather dramatic differences in MPH response. For example, S-1 (Figure 5.1, top) evidenced attentional and behavioral improvement as a direct function of increasing dose, peaking at the highest dose or 20 mg (i.e., linear dose–response effects). Alternatively, improvements in S-2's classroom behavior and performance were obtained up to the 15-mg dose, where peak effects were evidenced, followed by a decrement at the 20-mg dose. The latter is referred to as a "quadratic response" since there was one change in the slope of the dose–response curve. Finally, S-3 did not exhibit academic or behavioral change until a "therapeutic threshold" was attained at 10 mg, with little in the way of further enhancement at the higher doses (i.e., a threshold response). Thus, the dose–response profile and "optimal" or therapeutic dose differed for the three children.

Normalization of Classroom Functioning

Although the *statistical* significance of the behavioral effects of MPH have been demonstrated reliably, the *clinical* significance of behavioral changes for individual children with ADHD has been demonstrated less frequently. Some investigations have indicated that the task-related attention (Loney, Weissenburger, Woolson, & Lichty, 1979; Rapport, Denney, DuPaul, & Gardner, 1994; Whalen et al., 1978; Whalen, Henker, Collins, Finck, & Dotemoto, 1979) and aggressive behaviors (Hinshaw et al., 1989) of children receiving MPH is statistically indistinguishable from that of their normal peers. Abikoff and Gittelman (1985) found that 60% of children treated with MPH evidenced "normalized" behavior in attention span and impulse control in the classroom. In similar fashion, Pelham and colleagues (1993) found that approximately 60% of children receiving .6 mg/kg MPH were rated by teachers to behave "very much like a normal child" when interacting with peers and adults.

Rapport and colleagues (1994) examined the degree to which MPH normalized the classroom behavior and academic functioning of 76 children with ADHD based on comparisons with a normal control group of 25 children. Children with ADHD participated in a double-blind, placebo-controlled trial in which they received each of four doses (5, 10, 15, and 20 mg) of MPH and a placebo. Dependent measures included teacher ratings of social conduct, direct observations of classroom on-task behavior, and accuracy on independent academic tasks. Between 53% and 78% of the sample obtained scores within the normal range of functioning at one or more doses of MPH depending upon the specific measure employed (see Figure 6.2). Notably, teacher ratings of behavior control showed the most prominent improvements and normalization, followed by direct observations of task-related attention and academic efficiency. Approximately 47% of the sample did not show improvement in academic efficiency. Although these results provide further evidence of the strong therapeutic effects of stimulant medication, concomitant interventions (particularly those targeting academic performance) will be necessary for many children with ADHD, even for those whose classroom behavior is normalized by MPH.

Combination of Medication and Behavior Therapy

The two most common interventions for ADHD are stimulant medication and behavior modification strategies (Barkley, 1998). The largest scale and most comprehensive investigation of these two treatments was the Multimodal Treatment of ADHD (MTA) study completed at multiple sites in North America (MTA Cooperative Group, 1999). A sample of 579 7- to 10-year-old children diagnosed with ADHD was randomly assigned to one of four treatment groups. One group received stimulant medication that was titrated using state-of-the-art, multimethod, controlled trials, while a second group received multiple behavioral interventions across home, school, and summer camp settings. The school component of the latter protocol included (1) ongoing consultation with classroom teachers regarding behavioral interventions and (2) a paraprofessional working with the student with ADHD for half the school day on a daily basis for 12 weeks in the fall of the school year. The paraprofessional implemented behavioral interventions such as token reinforcement for appropriate classroom behavior. A third group received both carefully titrated medication and comprehensive behavioral intervention. Finally, a fourth group of participants received treatment as de-

FIGURE 6.2. Percentage of 76 children with ADHD exhibiting no change, clinically significant improvement, and normalized school behavior across three classroom variables as a function of placebo and MPH dose. From Rapport, Denney, DuPaul, and Gardner (1994). Copyright 1994 by the American Academy of Child and Adolescent Psychiatry. Reprinted by permission.

livered in the community (community-care control group). Approximately 67% of control group participants were receiving stimulant medication that was titrated using less-controlled and more typical procedures than was the MTA medication group. Dependent measures across multiple areas of functioning were collected at three time points during and immediately following the 14-month treatment protocol.

Participants in all four groups showed significant reductions in ADHD symptomatology during and following treatment. Significantly greater reductions in symptoms were obtained for the medication management and combined intervention groups relative to the behavioral-only and community-care control groups. Although carefully titrated stimulant medication clearly was the superior unimodal treatment, additional analyses shed light on the contribution of behavioral interventions. Specifically, the greatest improvement, particularly for problems associated with ADHD (e.g., oppositional behavior, social performance difficulties), was evidenced by children who received the combined intervention protocol (Conners et al., 2001; Swanson et al., 2001). Children in the combined intervention group required a lower mean dosage of medication than did the medication-only group. Using a relatively conservative definition of treatment "success," Swanson and colleagues (2001) found that 68% of combined intervention children were successfully treated relative to 56%, 34%, and 25% of the medication-only, behavioral intervention-only, and community-care control group children, respectively. Although, the effect size separating the behavioral intervention and community-care control group was small (Conners et al., 2001), it is important to note that most of the control group participants received stimulant medication as typically prescribed in the community. Thus, intensive behavioral programming appears equivalent to "medication as usual." Given the richness of the findings emanating from the MTA study, two journals have published special issues related to the results of this trial that should be of interest to school and mental health practitioners (*Journal of Abnormal Child Psychology*, 28(6), 2000; *Journal of the American Academy of Child and Adolescent Psychiatry*, 40(2), 2001).

Given the findings of the MTA study and prior less-comprehensive investigations, the combination of stimulant medication and behavioral interventions is now considered the "optimal" approach to treating ADHD for many children (Barkley, 1998). There are important shortcomings of each treatment when used alone, including a limitation of effects to the times when the interventions are "active," each is ineffective for a significant minority of children with ADHD, and the long-term effectiveness of both treatments has not been documented (Hoza, Pelham, Sams, & Carlson, 1992; Pelham & Murphy, 1986). Alternatively, the combination of behavioral and pharmacological treatments may minimize the limitations of each treatment while maximizing the chances of obtaining clinically significant changes (Pelham & Murphy, 1986).

Single-subject investigations have shown that "dosage" is an important variable in determining the response of individual children with ADHD to the combination of behavioral interventions and stimulant medication (Abramowitz, Eckstrand, O'Leary, & Dulcan, 1992; Hoza et al., 1992). For example, Abramowitz and colleagues (1992) evaluated changes in the classroom off-task behavior of three boys with ADHD as a function of varying dosages of MPH (placebo, .3 mg/kg, .6 mg/kg) combined with either immediate or delayed reprimands from the teacher. The results, displayed in Figure 6.3, indicate that response to the combination of interventions varied across children. Steven responded best to the combination of a low dose of MPH and a low "dose" of behavioral intervention (i.e., delayed reprimands), as displayed in the top graph of Figure 6.3. Alternatively, Tony evidenced an optimal response to the high dose of MPH in combination with either immediate or delayed reprimands (see middle graph in Figure 6.3). Finally, Kevin exhibited the least off-task behavior when treated with a low "dose" of behavioral intervention (i.e., delayed reprimands) combined with either a low or high dose of MPH (see bottom graph in Figure 6.3).

The results of the above and similar investigations indicate that some children will require a "low dose" of behavior modification (e.g., home-based daily report card) in combination with a low dose of MPH, while the ADHD symptoms of another child may be severe enough to warrant a high dose of MPH along with a "high dose" of behavior modification (e.g., classroom-based response cost system). Furthermore, the use of one treatment may result in an adjustment in dosage of another intervention. For example, the implementation of a behavior modification system may allow for a reduction in the amount of medication that a child may require. The titration of various strengths of each intervention must be conducted on an individual basis because the response to the combination of treatments will vary according to organismic (e.g., severity of ADHD-related behaviors) and environmental (e.g., classroom placement) factors (Pelham, 1989).

POSSIBLE SIDE EFFECTS OF CNS STIMULANTS

The most frequently reported acute side effects to MPH and other stimulants are appetite reduction (particularly at lunch) and insomnia (American Academy of Child and Adolescent Psychiatry [AACAP], 2002). The primary attribute of sleeping behavior affected by stimulants appears to

FIGURE 6.3. Off-task rates of three children treated with verbal reprimands and methylphenidate. D, delayed reprimands; I, immediate reprimands; Pl, placebo; Lo, 0.3 mg/kg MPH; Hi, 0.6 mg/kg MPH. From Abramowitz, Eckstrand, O'Leary, and Dulcan (1992). Copyright 1992 by Sage Publications, Inc. Reprinted by permission.

be a delayed onset of sleep rather than disturbance of sleep, per se (Stein & Pao, 2000). Other treatment emergent effects reported in the literature include increased irritability, headaches, stomachaches, and, in rare cases, motor and/or vocal tics (AACAP, 2002). Several research studies have explicated the percentage of cases experiencing possible side effects across a dose range of MPH (for a review, see Rapport & Moffitt, 2002). For example, Barkley, McMurray, Edelbrock, and Robbins (1990) examined the prevalence of parent- and teacher-reported side effects to two doses (i.e., 0.3 mg/kg and 0.5 mg/kg) of MPH in a large sample of children with ADHD. These investigators found that over 50% of the sample exhibited decreased appetite, insomnia, anxiousness, irritability, or proneness to crying with both doses of MPH. It should be noted that many of these apparent side effects (especially those associated with mood) were present during the placebo condition and may represent characteristics associated with the disorder rather than its treatment. Stomachaches and headaches were reported in about 33% of the participants. The severity of these side effects was mild in most cases, increased as a function of dose, and did not necessarily result in the discontinuation of treatment. Furthermore, it is apparent that the frequency and severity of possible side effects should be assessed during non-medication or pretreatment conditions to establish whether they are truly associated with drug ingestion.

Perceptions regarding the presence and severity of side effects may vary across parents, teachers, and students. DuPaul, Anastopoulos, Kwasnik, Barkley, and McMurray (1996) collected side effect ratings from a sample of parents, teachers, and adolescents in the context of a multiple dosage trial of MPH. Although teacher ratings of side effect severity did not vary systematically from placebo to active medication, parents reported side effect severity to be greatest during the *placebo* condition. Conversely, adolescents reported a greater severity of side effects during the two highest dosage conditions relative to placebo. Thus, side effects have to be considered from the "eye of the beholder." Several respondents should be consulted to provide different perspectives on this phenomenon. In our experience, parents will be the best reporter of the most common side effects such as appetite reduction and insomnia. Teachers can provide information regarding possible overfocused behavior, particularly during academic task conditions. Finally, children themselves may be the optimal reporters of possible medication effects on internalizing symptoms (e.g., anxiety) and are perhaps most sensitive to the overall severity of side effects.

Other possible treatment emergent effects that should be monitored include a "behavioral rebound" in the late afternoon and the onset or exacerbation of motor and vocal tics (AACAP, 2002). The "behavioral rebound" phenomenon is typically described as deterioration in conduct (exceeding that which is observed during baseline or placebo conditions) that occurs in the late afternoon and evening following daytime administrations of medication (Johnston, Pelham, Hoza, & Sturges, 1987). Studies that have examined this phenomenon have indicated that it occurs in about 33% of children treated with MPH and that the magnitude of the rebound varies considerably across days for individual children (Johnston et al., 1987). Furthermore, a late afternoon administration of a small dose of MPH may reduce the severity of rebound effects (DuPaul, Barkley, & Conner, 1998).

The degree to which stimulants induce motor tics and Tourette's disorder symptoms in children remains controversial. Some early studies indicated that a small minority of children may develop tics following stimulant treatment, and that tic frequency and severity did not diminish following termination of treatment (Bremness & Sverd, 1979). Alternatively, more recent investigations have indicated that the majority of children with ADHD and tic disorders will respond positively to stimulant treatment both in terms of behavior control and tic reduction (e.g., Castellanos et al., 1997; Gadow, Sverd, Sprafkin, Nolan, & Ezor, 1995). A minority of children may show exacerbation of tics, thus necessitating caution in prescribing stimulants for children exhibiting both ADHD and tic disorders. However, if monitored carefully, this class of medication may be viable for children with ADHD who have a personal or family history of tics.

Clinical observations have documented an increase in "overfocused" behavior among some children with ADHD treated with MPH (Solanto, 1984). This constriction of cognitive functioning may be demonstrated in a variety of ways, including persistence at a task for an abnormally long period of time, a disregard for relevant peripheral stimuli, or an inability to shift cognitive set to adapt to situational demands (Solanto & Wender, 1989). Empirical investigations have failed to document the occurrence of this phenomenon at a group level of analysis. However, at least one study has indicated that a subgroup of children with ADHD may demonstrate overfocused performance as a function of MPH (Solanto, 2000). This subgroup may include children who are less hyperactive and who demonstrate better baseline performance on cognitive testing relative to other children with ADHD. In similar fashion, Rapport and colleagues (1994) found that 47% of a large sample of children treated with MPH did not show improvement in academic efficiency at any dose. Presumably, the academic performance of some of these children was compromised by MPH-induced overfocused behavior, although direct measurement of the latter was not conducted. These findings provide a strong rationale for individualized assessment of academic and cognitive performance across doses when evaluating response to psychotropic medications. In fact, Rapport and Denney (2000) recommend that stimulant dosage be titrated on the basis of improvements in academic efficiency rather than the more typical reliance on changes in behavioral control. This argument is bolstered by the fact that when MPH improves academic performance, behavioral control tends to improve as well; however, the converse is rarely true.

The only long-term side effect of stimulant medication that has been well documented is suppression of height and weight gain. Studies examining this phenomenon have indicated that the probability of growth suppression increases with higher doses, is greater with dextroamphetamine than with MPH, and is higher during the first year of treatment (see AACAP, 2002). A rebound in growth following discontinuation of treatment or habituation to this effect seems to occur thereafter, with little appreciable alteration in eventual adult height or weight (Greenhill, 1984; Reeve & Garfinkel, 1991). Other possible long-term side effects that have been proposed, primarily in the popular media, include drug addiction, lower self-esteem, depression, or other emotional difficulties. These claims have no basis in the empirical literature and should not be considered actual treatment risks. For example, Biederman, Wilens, Mick, Spencer, and Faraone (1999) found that children treated with stimulants were *less likely* to have a substance use disorder as adolescents than were untreated children.

WHEN TO RECOMMEND A MEDICATION TRIAL

School psychologists and other educational professionals are in an ideal position to advocate for the appropriate treatment of a child with ADHD, given their opportunity to observe the student's functioning in a setting where the greatest problems with inattention, impulsivity, and overactivity typically occur (i.e., the school). The decision to initiate a trial of medication should not be an automatic response following the diagnosis of ADHD and obviously must be made in concert with a number of individuals, including the child's physician and parents. Prior to reaching this decision point, comprehensive physical and psychological examinations should be conducted to establish the presence and severity of ADHD symptomatology (see Chapter 2) as well as to identify any factors (e.g., heart condition) that may compromise the use of stimulant medication. In concert with the child's physician, the psychologist should consider the following factors (from DuPaul, Barkley, & Conner, 1998) prior to recommending a trial of medication:

1. *Severity of the child's ADHD symptoms and disruptive behavior.* As would be expected, the greater the severity of attention and behavior control difficulties, the more likely a medication trial will be necessary as a supplement to other treatment modalities (e.g., behavior modification program).

2. *Prior use of other treatments.* If other interventions (e.g., classroom behavior management program, parent training) have not been implemented, a trial of medication may be postponed, particularly if the severity of the child's ADHD is relatively mild. If other interventions currently are in place, one would want to assess their success and whether there is room for improvement (Power et al., 2003). Several questions must be considered including (a) have symptoms of the disorder improved as a function of the current intervention plan; (b) is the improvement considered sufficient by key individuals in the child's life; (c) are any adverse side effects present that would indicate discontinuation or modification of current treatments; (d) what are the effects of the current intervention on key areas of functioning; and (e) what is the likelihood that adding medication to the treatment plan will result in further, clinically significant, improvement? If limited success has been obtained with other interventions, then medication should be considered as an adjunctive treatment.

3. *Empirical support for medication.* The specific medication to be employed should be determined, in part, based on prior empirical studies of this treatment. As has been discussed in this chapter, CNS stimulants have a strong track record of success in treating this disorder. However, in practice, other medications may be used in isolation or in combination with stimulants, despite a minimal research literature to support such treatment decisions (Brown & Sammons, 2002).

4. *Parental attitude toward use of medication.* Parents who are strongly "anti-medication" should be offered the opportunity to research the advantages and disadvantages of pharmacotherapy. Specifically, they should be provided with literature that clearly describes the behavioral effects, side effects, and treatment-monitoring practices associated with medication (see Barkley, 2000). They *should not be coerced* into a medication trial given the higher likelihood of low treatment compliance in such cases.

5. *Adequacy of adult supervision.* The parents must be functioning at a level where they will adequately supervise the administration of the medication and guard against its abuse. Furthermore, all adults associated with the child's treatment program (i.e., physician, teacher, psychologist, parents) must make an ongoing investment of time necessary to determine the short- and long-term efficacy of the medication regimen.

6. *Child's attitude toward medication.* It is important that the use of medication is discussed with the child and that the rationale for treatment be fully explained, particularly with older children and adolescents. In cases where children are "anti-medication" or oppositional, they may sabotage efforts to use it (e.g., refuse to swallow the pill).

Regardless of whether stimulant medication treatment is employed and successful, the school psychologist is in a singular position to implement additional therapies for the child with ADHD. It is imperative that other interventions (e.g., behavioral and/or academic strategies) are utilized prior to or in addition to medication in an effort to optimize the child's classroom functioning (Barkley, 1998). In fact, as mentioned earlier, the concomitant use of behavioral strategies and stimulant medication may lead to additive behavioral effects, particularly on aggression and social interactions, thus minimizing the medication dose and/or the intensity of employed contingencies (Abramowitz et al., 1992; Hoza et al., 1992).

HOW TO ASSESS MEDICATION EFFECTS IN CLASSROOM SETTINGS

The methods used to monitor medication response in children with ADHD vary widely in content and quality. The results of the MTA study (MTA Cooperative Group, 1999) strongly indicate that controlled trials using multiple objective measures of drug response are optimal for titrating stimulant dosage. Unfortunately, all too frequently, titration of dosage and long-term assessment of efficacy are based solely on the subjective reports of parents, thereby increasing the chances of erroneous decisions (DuPaul, Barkley, & Connor, 1998). School professionals can have an impact on this practice to a large degree by communicating with physicians regarding changes in children's school performance associated with pharmacotherapy. In fact, recent guidelines published by the American Academy of Pediatrics (2001) and the American Academy of Child and Adolescent Psychiatry (2002) emphasize (1) the use of multiple outcome measures, (2) inclusion of school personnel in providing information about drug response, and (3) the need for ongoing monitoring via communication with schools and families.

Because the response to stimulant medication is frequently idiosyncratic and dose-specific, it is imperative to collect objective behavioral data across several doses, including a period of time when the child is not receiving active medication. Under ideal circumstances, a child's optimal dose should be established in the context of a double-blind, placebo-controlled assessment paradigm that includes multiple measures collected across several settings (e.g., home, school). This type of evaluation not only involves the aggregation of objective, quantitative data regarding a child's treatment response, but also controls for the biases inherent in some assessment measures (e.g., parent and teacher rating scales). Further details with respect to designing such an evaluation are discussed below and can be obtained by consulting several recent texts on pediatric psychopharmacology (Brown & Sawyer, 1998; Phelps, Brown, & Power, 2001; Werry & Aman, 1999).

In many instances, professionals do not have the resources and time to conduct elegant, placebo-controlled medication evaluations. Nevertheless, the school psychologist and physician can, as a team, collect objective data in a cost-effective fashion that would aid greatly in making medication-related decisions. Several steps are involved in this process including (1) designing a dosage sequence wherein the child receives one of several doses (including a baseline or nonmedication condition) every day for a week at each dose; (2) collecting objective measures of treatment response across dosage conditions; (3) assessing parent, teacher, and child perceptions of possible side effects across doses (including when the child is not medicated); and (4) communication between the physician and the psychologist both during and after the medication trial to determine whether a child responds positively, which dose optimizes his or her performance, and whether the severity of a possible side effect warrants discontinuing the trial. If possible, those adults who are directly evaluating changes in the child's performance (e.g., teachers) should be kept "blind" to the medication condition. For instance, even during a nonmedication phase the child may continue to go to the nurse's office for his or her noontime administration (and take a vitamin instead of short-acting MPH), thereby keeping the medication condition unknown from the teacher's perspective. With increased use of sustained-release stimulant compounds, it is easier to keep teachers and other school personnel "blind" to medication dosage.

Although the teacher is kept "blind" to the child's medication status, it is important to provide some information to the teacher about the positive effects and side effects usually associated with stimulants. A handout for teachers regarding stimulant treatment of ADHD is provided in Appendix 6.1. This information will help the teacher to focus on those behavioral changes that are most relevant to this treatment.

Measures of Medication Response

Several objective measures should be collected across medication conditions to assess treatment-related change, including teacher and parent ratings of behavioral control and side effects as well as direct observations of classroom behavior and academic performance. For youngsters with ADHD predominantly inattentive type, ratings and observations of changes in attention span and work productivity will suffice, as these children do not typically exhibit significant problems with behavior control (Carlson & Mann, 2000). The core components of a school-based medication trial are listed in Table 6.2 and discussed below.

Teacher Rating Scales

A plethora of teacher rating scales have been found to be useful in evaluating the effects of stimulant medication, including the Conners Teacher Rating Scale (Conners, 1997), ADD-H Comprehensive Teacher Rating

---

TABLE 6.2. Measures to Assess Medication Response

1. Teacher rating scales
   a. Conners Teacher Rating Scale (Conners, 1997)
   b. ADD-H Comprehensive Teacher Rating Scale (Ullmann et al., 1985)
   c. ADHD Rating Scale–IV (DuPaul, Power, Anastopoulos, & Reid, 1998)
   d. School Situations Questionnaire (Barkley, 1990) or School Situations Questionnaire—Revised (DuPaul & Barkley, 1992)
   e. Academic Performance Rating Scale (DuPaul et al., 1991)
   f. Side Effects Rating Scale (Barkley, 1990)

2. Parent rating scales
   a. Conners Parent Rating Scale (Conners, 1997)
   b. ADHD Rating Scale–IV (DuPaul et al., 1998)
   c. Home Situations Questionnaire (Barkley, 1990) and/or Home Situations Questionnaire—Revised (DuPaul & Barkley, 1992)
   d. Side Effects Rating Scale (Barkley, 1990)

3. Direct observations of school performance
   a. Classroom Observation Code (Abikoff et al., 1977)
   b. ADHD Behavior Coding System (Barkley et al., 1988)
   c. Behavior Observation for Students in Schools (Shapiro, 1996)
   d. On-Task Behavior Code (Rapport & Denney, 2000)
   e. ADHD School Observation Code (Gadow et al., 1996)

4. Academic performance measures
   a. Percentage of assigned work completed correctly
   b. Curriculum-based assessment

5. Self-report rating scales
   a. Conners–Wells Adolescent Self-Report of Symptoms (Conners et al., 2000)

Scale (Ullmann, Sleator, & Sprague, 1985), and the ADHD Rating Scale–IV (DuPaul et al., 1998). The inclusion of one of these questionnaires can provide a measure of treatment-induced reductions in the frequency and/or severity of behavioral control difficulties from the teacher's perspective. These brief rating scales are preferred to more comprehensive, broad-band measures (e.g., Child Behavior Checklist), as the former provide more circumscribed information about medication response and are more practical for teachers to complete on a repeated basis. Measures such as the School Situations Questionnaire (Barkley, 1990) and the School Situations Questionnaire—Revised (DuPaul & Barkley, 1992) can be included to assess changes in the pervasiveness of behavior problems and attentional difficulties across situations. Treatment-induced changes in academic productivity and accuracy can be assessed, in part, by using the Academic Performance Rating Scale (DuPaul, Rapport, & Perriello, 1991). All of these questionnaires have been found to possess adequate levels of reliability and validity. However, it is recommended that teacher questionnaires be administered twice during baseline conditions to assess possible "practice" effects that are frequently obtained with these measures (Barkley, 1998).

Parent Rating Scales

There are a number of parent questionnaires that have been documented to be sensitive to stimulant medication effects with this population such as the Conners Parent Rating Scale (Conners, 1997) and the ADHD Rating Scale–IV (DuPaul et al., 1998). The Home Situations Questionnaire (Barkley, 1990) and/or the Home Situations Questionnaire—Revised (DuPaul & Barkley, 1992) could be used to assess the situational pervasiveness of behavior control and attentional difficulties, respectively. As with the teacher questionnaires, all of these instruments have demonstrated reliability and validity for the purpose of assessing intervention effects (Barkley, 1998). Given the short-term behavioral effects of stimulant compounds, it is possible that parents will have limited opportunities to directly observe medication-induced changes in ADHD symptoms. Thus, teacher ratings may provide more sensitive treatment outcome data than do parent ratings.

Direct Observations of School Performance

School professionals are in a unique position relative to other mental health professionals because they have the opportunity to observe children in one of their most important natural environments. Thus, questionnaires completed by parents and teachers can be supplemented with behavioral observations that are presumably not subject to the possible biases associated with rating scales. A variety of coding systems have been developed for observing the behavior of students with ADHD (see Chapter 2) including the ADHD Behavior Coding System (Barkley, 1998; Barkley et al., 1988), the Hyperactive Behavior Code (Jacob et al., 1978), the Classroom Observation Code (Abikoff et al., 1977), the Behavior Observation of Students in Schools (BOSS; Shapiro, 1996), and the ADHD School Observation Code (ADHD SOC; Gadow et al., 1996). The use of such systems can provide valuable information regarding the frequency (usually in the form of percentages) of occurrence of various behaviors (e.g., on-task behavior, fidgets) over the course of the observation period. One alternative to the above coding systems is the simple recording of off- versus on-task behavior (i.e., visual attention to task materials) that has been found to be quite sensitive to the dose effects of MPH (see Rapport & Denney, 2000). The latter requires very little training and is likely to engender more than adequate levels of interobserver reliability.

Medication effects on children's social interactions should also be investigated. A variety of observational coding systems have been developed for this behavioral domain and have been adapted for evaluating stimulant medication effects (e.g., Pelham & Milich, 1991). For example, direct observations of social behavior using the ADHD SOC could be conducted in relatively unstructured settings such as the school lunchroom and/or playground. A variation of this observation code has been found to be sensitive to the effects of stimulant medication (e.g., Gadow et al., 1990) and allows one to document changes in both aggressive (e.g., physical aggression) and prosocial (e.g., appropriate social interaction) behaviors as a function of treatment.

Academic Performance Measures

Information regarding the child's academic performance should be gathered in conjunction with behavioral observations. For example, the percentage of work that the child completes relative to the amount assigned and the percentage accuracy of work could be calculated following the observation session. Such data are highly sensitive to MPH dose effects and can indicate when a medication-induced "cognitive decrement" or "overfocusing" phenomenon has occurred (Rapport & Denney, 2000). Under the latter conditions the child may show behavioral improvements but a diminishment of academic productivity and/or accuracy. Baseline stability and interobserver reliability should also be assessed for these measures. Curriculum-based assessment strategies (Shinn, 1998) are potentially appropriate techniques to assess medication-related changes in this functioning area as well. Several CBM probes per medication condition could be collected to determine treatment effects on the trajectory of skill acquisition (Roberts & Landau, 1995; Stoner et al., 1994). The collection of at least 10 data points per condition allows for more reliable estimation of CBM slope and is highly recommended (Shinn, 1998).

Self-Report Ratings

For older children (e.g., over the age of 9 years old) and adolescents, it may be helpful to obtain self-report ratings of treatment-related changes in behavioral control, academic performance, and self-esteem. Although the reliability of self-report data in this population may be suspect (Barkley, 1998), self-report ratings may serve two purposes. First, these data provide information about areas of functioning (e.g., depressive symptoms, self-esteem) that is not available through other modalities. Second, the student is directly involved in the medication evaluation process, thus increasing the chances of cooperation and compliance with the treatment regimen. Questionnaires that could be used for this purpose include the Conners–Wells Adolescent Self-Report of Symptoms (Conners et al., 2000). Self-report ratings of medication effects on ADHD symptoms appear to be sensitive to MPH effects, albeit less so than are parent and teacher ratings (DuPaul et al., 1996).

Assessment of Possible Side Effects

The child's teacher and parents should be asked to complete a brief Side Effects Rating Scale (Barkley, 1998) on a weekly basis. Older children (i.e., those over the age of 9 years old) should be asked to complete this questionnaire as well. These ratings provide information regarding the number and relative severity of possible treatment emergent effects (e.g., irritability, insomnia, appetite reduction). Parents can provide the most useful information in this domain because they have the greatest opportunity to observe the activities most likely to be affected (e.g., eating, sleeping). Sometimes, self-report ratings can be particularly critical in revealing side effects that are not observed directly by parents and teachers (DuPaul et al., 1996). As mentioned previously, it is crucial to obtain such ratings during a nonmedication condition as many behaviors that are possible side effects (e.g., irritability) could be occurring in the absence of treatment as well.

Medication Evaluation Procedure

Prior to the initiation of the medication evaluation, comprehensive physical and psychological evaluations are conducted to establish the need for a trial of stimulant medication, as outlined above. The steps to a school-based medication evaluation are presented in Table 6.3. Once a medication trial has been agreed upon, the school psychologist should contact the child's physician to discuss and establish the sequence of dosages that can vary as a function of the age of the child. Using short-acting MPH (Ritalin) as an example, the doses used would vary for preschoolers (2.5 mg, 5 mg, 7.5 mg), elementary schoolchildren (5 mg, 10 mg, 15 mg), and middle and high school students (10 mg, 15 mg, 20 mg). The dosage sequence should be randomized with the stipulation that the highest dose is never administered as the first dose. A nonmedication condition, preferably a placebo, is also included in this sequence. Both the physician and the school psychologist record the dosage sequence and store this information in a safe place until after the medication assessment is completed.

The physician prescribes 1-week's worth of medication at each of the doses, including a placebo, if possible. The parent then has the prescription filled at the pharmacy; if possible, the medication should be packaged in opaque, gelatin capsules. If the latter packaging is possible, the capsules are dispensed in vials that are labeled by week of the medication trial rather than by dosage to maintain the "blind." The parent and school nurse dispense the medication according to the schedule de-

---

TABLE 6.3. Steps to School-Based Medication Evaluation

1. Parent obtains prescription (e.g., Ritalin, 5 mg) from pediatrician.
2. Staff member not involved directly with evaluation (e.g., school nurse) and physician determine order of administration of several doses (i.e., 5, 10, 15, 20 mg), including a nonmedication trial.
3. Parent (or school nurse) administers dose according to predetermined schedule on a daily basis.
4. Assessment measures collected on a weekly (daily) basis:
   a. Teacher ratings
   b. Parent ratings
   c. Side effects ratings
   d. Observations of classroom behavior by independent observer during individual written seatwork.
5. Assessment measures must be taken to reflect the child's behavior during the active phase of the medication (i.e., 2–4 hours postingestion for short-acting preparations).
6. Are there "significant" changes in behavior (especially academic) at any dose?
7. If so, what is the lowest dose that brings about the greatest change with the fewest side effects?
8. Report results to child's pediatrician.

termined above. The typical dosing schedule for the short-acting preparations of MPH and dextroamphetamine is once in the morning and once at lunchtime, with approximately 4 hours between medication admininistrations. Although daily changes in dosage are recommended by some researchers in this area (e.g., MTA Cooperative Group, 1999; Pelham & Milich, 1991), it is often more practical to make these changes on a weekly basis. For instance, this would preclude asking teachers to provide behavior ratings on a daily basis.

Parent, teacher, and self-report ratings are completed on a weekly basis throughout the medication evaluation. Dosage changes should occur on Saturdays so that all ratings are completed on the last day of each dosage week (i.e., Fridays). If dosage changes occur on Saturdays, the parent is able to observe for possible side effects and contact the physician in a timely fashion. If observed side effects are severe enough, further administration of this dose would be omitted. It is optimal for the ratings to be completed with the parents, teacher, and child remaining "blind" to the medication dose to minimize measurement error due to rater bias. The best way to accomplish this is for the pharmacist to package the medication in opaque capsules and to use an inert placebo (e.g., lactose powder) during one of the "medication" weeks. If this is not possible, then the teacher and child may be kept "blind" by having the nurse dispense a vitamin tablet during the placebo or nonmedication week. Of course, the use of a sustained-release compound (e.g., Concerta) would preclude the need for "blinding" procedures at school; this is a chief advantage of such preparations. Pill counts should be used, whenever possible, to document compliance with medication administration. If the medication is not being dispensed in a consistent fashion at home, then both doses should be administered at school, if possible.

Regardless of the coding system employed, behavioral observations should be conducted at a time of the school day when the child is engaged in independent seatwork, because this is typically one of the more problematic situations for students with ADHD. Observations of social behavior in the school lunchroom and playground also may be helpful. Furthermore, observations should take place on as many days as possible during each dosage condition approximately 1.5–3 hours after medication ingestion to coincide with the time of peak behavioral effects. Observation periods should be between 15 and 20 minutes apiece. Also, observations should be conducted several times during baseline conditions to establish a stable "trend" (i.e., consistency in the data) prior to introducing treatment conditions. Interobserver reliability checks (e.g., conducted by a teacher aide or guidance counselor) should be obtained as frequently as possible, ideally at least once per dosage condition, throughout the medication trial to ensure the integrity of the data.

Academic performance data should be collected following each observation period. For example, the amount and accuracy of work completed during the observation session could be calculated before leaving the classroom. In addition, brief curriculum-based assessment probes could be conducted following an observation session. Care should be taken to collect such data from several students in the classroom so that the child with ADHD is not aware that he or she is being singled out for observation.

COMMUNICATION OF RESULTS
WITH PRESCRIBING PHYSICIAN

Throughout the course of the medication trial, the school professional should be in communication with the prescribing physician, especially when questions arise concerning possible side effects. At the conclusion of the treatment evaluation, it is best if a written summary of the results is forwarded to the physician to facilitate discussion during a follow-up telephone conversation (see Chapter 8 for additional discussion of communication with physicians). Two major questions should be addressed in the report: (1) are there clinically significant changes in the child's behavior control and academic performance at any active dose of the medication?; and (2), if so, what is the lowest dose (i.e., the minimal effective dose; see Fielding, Murphy, Reagan, & Peterson, 1980) that brings about the greatest change with the least side effects? These questions are addressed by systematically comparing assessment data collected during active medication conditions to those data obtained during nonmedication conditions. Significant changes are indicated when there is a change of 1 standard deviation from placebo to active dose conditions. Alternatively, reliable change indices (Jacobsen & Truax, 1991; Speer, 1992) could be calculated for each variable to determine statistical significance. Finally, comparison to a normative sample or to normal peers from the same classroom is helpful in determining the clinical significance of obtained treatment effects.

A sample summary of results for a 9-year-old girl with ADHD, Judy, who participated in a 4-week trial of MPH is presented in Table 6.4. Data are summarized across four dosage conditions (i.e., placebo and 5-, 10-, and 15-mg MPH) that were administered under double-blind conditions in a randomly determined sequence. Significant changes in objective ratings and direct observations of classroom behavior are identified by scores that are underlined (i.e., representing a change of 1 standard deviation from placebo or, in the case of direct observations, 10% change from placebo values). Judy evidenced appreciable improve-

TABLE 6.4. Sample Summary of Results for a Trial of Methylphenidate

Measure	Dose			
	Placebo	5 mg	10 mg	15 mg
Parent ratings				
CPRS-R[a]	7.0[b]	6.0	3.0[c]	2.0
Side Effects—Total	11.0	9.0	8.0	2.0
Side Effects—Severity	3.4	3.3	1.1	1.0
Teacher ratings				
CTRS[d]	14.0	15.0	9.0	4.0
SSQ[e]—Problem Settings	8.0	8.0	3.0	0.0
SSQ—Mean Severity	5.1	4.9	1.3	0.0
APRS[f]	49.0	51.0	58.0	67.0
Behavioral observations				
Percent on task	60.3	68.9	80.0	89.7
Academic completion[g]	49.7	59.8	95.0	98.0
Academic accuracy[h]	62.0	61.0	78.0	88.5

[a]Conners Parent Rating Scale Impulsivity Hyperactivity Factor.
[b]Values are raw scores for all variables.
[c]Underlined values represent change of greater than 1 standard deviation relative to placebo.
[d]Conners Teacher Rating Scale—Revised Hyperactivity Index.
[e]School Situations Questionnaire.
[f]Academic Performance Rating Scale Academic Productivity Score.
[g]Percentage of work completed relative to classmates.
[h]Percent correct on academic work.

ment in behavioral control across settings during both the 10- and 15-mg conditions, with no apparent increase in possible side effects. Her academic performance was optimally affected at the latter dose, which resulted in a recommendation for her to receive MPH at a 15-mg dose twice per day for the remainder of the school year.

The report to the physician should include a brief table of assessment results, with a one to two page report highlighting the changes in each area of functioning at each dose level. A summary paragraph should be used to indicate the dose, if any, that school personnel felt was most helpful in enhancing the child's school performance (see Chapter 8). Obviously, the ultimate course of treatment is determined by the physician and parents of the child. A week or two after sending the report to the physician, a follow-up phone call should be made in case the physician has any questions about the report or if additional school-based information is necessary before a final medication decision can be reached. Finally, a postassessment feedback session should be conducted with the child's parents and teachers to discuss the results of the medication evaluation and to answer questions about further treatment with medication (Gadow, Nolan, Paolicelli, & Sprafkin, 1991).

ONGOING MONITORING OF MEDICATION RESPONSE

Once a student's optimal dosage is established, the measures described above should be collected periodically throughout the school year to evaluate the need for dosage adjustments or the onset of side effects. The vast majority of the measures need to be readministered only every several months or so. It is usually a good idea for parents to complete the Side Effects Rating Scale on a monthly basis and submit this information to the physician.

Approximately every 6 months that a child is taking medication, the physician usually conducts a brief physical examination. During this time, the child's height, weight, blood pressure, and heart rate are recorded to determine potential side effects. Children receiving a tricyclic antidepressant (e.g., desipramine) should undergo a baseline electrocardiogram (ECG) with follow-up ECGs obtained with dosage changes or every few months, if normal, on a steady dose (Spencer et al., 1998). The school psychologist should attempt to collect relevant parent and teacher ratings prior to the 6-month checkup and relay any anecdotal information related to medication response to the physician.

When parents or teachers report that a previously effective dose "doesn't work anymore," the psychologist and the physician should work in tandem to determine possible factors for this apparent deterioration in response before making dosage adjustments. Behavioral changes could be related to medication factors (e.g., a switch from trade name to generic forms of the medication, poor compliance with treatment) or environmental events (e.g., family stress events, increase in difficulty of academic material). It is important to carefully assess possible nonmedication factors that could account for a decline in functioning. Often, parents and teachers of children with ADHD may be unrealistic in their expectations regarding the amount and consistency of behavioral improvements associated with pharmacotherapy. Thus, they should realize that even when medicated, children will experience occasional "bad days" regardless of the dosage being employed.

LIMITATIONS OF STIMULANT
MEDICATION TREATMENT

As with most treatment regimens, there are factors associated with psychotropic medications that limit their overall effectiveness. Some of these factors have been discussed above, including possible short- and long-term side effects as well as, in the case of the standard preparation stimulants, a relatively short duration of action on behavior. Furthermore, these medications do not "teach" the child to compensate for symptoms of his or her disorder and thus must be supplemented by skill-building strategies such as behavior modification programming (O'Leary, 1980). Of greatest concern is the lack of data supporting the long-term efficacy of stimulant medication treatment. In fact, most longitudinal studies conducted to date have not found significant differences between groups of children with ADHD who have or have not been treated with stimulants (e.g., Weiss, Kruger, Danielson, & Elman, 1975). Although these studies have been criticized for myriad methodological shortcomings (e.g., insensitive outcome measures), their results reinforce the fact that no single treatment modality, even one with demonstrated short-term efficacy, is sufficient in bringing about durable reductions in ADHD symptomatology. These older findings are counterbalanced by the results of the MTA study (MTA Cooperative Group, 1999) that documented consistent stimulant medication effects over a period of 14 months. With subsequent data collection on the MTA sample, more information is forthcoming regarding the long-term effects of these drugs on many areas of functioning.

Given the short intervals of behavior control resulting from a single or twice-daily dose of stimulant medication, much of the drug's influence has dissipated by the time the child is home from school. Furthermore, the family will witness the brunt of any side effects (e.g., insomnia) resulting from pharmacotherapy. As a result, families of children with ADHD will need more professional help to deal with the child's behavior problems at home (see Chapter 7). School professionals should be knowledgeable about the professional resources in the mental health community so that appropriate referrals on behalf of the family can be made (Barkley, 1998).

Although objective data are used to determine medication response, treatment decisions often rely heavily on "clinical judgment" (Gadow et al., 1991). For example, there are many times where treatment-related changes vary across areas of functioning or sources of data (e.g., parents, teachers). In such situations, the psychologist and the physician must decide which measures are most important to the decision. This can vary as a function of treatment priorities and the child's strengths and weaknesses. Specifically, those domains that address the child's greatest pretreatment difficulties are given the most weight in reaching decisions regarding dosage (Pelham et al., 1993). In addition, the child's response to other interventions and the degree to which additional improvement is necessary to move the child into the normal range of functioning is also taken into account (Pelham et al., 1991).

SUMMARY

Various psychotropic medications have been used to enhance the attentional, behavioral, and academic functioning of children with ADHD. CNS stimulant medications are the most effective medication for the symptomatic management of children with ADHD. Among positive treatment responders, stimulant medications significantly enhance the attention span, impulse control, academic performance, and peer relationships of children with ADHD, although effects on the latter two functioning areas must be replicated further. Side effects (e.g., insomnia, appetite reduction) are relatively benign and are more likely to occur at higher dose levels. Given that the behavioral effects of stimulants are moderated by dose and individual responsivity, each child's treatment response must be assessed in an objective manner across a range of therapeutic doses. School professionals can play a major role in evaluating stimulant-induced changes in the classroom performance of children with ADHD and providing objective outcome data to the prescribing physician. Because the overall efficacy of stimulant medication treatment is limited by a number of factors, other interventions (e.g., behavior modification) are likely to be necessary to optimize the probability of long-term improvements in the behavioral and academic status of children with ADHD.

APPENDIX 6.1

◆

Stimulant Medication Treatment of ADHD: A Teacher Handout

Children with ADHD exhibit significant problems with inattention, impulsivity, and overactivity. One of the most effective interventions for this disorder is the use of central nervous system (CNS) stimulant medications. The latter include Ritalin, Concerta, Metadate (all three are methylphenidate), Dexedrine (dextro-amphetamine), and Adderall (mixed amphetamine). Of these medications, methylphenidate is by far the most commonly prescribed. CNS stimulants purportedly increase the availability of certain neurotransmitters (i.e., dopamine and norepinepherine) in specific parts of the brain. This results in a greater level of CNS arousal, and hence increased attention and behavior control. It was once believed that these medications exerted a paradoxical (i.e., sedating) effect in children with ADHD and that this response was diagnostic. On the contrary, these medications act to stimulate brain activity not only in youngsters with ADHD but most other children and adults as well. Thus, one cannot diagnose a child as having ADHD based on his or her response to stimulant medication.

BEHAVIORAL EFFECTS

The primary behavioral effects of stimulants include enhanced attention, decreased impulsivity, and reduced task-irrelevant motor activity. Students are more likely to complete assigned tasks accurately, are more compliant with classroom rules, and evidence fewer aggressive behaviors. They may also show improved handwriting and fine motor skills, as well as greater acceptability by their classmates. In fact, some studies have shown that for a majority of treated children, stimulant medication can lead to changes in attention span and academic productivity such that levels of functioning in these areas are no different from those of their peers. It is important to note, however, that these medications do not "cure" ADHD and that a child with ADHD should be expected to evidence the usual "ups and downs" of behavior control even when a positive response has been obtained. Furthermore, these medications are never to be used as the sole treatment for ADHD. Often, when combined with other interventions (e.g., classroom behavior modification program), medication effects on behavior control are enhanced.

The behavioral effects of Ritalin and Dexedrine usually last between 3 and 4 hours after ingestion. Thus, most children take these medications twice per day (i.e., in the morning before school and at lunchtime). This effectively "covers" the school day, but teachers should be aware of a possible dropoff in effectiveness toward the latter stages of the morning. The other stimulants (e.g., Concerta, Adderall) typically are taken once per day, with behavioral effects lasting up to 8 hours. Some children do not respond as well to these sustained-release medications, however.

Approximately 70–80% of children with ADHD between the ages of 5 and 12 years old who receive stimulant medication evidence a positive response. For adolescents, the percentage of positive responders is somewhat lower (i.e., 60%). Thus, it can be assumed that the majority of students with ADHD who are treated with a stimulant will respond positively. Response to these medications varies as a function of the dose. Some children will respond to lower doses, while others will require higher doses to achieve the same effects. Dose–response to stimulants varies widely across individual children and cannot be predicted on the basis of a child's age or body weight. Specifically, the strength of obtained behavioral effects can range across children and doses from mild (i.e., minimal positive change in behavior) to strong (i.e., "normalization" of behavior control). Thus, most physicians will try a range of doses of a specific stimulant in an effort to determine a child's "optimal" dose.

In those instances when a child with ADHD does not respond to a particular stimulant, this is indicated by no change or, in some cases, a worsening of the core characteristics of ADHD (i.e., inattention, impulsivity, and overactivity). Usually, the physician will try an alternative stimulant when this occurs. For instance, some children who do not respond to Ritalin can be successfully treated with Adderall. If none of the stimulants work, some physicians may prescribe other medications such as antidepressants (e.g., bupropion). Thus, when a child's behavior is not affected by the first medication prescribed, there are other alternatives.

SIDE EFFECTS

The primary, acute side effects of stimulant medications are insomnia and appetite reduction. One of the latter side effects is likely to occur in about 50% of children treated with methylphenidate, particularly at higher doses and during the initial stages of treatment. In most cases, however, effects on sleep and appetite are quite mild and do not require discontinuing treatment. Other less common side effects include stomachaches, headaches, and increased anxiety or sad mood. Some children treated with methylphenidate will experience a "behavioral rebound" effect in the late afternoon when the medication is wearing off. The rebound effect is indicated by a worsening of the child's behavior and mood to an extent beyond what was evident prior to taking medication. The latter can be dealt with by reducing the dosage or by adding a late afternoon administration of the medication. A very small number (i.e., less than 5%) of children treated with stimulants will exhibit motor and/or vocal tics (i.e., repetitive motor movements or vocal noises). Usually, these will disappear after reducing the dosage or discontinuing the medication. In some cases, albeit very few, these tics will continue even when treatment is terminated.

One potential side effect that may be most prominent in school settings is an "overfocusing" effect. The latter refers to instances when a child may be exhibiting exemplary behavior control, but appears to be concentrating too hard on tasks with minimal output. In some children, this overfocused effect may be indicated by appearance (e.g., "glassy" eyes, restricted emotional expressions), while in others this may be signaled by a dropoff in academic performance (e.g., amount of work completed correctly). This reaction is usually a result of the child receiving a dose of medication that is too high.

Teachers and other school professionals should be cognizant of the possible side effects of stimulant medications. When these are noted to occur, the child's parents, physician, and/or the school nurse should be informed. This is especially the case when the child begins to exhibit tics or overfocused behavior. Care should be taken to evaluate possible side effects in comparison to the child's behavior without medication. In other words, sometimes what appears to be a side effect of medication is actually a behavior associated with ADHD that was evident prior to the initiation of treatment. For instance, some children with this disorder are prone to irritable moods regardless of whether they are receiving stimulant medication or not.

ROLE OF SCHOOL PROFESSIONALS IN TREATMENT

It is quite important that teachers and other school professionals are in communication with a child's parents and/or physician whenever stimulant medication is prescribed. This is true for at least two reasons. First, these medications are most active in affecting a child's behavior during the school day. In fact, many parents do not have the opportunity to see medication effects on their children's behaviors. Second, children with ADHD evidence their greatest problems in school settings, and thus the success of treatment is determined, in large part, by changes in a child's school performance.

School professionals can play a role in three stages of treatment. First, teacher input should be sought prior to initiating medication treatment. This is necessary to address whether the child has ADHD and, if so, whether medication treatment is needed. If this information is not actively sought by the child's physician, then someone from the school should contact the physician to provide school data. Second, changes in the student's behavior control and academic performance should be among the primary measures used to determine the best dose of medication. Objective information (e.g., rating scales completed by the teacher) about the child's classroom performance is invaluable in making medication-related decisions. Third, once a child's dosage is determined, teachers should communicate any significant changes in student performance that may occur during the school year. Although such changes are not always related to medication, sometimes a dropoff in behavior control may indicate that an adjustment in dosage is necessary. Thus, the school and the physician should be communicating throughout the various stages of medication treatment.

CHAPTER 7

◆ ◆ ◆

Adjunctive Interventions
for ADHD

◆

Children with ADHD often display problems with inattention, impulse control, and activity level across home, school, and community environments. Beyond the core behaviors that define ADHD, these children may exhibit difficulties in peer relationships, frequent noncompliance with authority figure commands, and conduct problems such as lying and stealing, as well as poor homework completion and study skills. Unfortunately, no single treatment modality, including psychostimulant medication, is sufficient for ameliorating the myriad problems related to ADHD. The chronic and potentially debilitating nature of difficulties associated with ADHD requires the use of multiple interventions implemented across settings over a long time period. In addition, treatment strategies should focus on multiple target behaviors to maximally impact the child's overall functioning. For many children with this disorder, a "prosthetic" environment must be engineered over the long term both at school and at home (Barkley, 1998). In keeping with this conclusion, the largest treatment outcome study conducted to date with this population (i.e., the MTA study; MTA Cooperative Group, 1999) included multiple components (parent training, school intervention, and summer treatment program) as part of its psychosocial intervention protocol.

Previous chapters have detailed the use of classroom-based behavioral procedures and psychotropic medications in the treatment of ADHD. Certainly, the combination of these therapeutic modalities represents the "optimal" intervention approach for ADHD at the current time. Nevertheless, adjunctive interventions will be necessary in many cases as a function of the severity of ADHD symptoms and the presence of additional behavioral difficulties. In this chapter, several therapeutic strategies that can supplement classroom behavioral programming and pharmacotherapy are delineated. First, school-based training of social skills is discussed. Peer coaching strategies also are delineated briefly. Next, home-based interventions such as parent training and behavioral family therapy are detailed, especially in relation to their impact on school performance. Strategies to promote success in completing homework assignments also are delineated. In the final section of the chapter, we review treatments for ADHD that have minimal or no demonstrated efficacy, yet often are touted as effective in the popular media. The implementation of these latter interventions often diminishes the time and resources available for proven treatments. Thus, it is important to make parents, teachers, and other school personnel aware of the relative support in the research literature for each of the therapies discussed in this book.

SCHOOL-BASED INTERVENTIONS

A variety of classroom-based interventions were described in detail in Chapter 5, including both proactive (e.g., peer tutoring) and reactive (e.g., token reinforcement) strategies. Several other treatment strategies can be useful in addressing problems related to ADHD. Social skills training techniques such as modeling, behavioral rehearsal, and reinforced practice have been proposed to ameliorate the social relationship difficulties often exhibited by children with ADHD. Although there is limited empirical support for social skills training with this population, we feel it is important for school practitioners to know what procedures might be most effective based on extant information.

Social Skills Training

As discussed in Chapter 1, children with ADHD frequently have difficulties getting along with their peers and sustaining close friendships with others. Their problems with inattention and impulse control disrupt the "social performance" of children with this disorder in a number of areas. First, they may enter ongoing peer activities (e.g., board or playground games) in an abrupt, disruptive manner that ultimately may lead to their peers becoming dissatisfied with the activity. For example, a child with ADHD is not likely to ask permission before trying to join a game and then may participate in a manner contrary to established rules. Second, they frequently do not follow the implicit "rules" of good conversation. A child with this disorder is likely to interrupt others, to pay minimal attention to what others are saying, and to respond in an irrelevant fashion (i.e., non sequitur) to the queries or statements of peers. Third, these children are more likely than their normal counterparts to "solve" interpersonal problems in an aggressive manner. This is not surprising, given the strong association between ADHD and physical aggression. Thus, arguments and fights with peers are common. In a related manner, children with ADHD are prone to losing control of their temper and becoming angry quite easily. Teasing and other forms of provocation that might be ignored or dealt with in an appropriate fashion by most children may be reacted to in a swift and violent manner by many youngsters with this disorder.

Given the variety of social performance problems that children with ADHD may display, they are more likely than their normal counterparts or even aggressive children to be rejected by their peers (Barkley, 1998). Of greater concern is the well-established finding that a child's rejected status often is stable over the course of development (Parker & Asher, 1987). Thus, interventions designed to address these myriad difficulties must be implemented for a sufficient duration to counteract the high risk for problematic outcome. What makes attempts to intervene in this area so difficult, however, is that children with ADHD do not appear to have deficits in social *skills* per se. They are able to state the "rules" for appropriate social behavior as well as their peers. What sets them apart from their typical peers is that they often do not act in accord with these rules. This performance deficit is consistent with the assumption that children with ADHD are impaired in delaying responses to the environment. Thus, in many interpersonal situations, they've behaved before they've had a chance to think about the consequences of their actions. These deficits in social *performance* are more difficult to ameliorate than skills problems for two primary reasons. First, most currently available social relationship interventions target deficits in skills rather than deficits in performance. Furthermore, because social performance problems occur across settings (e.g., classroom, playground, neighborhood), interventions addressing these difficulties must be implemented by a variety of individuals in a cross-situational fashion.

In similar fashion, interventions that target social knowledge and the acquisition of prosocial behaviors in group therapy formats (i.e., "traditional" social skills training) have not been found to lead to durable changes in interpersonal functioning for children with ADHD in "real-world" environments. Although impressive gains in conversation skills, problem solving, and anger control have been obtained during training sessions themselves, rarely do these improvements continue once the child leaves the therapy room (DuPaul & Eckert, 1994; Gresham, 2002).

The lack of maintenance and generalization of social skills training curricula has led to proposals for a more comprehensive approach to social relationship intervention for children with disruptive behavior disorders (for review of social skills strategies, see Gresham, 2002). For example, Sheridan (1995) has developed the Tough Kids Social Skills program for use in school settings. This program includes three possible levels of social skills training: small group, classwide, and schoolwide. Although all three training levels may be helpful for students with ADHD, it is likely that children with this disorder will require small-group training given their protracted relationship difficulties. Twelve, 60-minute group sessions are organized into three units: social entry, maintaining interactions, and problem solving. Training in social entry addresses conversation skills, joining peer activities, and expressing emotions. Two sessions are focused on maintaining interactions, including carrying on a conversation and playing cooperatively. Several problem-solving sessions are conducted to promote dealing with anger, maintaining self-control, and solving arguments. One or more booster sessions are used to promote maintenance of gains in social performance. Sheridan, Dee, Morgan, McCormick, and Walker (1996) have established preliminary empirical support for using the Tough Kids Social Skills program with students with ADHD.

Each Tough Kids session is conducted in a similar fashion. First, "homework" from the previous session is reviewed and discussed by the group. Group rules are also reviewed at the beginning of each session. Next, the specific social behavior targeted by that session is reviewed verbally and modeled by the group leader. Third, students role-play the specific social behavior using scenarios generated by participants and the group leader. It might be helpful to videotape role plays to facilitate review and feedback. The fourth component of the session is to have group members review each role play and provide feedback to participants. Students also can be asked to review their own performance before hearing feedback from other group members. Next, snacks are provided for those students who earned reinforcement by behaving in accord with group rules. Finally, each student is asked to set a goal for the coming week that is related to the specific social behavior covered during that week's session. These goals should be individualized as much as possible. A behavioral contract is then used to identify reinforcers that will be available contingent upon students' reaching their stated goals.

Generalization Programming

Although the skills training package described above may lead to appreciable gains in socially appropriate behaviors exhibited in the training setting, such changes do not necessarily transfer spontaneously to the real world (e.g., playground, neighborhood, classroom). Thus, a comprehensive peer relationship intervention program *must* include direct steps to promote maintenance and generalization of acquired social behaviors. Generalization programming can entail within-training strategies as well as structuring the environment to support enactment of prosocial behaviors (Hoff & Robinson, 2002).

Various procedures should be incorporated into the social skills training sessions themselves to increase the probability of generalization to real-world settings. As exemplified in the Tough Kids Social Skills program, these strategies include (1) using real-life vignettes generated by the group participants for role plays; (2) employing multiple exemplars and diverse training opportunities during modeling and role plays; (3) assigning homework that incorporates self-monitoring and self-reinforcement procedures; and (4) having periodic booster sessions to reinforce and extend previous training.

One of the major reasons that appropriate social behaviors do not generalize to real-world environments is that adults (e.g., parents, teachers) and peers do not necessarily prompt and/or reinforce the desired behaviors on a consistent basis. Under typical circumstances, continued use of newly acquired skills is unlikely to occur. Therefore, changes must be made to the child's natural environment such that the latter supports the ongoing use of appropriate interpersonal behaviors. Components of environmental programming might include (1) instructing parents and teachers to prompt children to enact the behaviors trained in the social skills sessions; (2) developing contingency management programs at home and at school to reinforce trained skills and decrease the probability of verbal and physical aggression (e.g., token reinforcement plus response cost for specific social behaviors); and (3) teaching children to elicit reinforcement from others in the environment, based on their engaging in prosocial behaviors (DuPaul & Eckert, 1994). Thus, parents and teachers are integral members of the "social skills treatment team" by serving as agents for generalization.

Strategic Peer Involvement

In addition to the child's parents and teachers, his or her peers should be enlisted to support the generalization of prosocial behaviors across settings. The inclusion of peers is quite important, as they often are present in settings where adult monitoring and attention is remote (e.g., neighborhood games). Moreover, peers are the crucial determinants of whether changes in social behaviors are clinically significant (i.e., enhanced social acceptance and increased friendships). Peers could be involved in all phases of social skills intervention. First, nonhandicapped peers can participate as "role models" in the skills training sessions. Through their participation in role plays and providing feedback, they could serve in a "cotherapist" role. In fact, behavior change is significantly greater in social skills training that includes a diverse peer group relative to the use of groups of children who all have antisocial behavior difficulties (Ang & Hughes, 2002). Second, peers could serve as social skills "tutors" in the natural environment by prompting and reinforcing the enactment of social behaviors that have been targeted in the training sessions. Once again, this would require training the non-ADHD peers in the parameters of acting as cotherapists. Cunningham and Cunningham (1998) have developed a student-mediated conflict resolution program that involves peers acting as playground monitors. The use of peer-mediated programs is associated with schoolwide reductions in playground violence and negative interactions. Finally, parents can structure home-based friendship training experiences by supervising their child with ADHD in the context of highly structured, noncompetitive activities with a small group of peers (Guevremont, 1990). In many cases, this would be preferable to encouraging children with ADHD to participate in community-based activities such as athletic teams or scouting, which may be less closely supervised and inherently more competitive.

Coaching Teens with ADHD

Students with ADHD frequently experience difficulties planning their activities and completing tasks within reasonable amounts of time. For this reason, they may benefit from support strategies that promote goal setting, self-monitoring, and timely task completion. One possible way to accomplish this is through the use of coaching strategies wherein an adult or peer works with the student with ADHD to prompt and reinforce appropriate goal-setting and time management behaviors. Dawson and Guare (1998) have developed a program for coaching teens with ADHD. There are two major phases to their coaching program. In the first phase, the teen with ADHD works with a coach to (1) identify possible long-term goals, (2) determine criteria that defines successful goal attainment, and (3) delineate potential barriers to reaching a goal. For example, a student may wish to obtain a successful grade in a particular subject area. The criterion for success would be the specific grade (e.g., a "B" or better) and, perhaps, teacher judgment that the student has mastered the material. Possible barriers to success could include a lack of understanding of some of the subject matter, distractions present in the home environment (e.g., CD player, video games) that could get in the way of studying, and poor note-taking skills.

In the second phase of the coaching program, the student and coach meet on a regular basis to design strategies and review progress toward goals. These sessions include four components (denoted by the acronym REAP): (1) Review, (2) Evaluate, (3) Anticipate, and (4) Plan. The coach and student review what the latter has accomplished between sessions and evaluate whether progress is being made toward the long-term goal. Many times, this process is aided by setting interim short-term goals to provide reinforcement for successive approximations toward the long-term goal. Possible hurdles toward further goal attainment are anticipated and a plan is developed for how the student will negotiate these hurdles while implementing strategies designed to help with goal attainment. Sessions are conducted on at least a weekly basis and are relatively brief (30 minutes).

Although Dawson and Guare (1998) do not present outcome data regarding their coaching model, it does seem to be a promising approach to helping adolescents with ADHD. In particular, students who have made significant behavioral improvement through other treatment strategies (e.g., stimulant medication and behavior contracting) may be amenable to taking the next step toward self-control. A student needs to be motivated and willing to work with an adult or peer in order to profit from the coaching program. Thus, school practitioners should consider the match between the student and the program approach, as well as who might best serve as a coach for the student. In some cases, an adult (e.g., teacher, counselor, or older sibling) might be the best "fit," whereas in other situations a student may work best with a peer or a higher achieving classmate.

HOME-BASED INTERVENTIONS

Parent Training

It often is important for parents of children with ADHD to receive supportive instruction in behavior management strategies designed to enhance their children's attention to household tasks and rules. In some instances, school psychologists or social workers provide parent training services in the school setting, especially when these services are not available in the community (e.g., with a clinical child psychologist). When school-based parent training is provided, there usually is an emphasis on helping parents to supervise the completion of academically relevant tasks such as homework and studying for tests. A number of programs for providing parent training in behavior modification strategies have been developed (e.g., Webster-Stratton, 1994).

Barkley (1997b) has adapted the Forehand and McMahon (1981) parent training program to more specifically address the core problems related to ADHD. This training program, as described below, can be conducted with individual parents or in a group format. Usually the child does not participate in the training, except in cases where the therapist wants the parent to practice management skills *in vivo*. Training sessions last 1–1.5 hours for an individual family and 1.5–2 hours for groups of parents.

Each training session follows a similar sequence of activities, including a review of the information covered the previous week, a brief assessment of whether any critical events occurred since the previous meeting, and a discussion of homework activities that were assigned at the end of the last session. The therapist then provides instruction with respect to particular management methods that the parents are to practice during the subsequent week. Following didactic instruction, the therapist models the appropriate behavior(s). The parents rehearse the management strategies and receive feedback and further guidance from the therapist. At the end of the session, additional practice of management skills is assigned as homework for the coming week. Written handouts detailing the session's techniques and procedures are distributed for review.

Parent training is usually provided over the course of nine weekly sessions. Session topics include a discussion of why children engage in disruptive behavior, strategies for attending to child behavior, methods to increase compliance and independent play, development of a token reinforcement program, use of response cost and time-out from positive reinforcement, strategies to manage child behavior in public places, use of a home–school communication program, and how to handle future behavior problems. At the conclusion of the initial course of training, follow-up meetings are scheduled every several months to provide "booster" sessions in management techniques and to support maintenance of acquired skills. For more detailed information regarding parent training, the reader should consult Barkley (1997b) and Anastopoulos and colleagues (1998).

Despite the substantial empirical support of parent training for the treatment of noncompliance in children (Brestan & Eyberg, 1998), less data have been gathered regarding the effects of this intervention specifically with children who have ADHD. Several investigations indicate that this treatment approach is effective (e.g., Anastopoulos, Shelton, DuPaul, & Guevremont, 1993; Horn, Ialongo, Popovich, & Peradotto, 1987);

however, many questions remain given the relatively small number of empirical studies and the numerous differences in methodology that exist across investigations. In particular, future research will be necessary to examine the durability over time and the generalization across settings of obtained treatment effects with this population. Furthermore, this training paradigm may be useful in training teachers to use behavior management principles. Despite the need for further research, parent training in behavior modification strategies is an integral and often necessary component of a multimodal treatment program for ADHD. Indeed, one of the major components of the behavioral intervention arm of the MTA study was an intensive parent training program (Wells et al., 2000).

Behavioral Family Therapy for Adolescents

Teenagers with ADHD often exhibit higher rates of disruptive noncompliant behavior, rebelliousness, conduct problems, and conflicts with family members than non-ADHD adolescents (Barkley, Anastopoulos, Guevremont, & Fletcher, 1991; Robin, 1998; Weiss & Hechtman, 1993). Interpersonal conflict is particularly prominent in families of adolescents with both ADHD and oppositional defiant disorder because these families are more likely to exhibit aversive behaviors (e.g., insults, complaints) in discussions than are parent–teen dyads in groups of ADHD-only or normal control adolescents (Edwards, Barkley, Laneri, Fletcher, & Metevia, 2001). Possible treatment approaches to address parent–adolescent conflict include the most common interventions for ADHD (i.e., stimulant medication and contingency management) and various forms of family therapy (e.g., structural family therapy; Minuchin, 1974).

A behavioral family therapy approach known as "problem solving and communication training" (PSCT; Robin & Foster, 1989) combines elements of contingency management training and structural family therapy. Specifically, PSCT involves skill-building techniques such as instruction in problem solving and appropriate communication behaviors, as well as prescribed changes in family systems and coalitions. In many cases, cognitive therapy procedures are employed to restructure the irrational belief systems of family members (Robin & Foster, 1989).

Two investigations have evaluated the effectiveness of PSCT in treating adolescents with ADHD and oppositional defiant disorder. Barkley, Guevremont, Anastopoulos, and Fletcher (1992) found PSCT to be as effective as contingency management training and structural family therapy in reducing the number of conflicts and the intensity of anger during conflict discussions at home. In addition, PSCT significantly improved the quality of parent–adolescent communication according to the independent reports of 21 teenagers with ADHD and their mothers. Improvements also were reported by parents with respect to their adolescent's school adjustment and in the broad-band dimensions of both internalizing (e.g., depression) and externalizing (e.g., conduct problems) symptomatology. This treatment was rated positively by all family members on consumer satisfaction questionnaires and obtained improvements were maintained at a 3-month follow-up. Unfortunately, treatment effects were not obtained on direct observations of parent–adolescent conflict, did not result in clinically significant change for most of the sample, and PSCT appeared to worsen the degree of irrational beliefs that some mothers held about their teenagers' conduct problems.

Barkley and colleagues (2001) replicated these findings while also determining whether combining PSCT with contingency management procedures would enhance outcomes. Behavioral effects were equivalent for PSCT alone and in combination with contingency management training, although families were more likely to drop out of the PSCT alone group. Family functioning was normalized in up to 70% of the families across the two treatment conditions. These findings provide at least preliminary support for the use of PSCT for treating adolescents with ADHD and their families. More research is needed to determine which families are most likely to profit from this treatment approach and whether other intervention components (e.g., contingency management) are necessary for a given family.

Homework Interventions

Given the academic and behavior difficulties experienced by students with ADHD, it is not surprising that many of these students have problems completing homework in a timely successful fashion (Karustis, Power, Rescorla, Eiraldi, & Gallagher, 1998). Specific difficulties include not writing down assignments, not bringing assignments home, not completing assignments in an accurate fashion, arguing with parents about completing homework, and failing to turn in assignments on time (Power et al., 2001). Problems with homework completion are critical because of the connection between homework and academic achievement (Cooper, Lindsay, Nye, & Greathouse, 1998). Thus, over the years, intervention programs have been developed to address homework difficulties (e.g., Olympia, Jenson, & Hepworth-Neville, 1996).

Power and colleagues (2001) have developed and pilot-tested a very promising homework intervention program specifically for students with ADHD. Their Homework Success program involves seven, 90-minute sessions conducted with parent groups. As such, this program could be incorporated into an ongoing parent training program (as described above) or could be a stand-alone program. There is a strong collaborative component to this program, in which teachers and children are also included at appropriate points in treatment. For example, a parent–teacher conference is facilitated at the outset of the program to identify specific homework problems and emphasize the importance of home–school collaboration.

The core component of this program is the use of goal-setting and contingency management procedures to encourage more consistent homework performance. Topics of the Homework Success sessions include introducing the program, establishing a homework ritual, providing positive reinforcement, managing time and goal setting, using aversive procedures appropriately, anticipating future homework problems, and providing follow-up support. This is a skills-based program wherein parents are instructed in new strategies during each session. Parents are expected to complete their own homework between sessions and their success in implementing strategies is reviewed at the beginning of each session. Power and colleagues (2001) emphasize the use of data to track changes in homework performance over time and they provide several measures to facilitate feasible data collection. Although extensive controlled research has yet to be conducted with this program, controlled case study data indicates that Homework Success leads to improvements in homework completion and accuracy (Daniel, Power, Karustis, & Leff, 1999).

Parent Support Groups

It usually is quite helpful for parents of children with ADHD to interact with other parents of similar children to share their frustrations, successes, and advocacy strategies. A number of national parent organizations have been founded to play a supportive role, to serve as a clearinghouse for information relative to ADHD, and to lobby political groups to supply greater services for this population. One of the most prominent national parent organizations is the Children and Adults with Attention-Deficit/Hyperactivity Disorder (CHADD) organization based in Landover, Maryland.[1] CHADD was founded in 1987 and has local chapters in virtually every state. In addition to publishing a quarterly magazine, this organization sponsors an annual confer-

---

[1]Information about joining CHADD or a local chapter of this organization can be obtained by contacting the CHADD national office at 1-800-233-4050, by writing their office at 8181 Professional Place, Suite 201, Landover MD 20785, or by visiting their website: *www.chadd.org.*

ence on ADHD that draws a national audience. CHADD members include not only parents but teachers and health care professionals working with children with ADHD. Organizations such as CHADD serve an important role in the overall treatment of ADHD as they provide valuable information about the disorder as well as guidance for its members in advocating for proper educational and therapeutic intervention for their children.

INTERVENTIONS WITH LIMITED OR NO EFFICACY

A number of treatments for ADHD have been proposed and promoted over the years that have been found, via controlled research, either to have minimal efficacy in ameliorating attention deficits or have not been subjected to controlled empirical investigation. Despite a lack of demonstrated efficacy, many of these interventions (e.g., dietary management) are quite popular and are commonly employed. In general, continued support for these treatments is derived from theory, "expert opinion," and/or face validity (i.e., the approaches appear to make great intuitive sense and consequently have tremendous consumer appeal). Although ineffective treatments are rarely physically harmful, their use diverts valuable time, energy, and resources from the implementation of more effective therapies. Thus, it is important for school practitioners to be aware of ineffective treatment modalities and to discourage their use whenever necessary. Of course, this should be done in a sensitive manner, while offering alternative, better supported, interventions.

Treatments that have minimal or no established efficacy for children with ADHD include relaxation training, play therapy, prescription of megavitamins, amino acid supplementation, electroencephalogram (EEG) biofeedback training, herbal medicines, ocular motor exercises, and specialized diets (e.g., Feingold diet).

Factors to Consider before Recommending a Treatment

Due to the plethora of proposed treatments for ADHD, it is not possible to discuss the relative merits of every one of these techniques. Nevertheless, it is important to enumerate several guidelines that can be employed when considering the use of a "new" or "alternative" therapy for ADHD because the use of the latter may detract from treatment efforts in more effective directions (Ingersoll & Goldstein, 1993).

1. If the developer or a proponent of a particular therapy states that the treatment "cures" ADHD or that it can be used alone to treat

this disorder, then an automatic red flag should be raised. Even well-researched, effective treatments for ADHD (e.g., stimulant medication) do not lead to irreversible improvements in children's functioning and must be supplemented by a variety of treatments implemented across settings. Thus, claims for "cures" must be met with a high degree of caution.

2. Treatments that are touted as effective and potentially curative for a variety of disorders (e.g., ADHD, learning disabilities, autism, depression) should be met with caution. It is highly unlikely that one specific therapy would lead to clinically significant results in treating children with a variety of disorders. Such claims should lead to an automatic red flag and further information regarding the empirical underpinnings of the therapy should be obtained.

3. It is incumbent upon the developer or proponent of a novel treatment to demonstrate its therapeutic efficacy in the context of a controlled, experimental design using reliable and valid dependent measures. It is not enough to offer case study data or testimonials from satisfied clients. Furthermore, data should be available that allow direct comparison of the effects of novel therapies relative to those associated with established effective interventions. Thus, one of the first questions to ask proponents of a new treatment for ADHD is "Where are the data?"

4. The quality of experimental research investigating a novel treatment can be assessed by asking several questions. Were the participants classified as ADHD using reliable and valid indices of the disorder? Were the dependent measures collected in such a fashion as to reduce possible biases (e.g., behavioral observations conducted by individuals who were unaware of the clinical population being studied and the treatment being investigated)? Are threats to the internal validity (e.g., maturation) of the treatment controlled for? How generalizable are the obtained results to other children with ADHD? Was the clinical significance (e.g., normalization) of the obtained findings assessed? Did the investigators examine the generalization of treatment effects across settings (e.g., home and school) and over time (e.g., follow-up assessment)?

5. Whenever school professionals encounter novel treatments that are not substantiated by empirical evidence, it is important to communicate their skepticism to parents and educators of children with ADHD. Parents of these children may be particularly prone to "buying into" new therapeutic approaches given their frustrations in dealing with ADHD-related difficulties and their knowledge of the limitations of currently available treatments. Furthermore, in our experience, these parents often lack a clear understanding of the necessity and requirements of the scientific study of treatments.

SUMMARY

The chronic exhibition of ADHD-related behaviors across settings and caretakers necessitates the implementation of a multimodal treatment program over several years or longer. A number of adjunctive intervention approaches can supplement the use of classroom behavior support strategies and psychotropic medications. Additional school-based treatments may include social skills training and peer coaching. Home-based treatments include parent training in behavior modification techniques, behavioral family therapy for adolescents with ADHD, homework interventions, and parental participation in support organizations (e.g., CHADD). Over the years, a number of therapies for ADHD (e.g., Feingold diet) have been proposed that either have not been subjected to empirical investigation or have been found ineffective in the treatment of this disorder. Given the popularity of some of the latter therapies, it is important that the school-based professional is cognizant of both empirically sound and less efficacious interventions in order to more effectively advocate for the appropriate treatment of students with ADHD.

CHAPTER 8

◆◆◆

Communication with Parents,
Professionals, and Students

◆

Clear and accurate communication is a foundation of all professional service delivery in education, psychology, medicine, and related professions, and is a cornerstone of high-quality service delivery in support of students with ADHD, their parents, and their teachers. There are several reasons why communication is so critical. The assessment of ADHD and related problems is a process involving multiple informants and multiple methods across multiple settings. This process involves the communication of information, observations, opinions, and professional judgments among parents, teachers and other school-based professionals, students, psychologists, and physicians (also see Chapter 2). The design, implementation, and evaluation of interventions for ADHD involve similar processes and communications. Consequently, clear and ongoing communication with parents, teachers, and other professionals involved with identified children is warranted, and will necessarily involve discussions of issues critical to assessment, diagnosis, instructional planning, intervention management, and professional service delivery in general.

For example, concerns regarding a child's problem behavior(s) typically are raised first by school professionals and/or parents. Furthermore, medical professionals (e.g., pediatricians, psychiatrists) are involved with students who are diagnosed with ADHD quite frequently. Together, these persons will make screening, referral, classification, and intervention selection and outcome decisions. Productive interactions among these persons rely on clear and specific communications despite differing vocabularies, perspectives, and backgrounds.

Consider also that the diagnosis of ADHD is based on a psychiatric classification system (DSM-IV), yet the identified children and their parents interact most frequently with school-based education professionals, while also being served in many cases by community-based physicians and mental health professionals. Education professionals typically are less familiar with DSM than they are with the special education classification system contained in the Individuals with Disabilities Education Act of 1997 (IDEA, 1997). Equivalent understanding of these two classification systems across involved individuals cannot be assumed, thereby necessitating explanatory communications (and, in some cases, professional training) regarding the systems and their foundations (e.g., research, policy), terminology, implications for treatment planning, and related issues.

Clearly, effective design, implementation, and evaluation of medical, behavioral, and educational interventions for children with ADHD rely a great deal on effective communication, given the inherent differences of beliefs, opinions, and knowledge of the professional literature across the persons involved. Of particular concern here is that the development of interventions often is a clinic-based or office-based activity, while an intervention's implementation, positive behavioral effects, and any undesirable effects are experienced in home, classroom, and community settings. Thus, the evaluation of interventions and their effects requires communication among physicians, parents, teachers, students, and other professionals.

Last but not least, the ethical principles and standards for practice of the National Association of School Psychologists[1] (NASP; 2000) indicate that professional communication with parents, students, and other professionals is an expected component of appropriate school psychology practice. These guidelines for professional conduct specify that the purpose(s) and possible consequences of the professional's involvement, as well as intervention options and alternatives, be discussed with parents and students in a manner that is understandable to them. Guidelines also are provided regarding the development of relationships between professionals (e.g., school psychologists and pediatricians) when such relationships are in the best interest of the students being served. In the latter sections of this chapter pertinent examples of these guidelines are provided as introductory statements for those sections.

---

[1]The American Psychological Association, the Council for Exceptional Children, and other professional organizations have similar ethical guidelines.

The purpose of this chapter is to identify and discuss several important issues related to ADHD for communication among and between school professionals and others involved with identified students, including parents, other professionals, and the students themselves. Although each topic in this volume is worthy of discussion and consideration, primary attention here is given to (1) the relationship between a diagnosis of ADHD and educational services; (2) the responsibilities of education professionals; (3) issues surrounding stimulant medication treatment; and finally, (4) issues specific to communication with parents, physicians and other professionals, and students. Perhaps we are stating the obvious. However, we believe that by discussing and clarifying these issues, professional and parental decision making and actions can be facilitated, resulting in improved outcomes for children.

DSM DIAGNOSES AND EDUCATIONAL SERVICES

Where ADHD is a concern, professionals and parents will need to discuss a range of answers to the question, "How does a DSM diagnosis or other classification relate to educational service delivery?" The usefulness of diagnostic classification systems of childhood problems has been debated for years (Garmezy, 1978; Gresham & Gansle, 1992a, 1992b; Hynd, 1992; Martens, 1992; Reynolds, 1992; Schact & Nathan, 1977; Shapiro, 1992), yielding a wide range of professional opinions. In fact, the DSM-IV-TR (American Psychiatric Association, 2000) states that a diagnosis is merely a starting place for planning services:

> Making a DSM-IV diagnosis represents only the first step in a comprehensive evaluation. To formulate an adequate treatment plan, the clinician will invariably require considerable additional information about the person being evaluated beyond that required to make a DSM-IV diagnosis. . . . The clinical and scientific considerations involved in categorization of . . . conditions as mental disorders may not be wholly relevant to legal judgments, for example, that take into account such issues as individual responsibility, disability determination, and competency. (pp. xxxiv–xxxv, xxxvii)

From an *educational* decision-making standpoint, it must be recognized that the DSM system of classification is tied to assessment tools and procedures that are *nomothetic* in their foundations and assumptions. In psychology and education, reliable and valid nomothetic assessment yields information useful for comparing children with one another along the measured dimension or construct (e.g., intelligence). For example, a child who earns a score at the 37th percentile on an intelligence test has performed less well than a peer who earns a score at the 78th percentile. Developing an instructional intervention or planning an educational program for either child based solely on this information is not defensible. However, information based on nomothetic assessment procedures can be used in a reliable and valid manner for making screening, referral, and classification decisions.

By comparison, intervention planning and effectiveness decisions are more readily linked to other types of assessment tools and procedures that are *idiographic* in their foundations and assumptions. Idiographic assessment does not focus on the relative classification of individuals vis-à-vis their behavioral presentations (e.g., Anna meets criteria for ADHD, while James does not), but rather is concerned with relative comparisons of the behavior of an individual over time (e.g., Sam's reading achievement in March is much improved relative to his reading achievement in November) as a result of intervention, development, change in programs, and the like.

When the idiographic assessment measure possesses the characteristics of accuracy and utility, it can yield information useful for the development of effective instructional and intervention programs. For example, accurate assessment information regarding a child's ongoing and differential performance in two different reading curricula could be directly relevant to instructional planning decisions (for a thorough comparison of nomothetic and idiographic approaches to assessment, see Barrios & Hartmann, 1986; Cone, 1986; Merrell, 1999). Based on the child's reading performance, a decision to provide instruction within the curriculum yielding higher rates of success would seem warranted. Intervention outcome evaluations, that is, comparing a child's behavior or performance over time, also need to be grounded in idiographic assessment information, although supplemental information regarding peer comparisons might also be useful.

A primary limiting factor preventing direct linkages between diagnosis and intervention is the large degree of variability in the behavior of children diagnosed with ADHD (Barkley, 1998; Frick & Lahey, 1991). That is, all children diagnosed with ADHD do not display the same problem behaviors, nor do they experience the same difficulties, if any, in school. In assessment terms, Haynes (1986) has referred to the variability among persons classified in the same manner as an issue of "diagnostic homogeneity." Specifically, Haynes noted that "if individuals placed in a particular classification category . . . are homogeneous on dimensions of topography, etiology, and response to treatment, categorization is sufficient for description and intervention design, and the benefits of additional preintervention assessment are reduced" (p. 391). Given the variability in behavioral topography and response to treatment of children with ADHD (Barkley, 1998), intervention design, implementation, and evaluation will require even more professional effort than that required for diagnosis or classification. In part, the focus of this effort must depend on professional training and responsibilities.

These issues should be discussed openly at various stages of the assessment process. When a child is exhibiting significant attention and/or behavior control problems, the first step is to collect screening information (see Chapter 2). Sometimes, at this stage, the child's parent or teacher specifically questions the presence of ADHD, as though this is all that needs to be determined. This situation provides an opportunity to put the diagnostic process into perspective. Specifically, it should be communicated clearly that evaluation data are being collected not simply to derive a diagnosis, but also to gather information that will lead to effective intervention. Similarly, when the multimethod assessment of ADHD (i.e., Stages II and III; see Chapter 2) is concluded, it is helpful to reiterate that a diagnosis is actually a "way station" between the referral and the design of an intervention program. Furthermore, it should be stated that the informational value of the diagnosis lies in its usefulness in directing further assessment activities, suggesting risks for associated behavior or learning difficulties, and increasing the probability of choosing effective treatment strategies. Finally, it must be stressed with school team members that ongoing assessment of the child's functioning will be necessary to evaluate the relative efficacy of intervention procedures. When these points are communicated effectively, the focus of the evaluation team can be *balanced* across efforts at multimethod assessment, diagnostic decision making, and the development of a potentially successful treatment protocol. This balance is important, as we see it, as all too often the bulk of professional efforts are aimed at diagnosis, with comparatively small amounts of intervention effort.

Discussions of these issues can help to identify and clarify the expectations held by parents, teachers, and others regarding the utilization and benefits of various assessment procedures. An excellent tool that can prompt and facilitate these types of discussions, as well as discussions of treatment approaches for ADHD, is the Attention Deficit/Hyperactivity Disorder Knowledge and Opinion Survey (AKOS), published by Power and colleagues (2001). The AKOS consists of 43 items answered in either a true/false or Likert-type fashion to determine degree of parent/ teacher expectations, knowledge, and opinions about various assessment and intervention strategies pertinent to ADHD. Identifying and clarifying these expectations should result in improved understanding of the need for linkages between assessment, intervention, and education in serving students with ADHD.

EDUCATIONAL TRAINING AND RESPONSIBILITIES

The primary professional responsibilities of education professionals involve the development and delivery of curricula and instruction. As such, educators make decisions and take actions regarding *what* to teach (i.e., selecting curricula and instructional objectives), *how* to teach (i.e., identifying which materials, procedures and methods to use), *when* to teach (i.e., instructional design and organization), *who* will teach, and *where* to teach (instructional environment). Decisions surrounding these issues are important for *all students*, including those identified with ADHD, and arguably define the domain of education. Therefore, these issues should be paramount in the decision making of educators responsible for students with ADHD vis-à-vis the child's learning and achievement. In addition, because the diagnosis and treatment of ADHD nearly always involves pediatricians, psychiatrists, clinical psychologists, and other support professionals, collaborative efforts at assessment and treatment will need to be developed and maintained.

The wide range of issues and concerns requiring professional involvement where children diagnosed with ADHD are concerned, clearly warrants interdisciplinary collaboration. Also warranted are frank discussions about appropriate roles and responsibilities for the professionals involved. School psychologists and special educators, in particular, may be faced with challenging demands for service delivery in light of the eligibility for special education services of children identified with ADHD under the "Other Health Impaired" category of the Individuals with Disabilities Education Act of 1997 (IDEA, 97; Hakola, 1992). For example, these professionals and their colleagues are likely to need professional development activities to help them obtain knowledge and skills in the DSM psychiatric classification system, developmental psychopathology, psychopharmacology, and the methods and models of clinical psychology and psychiatry.

Additionally, professionals need to be prepared to discuss with parents and others available educational service delivery models and options for students with ADHD. For example, questions will be raised regarding (1) whether or not a child is eligible for special education services, (2) whether or not a child should have a "504 accommodation plan," and (3) in what manner is the school system providing appropriate support for this student with ADHD?

Many children with ADHD may be eligible for special education services within their public school systems under the provisions of IDEA 1997 (see Telzrow & Tankersley, 2000, for a thorough review of this legislation). However, children with ADHD do not automatically qualify for services under IDEA by virtue of their ADHD diagnosis. The IDEA legislation and its predecessors intend that U.S. students with disabilities should receive a free and appropriate public education, in the least restrictive environment, and have the benefit of an individualized educational program (IEP). Eligibility for special education services under IDEA is contingent on meeting each of two criteria. The first is having a disability as defined in the IDEA legislation. Children with ADHD are most likely to meet this criterion within the categories of "specific learning disability," "other health impaired," and in some cases "emotional disturbance." The second criterion is that a child with an identified disability must have a *demonstrated need for special education services.* This latter criterion often is met through a documented lack of student responsiveness to interventions/supports implemented through general education programs and staff. In many instances parents and in some instances professionals are unaware of the second of these criteria, and therefore could benefit from a discussion of the eligibility requirements.

Another legal consideration relative to students with ADHD in the schools is Section 504 of the Rehabilitation Act of 1973 (see Zirkel & Aleman, 2000, for a review of this legislation and its implications for educational practice). In general, this legislation prohibits discrimination on the basis of disability by recipients of federal funds, such as school systems. Section 504 stipulates that students with a mental or physical disability that impairs a major life activity (e.g., education) to a substantial degree are entitled to supports/adjustments to accommodate their participation in either general or special education programs (see Chapter 3 for a thorough discussion of IDEA and Section 504). Efforts will need to be made to help parents and professionals become knowledgeable of the distinctions between IDEA and Section 504 eligibility and supports.

One further consideration in this arena is that the fields of school psychology, special education, and to some degree general education recently have been discussing and in some cases adopting noncategorical, intervention- and outcomes-oriented models of service delivery (Bardon, 1988; Reschly, 1988, 2000; Reschly, Tilly, & Grimes, 1999; Stoner & Green, 1992b). To date, however, how such models might accommodate children with ADHD has received limited professional consideration (cf., e.g., Hakola, 1992, with Stoner & Carey, 1992).

Noncategorical service delivery is intended, in part, to prevent an overemphasis on the diagnosis and classification of children, which may preclude school psychologists from taking more active roles and responsibilities in developing and implementing effective interventions. To further illustrate this point, suppose that school professionals are involved with a child who is accurately diagnosed with ADHD. Does this disability necessarily represent a handicapping condition and therefore warrant special services? It has been argued that a recognizable disability, such as ADHD, only becomes a handicap in a nonaccommodating environment (Kameenui & Simmons, 1990; Shinn, 1998). That is, if a school is providing instructional and social support such that a student with a recognized disability is not considered to be handicapped (i.e., his or her performance meets or exceeds expectations, and is commensurate with same-age, typical peers), that school should be recognized as providing exemplary services. Of course, given evidence that a student is not meeting the expectations of his or her current environment, reasonable accommodations should be made in attempts to support the student (and teacher) toward meeting those expectations (e.g., matching instructional materials with current academic skills, providing more frequent positive and corrective feedback, enhancing motivation to engage in academic work, increasing opportunities to practice newly acquired skills and knowledge) and achieving academic success. The emphasis here is on encouraging schools to allocate limited resources primarily to procedures that monitor and foster the individual social and academic progress of all students (Reschly, 1988, 2000).

These service delivery issues will need to be discussed among all interested parties so that the expectations and responsibilities of each team member may be clarified, and so that parents understand what to expect from the school system personnel with whom they are working. Clarification of team member expectations and responsibilities must be established at a minimum of three points in the evaluation and treatment process. Prior to conducting a multimethod evaluation of ADHD (i.e., Stage II of the assessment process; see Chapter 2), the specific responsibilities of each school-based professional should be delineated clearly. Furthermore, the theoretical and professional "biases" of each team member should be elicited openly and discussed. For example, in some instances teachers and parents may question even the existence of attention-deficit/hyperactivity disorder itself, and a discussion of the recently published International Consensus Statement on ADHD (Barkley, 2002) may be warranted. Although discussion of this type will not necessarily lead to a complete resolution of potential conflicts and disagreements, it will increase the awareness of similarities and differences among the positions of all team members. This is, at least, the first step in promoting greater collaboration in team-based service delivery.

The second point where service delivery issues will need to be discussed is when the intervention plan is designed (Stage IV of the assessment process; see Chapter 2). At this point, decisions must be made not only as to which treatments to recommend, but also with respect to who will implement each intervention. There may be initial confusion among some team members as to what ADHD is and the most effective treatments for this disorder. In particular, questions surrounding the use of stimulant medication may arise. It may be helpful to provide written information (e.g., see Appendix 6.1) and/or suggested readings (see Appendix 8.1) about ADHD and its treatment to all interested parties. The appointment of a case manager (see Chapter 9 for further discussion of the role of a case manager) will facilitate treatment planning as well as enhance the maintenance of consistent service delivery. Given that some treatments for ADHD (e.g., stimulant medication) are provided by community-based professionals, the need for the school to "speak with one voice" is particularly crucial. Potential disagreements among team members should be elicited actively and resolved prior to implementing treatment procedures. It has been our experience that although the latter may delay service delivery, it often prevents more serious and time-consuming conflicts once treatment has begun.

Service delivery expectations and responsibilities should be discussed periodically in the context of ongoing evaluation of the treatment strategies. Several meetings per year should be held for the school-based team, including the parent(s), to discuss the efficacy of each specific intervention and the need for adjustments in programming. This provides the opportunity to make changes in specific responsibilities among team members, if necessary. It is particularly important for those team members (i.e., teachers and parents) who are performing the bulk of the direct intervention to receive reinforcement and support for their efforts. Furthermore, if possible, responsibilities should be rotated among team members to enhance collegiality and prevent the potential "burnout" of a specific individual.

ISSUES SURROUNDING STIMULANT MEDICATION TREATMENT

As discussed in Chapter 6, the most frequent intervention for ADHD is stimulant medication, typically methylphenidate (MPH). By all accounts, the use of stimulant medication in the treatment of ADHD-related problems is common and affects the lives of a significant number of school-age children. Furthermore, stimulant medication treatment needs to be undertaken with caution because beneficial effects do not occur for all treated children. Moreover, for those who do benefit, medication response will be dose- and behavior-specific. Finally, some children will experience adverse effects related to stimulant treatment.

The use of stimulant medication treatment (SMT) for problems of children's inattention, overactivity, and impulsivity has not been without controversy. Concerns that have arisen around SMT primarily involve discrepancies between defensible professional practices and the personal beliefs of involved parents, educators, and other professionals regarding several key issues including (1) the potential benefits of treatment; (2) the potential harmful effects of treatment; and finally, (3) the values of parents, educators, and other professionals involved in intervention decision making. Communication and discussions of each of these issues will be critical where stimulants and other psychotropic medications are being considered in the treatment of a child with ADHD.

Potential Benefits of Stimulant Medication Treatment

Numerous research investigations conducted since the 1960s have documented positive, short-term benefits of stimulants for *most* children diagnosed with hyperactivity and/or attention problems. These outcomes have been demonstrated in the areas of (1) academic performance, (2) social interactions, and (3) on individually administered, performance assessment tasks (see Chapter 6). However, it also has been demonstrated that response to stimulants varies from child to child (even those of the same body weight) and across target behaviors for any given child (Rapport & Denney, 2000). As such, the determination of stimulant treatment outcomes for individual children must be made cautiously, and will require the generation and analysis of individual outcome data (see Chapter 6 for details of school-based medication evaluation).

Potential for Adverse Effects of Stimulant Medication Treatment

Of concern to parents and professionals considering stimulant treatment for children are potential adverse effects of medication. Children treated with stimulants may experience adverse physical side effects such as appetite suppression, nausea, headaches, irritability, insomnia, growth suppression, and, in rare instances, motor or vocal tics (see Chapter 6). Furthermore, in a minority of cases, stimulant treatment may result in an "overfocused" child who appears to be overly attentive to specific stimuli and is slow to orient to alternative activities or tasks. Although problems such as these typically have been reported at relatively high doses of medication, the potential for their occurrence is present at low doses as well. These possibilities and monitoring systems aimed at detecting potential adverse outcomes need to be discussed among professionals and parents.

Values Conflicts or Assumptions on Which Treatment Is Based

From a personal values standpoint, some parents and professionals are resolute in their opposition to using stimulant treatment with children. These values take various forms and are difficult to attribute to any single source or concern. Rather, support for a values position against the use of medication can be found in a variety of professional and popular publications. For example, one researcher (O'Leary, 1980) has argued that identified children need to learn social and self-management skills rather than to be chemically quieted. Similarly, a popular book published in the 1970s (Schrag & Divoky, 1975) asserted that stimulant medication, along with widespread testing, labeling, and "behavior modification" with all children, were all methods of inappropriate institutional control of human rights. More recently, legal suits against prescribing physicians and the picketing of professional conferences have been supported by an organization within the Church of Scientology, the Citizens Commission on Human Rights. This group alleges that the use of stimulants and other psychotropic medications for childhood problems are turning schoolchildren into drug addicts. As discussed in Chapter 6, these criticisms of stimulant medication are not supported by the empirical literature. Unfortunately, these value-laden critiques are unlikely to be influenced by objective outcome data. However, from an empirical perspective, reliable and valid data regarding meaningful treatment outcomes can and should be critical determinants of parent and professional decision making about the therapeutic usefulness of stimulant medications.

Outcome data have the potential to allow for reasoned judgments to be made regarding the benefits and costs of stimulant medication treatment for any given child. Furthermore, with a focus on a range of carefully measured outcomes (e.g., academic performance, social behavior, adverse physical effects) both the misgivings and the goals of involved parents and professionals may be addressed. Thus, if a child's physician and the school-based evaluation team agree that stimulant medication may be warranted, the student's parents should be provided with accurate and unbiased information regarding the costs and benefits of this treatment as well as how its efficacy will be evaluated. For example, the parents could be provided with a handout, similar to the one designed for teachers in Appendix 6.1, delineating the potential benefits and side effects of stimulants (see Barkley & Murphy, 1998, for a parent handout on stimulant medication).

The parents' decision about medication treatment should be placed in an appropriate context. The initial decision is whether or not to conduct a *controlled trial* of stimulants (or other medication), not a decision to permanently and irrevocably place a child on medication. Also, the parents should be aware of the need for ongoing assessment of medication response to occur on at least an annual basis. Thus, even if the initial trial of medication is successful, professionals are not communicating to the parents that pharmacological treatment is a permanent part of the treatment plan. Nevertheless, given the chronicity of ADHD symptoms, it is realistic to assume that medication may be necessary for at least a year or more.

School Involvement

Management and evaluation of stimulant treatment often involves activities within the school and the classroom. Suggestions for school involvement and collaboration with prescribing physicians have been discussed fully in other places (see Chapter 6; see also Brown & Sawyer, 1998; Gadow, 1993) and include (1) establishing district- or schoolwide policy and communication systems for collaboration with community physicians, (2) establishing a systemwide outcome evaluation system for use with children being treated with stimulant medications, (3) delineating the specific roles of school system personnel in the implementation and monitoring of medication trials, and (4) ensuring that all staff are appropriately trained to fulfill their responsibilities. School psychologists and school nurses should be qualified to facilitate the coordination and implementation of each of these suggestions within their districts.

In addition to discussions of assessment and diagnosis, educational responsibilities, and stimulant medication, involvement with children with ADHD requires education professionals to communicate specific information, requests (e.g., referrals for evaluation), and expectations to parents, other professionals, and children. These person specific communications are the focus of the remainder of this chapter.

COMMUNICATION BETWEEN EDUCATION PROFESSIONALS AND PARENTS

The following excerpts outline the ideal approach for school practitioners (National Association of School Psychologists, 2000):

> *Ethical guideline C1.* School psychologists explain all services to parents in a clear, understandable manner. They strive to propose a set of options which takes into account the values and capabilities of each parent.

Ethical guideline C3. School psychologists encourage and promote parental participation in designing services provided to their children. When appropriate, this includes linking interventions between the school and the home, tailoring parental involvement to the skills of the family, and helping parents gain the skills needed to help their children.

Ethical guideline C4. School psychologists respect the wishes of parents who object to school psychological services and attempt to guide parents to alternative community resources.

Ethical guideline C5. School psychologists discuss with parents the recommendations and plans for assisting their children. The discussion includes alternatives associated with each set of plans, which show respect for the ethnic/cultural values of the family. The parents are informed of sources of help available at school and in the community.

Communication with parents regarding the education of children with ADHD can be conceptualized broadly as intended to involve parents, and support them, in a variety of activities that contribute to educational decision making. The time and effort necessary for these communications and activities will vary widely. For example, compare issues of due process notification and consent for assessment with completing a behavior rating scale or participating in a structured interview to derive goals for educational planning. Regardless of the time required, our goals should be to communicate as directly and clearly as possible with parents, and to facilitate their involvement and understanding to the fullest extent possible. Particular attention is warranted to issues of due process notifications, parent involvement in educational decision making, and parent roles in educational program implementation.

Due Process Notifications

The Individuals with Disabilities Education Act of 1997, its predecessors, and related public laws ensure the rights of all children to a free and appropriate education, regardless of disability or handicapping condition. These laws require that parents be notified of and give consent to initial placement of children into special education programs, as well as to assessment activities that might lead to such changes (Bersoff & Hofer, 1990). Parental notification also is required as to when a conference will be held for purposes of discussing these decisions. Bersoff and Hofer (1990) note that informed consent involves parental *knowledge* of the action(s) to be taken, *voluntariness* or freedom from coercion, and *capacity* or competence to provide consent. These procedural requirements can best be met via open and informative communication, as can involvement in educational decision making.

Involving Parents in Educational Planning and Decision Making

Five distinct and related types of educational decisions that can be facilitated by careful assessment have been delineated by Salvia and Ysseldyke (1998). They are screening, referral, classification or eligibility, instructional program planning including placement decisions, and program evaluation (including student progress evaluation). It is incumbent upon professionals to clarify and discuss with parents the issues and procedures involved in assessment for each these purposes, as well as how they relate to educational decision making. These discussions can help parents to be truly informed and knowledgeable consumers who can better act in the best interest of the child(ren) being served.

As part of these discussions, professionals likely will want to clarify several aspects of their work for parents by providing information along some or all of the following dimensions. For example, what is your model of (or general approach to) professional practice, and, based on the assumptions of that model, what are the implications for service delivery? With respect to assessment, what activities do you and your organization typically engage in when addressing issues of screening, referral, classification, and eligibility for programs? How will you convey to parents the concept that there is no "litmus test" for diagnosing ADHD, especially when faced with parents, teachers, and other professionals saying "We really need to know whether or not this child has ADHD"?

When issues and questions regarding a diagnosis of ADHD are at hand, parents will need to be informed as to the nature and implications of an ADHD diagnosis. For example, how was this diagnosis arrived at? How should parents view this problem? Should they view this as a medical disorder, a developmental disorder, an educational problem, or some combination of the three? What is the prognosis for children diagnosed with ADHD? In our experience, it is helpful to convey to parents of children with ADHD that in a general sense they face two primary problems: first, their child is likely to present with *difficult-to-manage behavior*; and second, their child is likely to be *difficult to teach*. Intervention strategies and options for child management by parents and teachers, as well as by self-management and medication, may be appropriate to discuss at this point. Also, with respect to interventions, the importance of careful planning, implementation, and evaluation of intervention strategies should be conveyed to parents. Finally, professionals should do their best to expose myths regarding ADHD. For example, commonly held beliefs such as ADHD is caused by food allergies or that medication response is a diagnostic indicator of ADHD can be discussed in the course of communications around the appropriate topic (e.g., etiology, assessment, intervention). Discussion of these issues can be facilitated by providing the parents with a brief fact sheet about ADHD (see Barkley, 1998) and/or a list of suggested readings (see Appendix 8.1).

Parent Involvement in Educational Programming

Professional–parent partnerships, within which collaborative efforts to foster a shared responsibility for student learning, are part of the spirit and the letter of IDEA 1997 and related public laws. Furthermore, parent involvement in educational and school-related activities has been documented to enhance student achievement (Christenson, Rounds, & Gorney, 1992; Christenson & Sheridan, 2001). However, as Epstein (1986) has pointed out, although parents want their children to succeed in school, in general, parents are unclear as to how to assist their children to achieve that success. Christenson and Sheridan (2001) provide an excellent review of literature on those family/parent influences on achievement that have been documented to be both positively correlated with student achievement and are manipulable. Of particular relevance here are parental influences involving school–home communications and the structuring of and participation in learning-related activities at home.

A variety of home–school communication strategies are available for consideration. For example, Turnbull and Turnbull (1986) and Christenson and Sheridan (2001) describe and discuss the organization and utility of conferences, informal school visits, telephone calls, log books or notes (see Chapter 5 for a discussion and examples of home–school notes), newsletters, and report cards as viable strategies. In addition, they suggest that school professionals solicit input regarding parent preferences for method and frequency of home–school communication. These strategies can be utilized to foster parental understanding of school programs, as well as to facilitate parental monitoring of student behavior and achievement. In addition, their use can facilitate parental ability to specifically discuss aspects of their children's schooling at home, and to incorporate motivational and feedback strategies around schooling into their routines. Additionally, informed parents can recognize and celebrate student accomplishment(s) on a regular basis, as well as prevent problems and/or manage problems as they arise (see Eddy, Reid, & Curry, 2002, for a discussion of the critical nature of parental monitoring in preventing patterns of antisocial behavior). An important aspect of these activities is their ability to help parents communicate to and teach children that education, learning, and socially appropriate behavior are valued in their homes.

Home-based learning activities also teach children that education and learning are valued. For example, parents can be involved in activities such as monitoring homework completion and discussing school work that are linked to children's classroom assignments and responsibilities. Additionally, parents can foster learning by ensuring that books are available at home; that they themselves spend time reading, enjoying, and discussing books and other reading material; and by providing a variety of opportunities for learning. However, it is quite likely that parents will need assistance in organizing and structuring such activities (for useful information and materials, see Christenson & Sheridan, 2001; Epstein, 1986; Power et al., 2001. Also, it should not be assumed that teachers are familiar with strategies to recommend to parents or comfortable with actually making such recommendations. Working together with parents, however, school psychologists, teachers, and administrators can help to promote parent involvement in activities likely to foster learning and achievement.

COMMUNICATION WITH PHYSICIANS
AND OTHER PROFESSIONALS

The National Association of School Psychologists (2000) *Professional Conduct Manual* reads as follows:

> *Ethical guideline E1.* To best meet the needs of children and other clients, school psychologists cooperate with other professional disciplines in relationships based on mutual respect.
> *Ethical guideline E2.* School psychologists recognize the competence of other professionals. They encourage and support the use of all resources to best serve the interests of children and other clients.
> *Ethical guideline E3.* School psychologists should strive to explain their field and their professional competencies, including roles, assignments, and working relationships to other professionals.
> *Ethical guideline E4.* School psychologists cooperate and coordinate with other professionals and agencies with the rights and needs of children and other clients in mind. If a child or other client is receiving similar services from another professional, school psychologists promote coordination of services.

In our experience, where ADHD is of concern, educators' communication with and referrals to physicians center around two primary issues: the diagnosis of the disorder and medication treatment. In these instances, families should be involved in the decision-making process (e.g., to make a referral) and should always be treated with dignity and respect. In doing so, the person(s) making the referral should patiently help parents to understand the purpose of the referral. For example, it might be communicated to parents that "I am [we are] concerned about your son, and believe that he may be diagnosable with ADHD. In many instances where professionals have such concerns, it is helpful to have the input and opinion of physicians. As such, we would like to refer you to your family pediatrician [or other medical professional] for a professional opinion regarding our concerns." If parents are in agreement with a referral, assistance should be offered to them in the form of a letter (or in some cases, a phone contact) to the referee conveying both the specific concerns being raised and what questions the person making the referral would like to have answered (e.g., diagnostic classification). A sample referral letter is included as Appendix 8.2.

For children who already have been diagnosed with ADHD, a referral might be made to inquire about the appropriateness of a medication trial (see Appendix 8.3). Here, the referral might include information about other interventions that have been attempted or that are in place. In addition, school-based professionals might offer to systematically gather information that could be used to evaluate and monitor medication effects (e.g., using side effects questionnaires, academic performance information, behavior rating scales). In Appendices 8.4 and 8.5, we have included two sample letters discussing the evaluation of a medication trial and its results, respectively. In making professional referrals, it is important to keep in mind appropriate referrals do not prescribe or dictate to other professionals how to practice. Rather, referrals are requests for professional assistance in producing information to answer particular questions; the manner of producing the information or answering the question remains the professional's prerogative.

Finally, when school-based professionals are responsible for children who are being treated with psychoactive medications, a number of issues and questions should be discussed with parents and physicians. For example, who should be responsible for ensuring that a student takes his or her medication, and what happens if a student refuses to take prescribed medication? Who is responsible for assessing side effects and for monitoring medication effects on a student's social, academic, and physical functioning? Who will be making decisions about changes in the medication regimen? How will these tasks be accomplished? How will changes in the student's physical, social and academic functioning be measured in valid and reliable ways? (See Chapter 6, as well as Gadow, 1993, and Brown & Sawyer, 1998, for some suggested answers to these questions.)

COMMUNICATION WITH STUDENTS

The following excerpts outline appropriate communication with students (National Association of School Psychologists, 2000):

Ethical guideline B2. School psychologists explain important aspects of their professional relationships (i.e., to students) in a clear, understandable manner that is appropriate to the child's or other client's age and ability to understand. The explanation includes the reason why services were requested, who will receive information about the services provided, and the possible outcomes.

Ethical guideline B4. Recommendations for program changes or additional services will be discussed with appropriate individuals.

As with parents and physicians, students also should be treated with dignity and respect as they are involved in discussions and communications regarding assessment, diagnosis, and interventions, as well as the actual activities. First, in communicating the results and implications to a student diagnosed with ADHD, care should be taken to utilize language the student is likely to understand. Rather than telling a child that he or she has a disorder, the focus of the discussion should be on individual strengths and weaknesses. The student should be told what strengths and weaknesses were indicated by the evaluation. It should be pointed out that all of his or her classmates have individual strengths and weaknesses, so that he or she is not unique in this regard. Behaviors and weaknesses related to ADHD should be discussed in terms of problems sustaining attention, inhibiting impulses, and controlling activity level especially in certain situations, such as during independent seatwork. The student might be asked to enumerate specific examples of when, where, and how these problems are experienced on a daily basis. It should be emphasized that many students have weaknesses in these areas and that there are some ways to help with these difficulties. Discussion of various treatment modalities would ensue in language that the child will understand. For example, the use of stimulants would be framed in the context of trying to see whether medication would help the student to pay attention better and get more work done. If positive changes occur, the student is reminded that he or she was responsible for these improvements and that the medication merely helped to make these changes possible.

With older adolescents (e.g., high school students), more specific information about ADHD should be communicated (see Barkley & Murphy, 1998, for useful materials). Depending upon the cognitive abilities of the specific student, the handouts and readings recommended for parents and teachers might be provided. Several counseling sessions may be necessary to accurately communicate this information, answer student questions, and provide emotional support. As with younger children, the emphasis of these discussions is not on what the student does wrong, but rather that these weaknesses must be addressed in a long-term fashion with the help of teachers and parents.

Other important issues to discuss with adolescents with ADHD will be ones related to current and future academic support (e.g., test accommodations, adjustments to workload), and planning for postsecondary education, employment, and/or other goals. For students participating in special education services, postsecondary school planning is a required part of such services by law. This type of planning is likely to include parents and take the form of family counseling around issues of future planning for the student (see Robin, 1998, for a thorough discussion of working with adolescents with ADHD and their families), as well as issues of self-advocacy, and knowledge and understanding of available and potential educational and vocational options.

Regardless of the individual focus, in an ongoing fashion, time should be taken to involve students in service delivery decisions (e.g., intervention development and choices when possible) as appropriate. As a general rule for educating students diagnosed with ADHD, in every possible way we will want to convey encouragement, reinforce effort, plan for success, and provide constructive feedback and formative evaluation to promote success.

A primary consideration with children diagnosed with ADHD is the attributions that they develop for their behavior, achievement, and academic progress, especially when they are being treated with stimulant (or other) medication. A small, developing literature in this area (DuPaul et al., 1996; Pelham et al., 1992) suggests that children with ADHD rate both current and predicted behavior more favorably when they have taken medication. Although further work is needed in this area, the reported findings suggest that it is important to consider and evaluate what "messages" children are receiving or sending to others with respect to attributing their behavior to medication or to their own competence. Thus, regardless of whether they have taken their medication or not, all students with ADHD must feel that they themselves are responsible for their own behavior.

SUMMARY

Taking the position that child advocacy and student outcomes should drive professional practice has several implications for the services provided by school psychologists to students who are, or may be, diagnosed with ADHD. It requires a focus on the identification and definition of problems and concerns, in addition to diagnoses. Thus, careful communication with parents, physicians, children, and others set the agenda for assessment procedures and intervention activities.

Our comments regarding educational services for children diagnosed with ADHD have focused briefly on the linkages between diagnosis and educational programming, professional responsibilities, stimulant medication use, and communications with a parents, physicians, and children. Other perspectives and issues are relevant and certainly will arise to challenge professionals, parents, and children alike. The challenge for those involved will be to balance/divide their attention appropriately between the often competing needs to focus not only on legal or procedural requirements related to diagnosis and classification, but on student outcomes. The communication challenge will be to overcome the potential barriers raised by a lack of common vocabulary, training, and perspectives, while building effective interventions through collaboration. However, by initiating and promoting the discussions identified herein, parents, students, and professionals can contribute to improving meaningful student outcomes.

Suggested Readings on ADHD and Related Difficulties for Parents and Teachers

Barkley, R. A. (2000). *Taking charge of ADHD: The complete, authoritative guide for parents* (rev. ed.). New York: Guilford Press.

Christenson, S. L., & Sheridan, S. M. (2001). *Schools and families: Creating essential connections for learning.* New York: Guilford Press.

Forgatch, M. S., & Patterson, G. R. (1989). *Parents and adolescents living together: Part 2. Family problem solving.* Eugene, OR: Castalia.

Fowler, M. (1992). *C.H.A.D.D. educators manual: An in-depth look at attention deficit disorders from an educational perspective.* Plantation, FL: CHADD.

Ingersoll, B. D. (1997). *Daredevils and daydreamers: New perspectives on attention-deficit/hyperactivity disorder.* New York: Doubleday.

Parker, H. C. (1992). *The ADD hyperactivity handbook for schools: Effective strategies for identifying and teaching ADD students in elementary and secondary schools.* Plantation, FL: Impact.

Patterson, G. R., & Forgatch, M. S. (1989). *Parents and adolescents living together: Part 1. The basics.* Eugene, OR: Castalia.

Power, T. J., Karustis, J. L., & Habboushe, D. F. (2001). *Homework success for children with ADHD: A family–school intervention program.* New York: Guilford Press.

Robin, A. L. (1998). *ADHD in adolescents: Diagnosis and treatment.* New York: Guilford Press.

Referral Letter to a Physician

Dr. Janet Williams
755 E. 45th Street
Anywhere, USA

Dear Dr. Williams:

We are writing with a referral question regarding one of your patients, Michael Winston. Michael is a first-grade student with us here at Edgars Elementary, and we have concerns as to whether he might be a child with attention-deficit/hyperactivity disorder. Michael's teacher and our school psychologist have completed systematic observations of Michael's classroom behavior. As compared to his peers, Michael was observed to spend significantly less time engaged in assigned classroom tasks and significantly more time out of his seat and fidgeting while in his seat. At this point, Michael is keeping up with his peers academically, but we are concerned that he frequently does not complete in-class assignments or he completes them quite quickly with little attention to detail. Although, as yet, we have not developed a systematic intervention program for Michael, we are considering developing one. Before doing so, however, we would like your professional opinion as to whether Michael might be diagnosable with ADHD, and, if so, we would appreciate your input as to potential directions for intervention. We would be pleased to provide other information at your request. Thank you for your assistance in this matter.

Sincerely,

School Psychologist   Teacher   School Principal

Referral to Physician
for Possible Medication Trial

Dr. James Smith
The Anytown Clinic
1162 Willams Street
Anytown USA 99999

RE: Billy Buck

Dear Dr. Smith:

As you are aware, we have been working with the above-named student to address his problems with inattention, impulsivity, and overactivity in the classroom. Previously, you had identified Billy as having ADHD. We are writing to provide an update of his progress and to request your input regarding the need for additional intervention (e.g., stimulant medication).

Over the past several months, we have implemented a number of interventions designed to enhance Billy's academic performance and behavior control. These have included a token reinforcement program in the classroom, a home–school communication protocol, and the use of peer tutoring for certain subject areas (e.g., math, spelling). Although these interventions have been helpful, Billy continues to display attentional difficulties throughout the school day and also is very disruptive on the playground and in the lunchroom. We plan to modify and continue these interventions for the remainder of the school year. Nevertheless, we are requesting that you evaluate the need for a stimulant medication trial.

We have discussed the need for this referral with Mr. and Mrs. Buck. They are in agreement with us that further treatment appears necessary. Of course, as with previous cases, we are willing to provide objective data to you regarding Billy's response to stimulant medication.

If you need further information about Billy's school program, please do not hesitate to contact us at any time. We look forward to hearing from you in the near future.

Sincerely,

School Psychologist   Teacher   School Principal

APPENDIX 8.4

♦

Description of Medication
Trial to Physician

Dr. James Smith
The Anytown Clinic
1162 Willams Street
Anytown USA 99999

Dear Dr. Smith:

We are pleased to be working with you and your patient, Thomas Jones, in evaluating the effects of stimulant medication on Thomas's academic and social functioning in school. Enclosed you will find a brief description of the project, its purpose, and goals. I am writing to ask your cooperation in prescribing the medication for the trial. Joan Williams, head pharmacist at the Health Center, has agreed to facilitate packaging of medication for the trial. Joan has agreed to label the separate bottles of medication with a code letter and dates (e.g., methylphenidate, dose A, week of April 14). Of the people involved in administering the medication trial, only you and I will be aware of the actual dose on any medication day. Please write four separate prescriptions as follows, and specify that the prescription is to be filled by the Health Center:

Methylphenidate 5 mg; dispense 6 doses.
Methylphenidate 10 mg; dispense 6 doses.
Methylphenidate 15 mg; dispense 6 doses.

Mrs. Jones will pick up the prescriptions from your office when they are ready. The dates and doses (randomly assigned) of Thomas's medication trial will be as follows:

Dates	Dose
Week of April 7	Baseline
Week of April 14, Monday thru Saturday	10 mg
Week of April 21, Monday thru Saturday	5 mg
Week of April 28, Monday thru Saturday	15 mg

We will provide you with a summary of the results of this evaluation upon completion of the trial. We look forward to working with you. Please contact us if you have any questions.

Sincerely,

School Psychologist   Teacher   School Principal

♦

Report of Results of Medication Trial to Physician

Dr. James Smith
The Anytown Clinic
1162 Willams Street
Anytown USA 99999

Dear Dr. Smith:

We have now completed the methylphenidate evaluation trial for your patient, Thomas Jones. The conditions and dates of the trial were as follows:

Dates	Dose
Week of April 7	Baseline
Week of April 14, Monday thru Saturday	10 mg
Week of April 21, Monday thru Saturday	5 mg
Week of April 28, Monday thru Saturday	15 mg

Ongoing measures consisted of Thomas's reading performance in passages sampled from his curriculum, math performance in basic math skill probes, teacher ratings of classroom behavior and performance, parent ratings of behavior, and side effects ratings completed by Thomas and his mother. A graph of Thomas's reading data is attached. The overall results of the trial are summarized in the table that follows.

Measure	Optimal dose(s)
Daily curriculum-based reading performance	15 mg
Daily math performance	15 mg
Teacher ratings of classroom behavior	10 mg/15 mg
Parent ratings of behavior	15 mg/5 mg

With respect to side effects, some dizziness, irritability, stomachaches, and difficulty sleeping were reported by both Thomas and his mother at both the 10-

---

mg and 15-mg doses. These problems were reported as minor-to-moderate in severity, and tended to diminish over the course of each of these weeks.

The results of this evaluation indicate that the 15-mg dose of methylphenidate optimally enhanced Thomas's behavior across social and academic performance measures. Should methylphenidate be prescribed for Thomas at this dose, side effects should be carefully monitored. We hope that you find the results of this evaluation to be useful to you in your work with Thomas and his family. If we can be of further assistance with Thomas or other children, please do not hesitate to contact us.

Sincerely,

School Psychologist   Teacher   School Principal

THOMAS J.: READING PERFORMANCE

CHAPTER 9

◆ ◆ ◆

Conclusions and
Future Directions

◆

Meeting the needs of students with ADHD presents significant challenges to educational personnel. The hallmark characteristics of this disorder (i.e., inattention, impulsivity, and overactivity) often lead to disruptions of classroom decorum, academic underachievement, and difficulties making and keeping friends. Each of the characteristics comprising ADHD appears to exist on a continuum (i.e., normal curve) within the population such that the upper 2–5% of children in a given age and gender group could be diagnosed with the disorder. Furthermore, there is an additional 5% of children in a given population who are just out of the range of "clinically diagnosable" ADHD who present with significant, albeit less severe, attention and behavior control problems. Thus, in a general education classroom of 25 children, a teacher would be faced with at least two or three students who have notable difficulties attending to instructional activities and complying with classroom and school rules.

The academic performance of most children with ADHD is deficient due to their poor study habits, lack of work completion, and inconsistent accuracy on seatwork, homework, and tests. In addition, about one-third of these students are significantly below average in academic skills, and therefore are identified as having a learning disability. Over the past decade, changes to federal guidelines have allowed for the provision of special education services to children with ADHD solely on the basis of this disorder limiting their educational performance. Special education eligibility decisions should be made by conducting a reliable and valid assessment of ADHD and related problems, determining the degree to which the child's ADHD impacts his or her academic and social functioning, and evaluating the success of interventions in general education classrooms for ameliorating behaviors related to the disorder.

The first step in addressing the needs of children referred for problems consistent with ADHD is to conduct comprehensive psychological and, if necessary, educational evaluations. The school-based assessment of ADHD is comprised of multiple techniques utilized across a variety of settings (e.g., classroom, playground) and sources of information (e.g., parent, teacher, and child). Following a teacher referral for possible ADHD, five stages of assessment are conducted, including initial screening for ADHD symptoms, multimethod assessment, interpretation of results to reach a classification decision, development of a multimodal treatment plan, and ongoing monitoring of progress resulting from intervention(s).

Reaching a diagnosis of ADHD does not signal the end of the evaluation process, nor is it the ultimate goal of an assessment. Rather, the value of the initial assessment lies in the determination of an intervention plan whose success is linked to the information gathered in the evaluation process. The use of behavioral methodologies, including parent and teacher interviews, parent and teacher rating scales, direct observations of school behavior, and collection of academic performance data, is the optimal way to address both goals of the evaluation. These assessment data continue to be collected throughout treatment to determine the efficacy and/or limitations of the various components of an intervention program.

The most effective psychosocial interventions are those based on principles of operant conditioning and social learning theory. Typically, these include reactive or consequence-based strategies such as token reinforcement systems, response cost, and self-management interventions. We have articulated a need to develop balanced intervention plans that include both reactive and proactive procedures. The latter include strategies (e.g., choice making and peer tutoring) that involve changes to antecedent conditions in order to prevent disruptive or inappropriate behaviors. Treatment targets include maladaptive behaviors (e.g., inattention to task) to be reduced, as well as competencies (e.g., academic performance, social acceptance) to be enhanced. In fact, when adaptive behaviors are increased, disruptive actions usually are diminished in frequency due to the inherent incompatibilities between these two classes of behavior. Therefore, proactive and positive reinforcement procedures are emphasized, with the realization that mild punishment strategies will be necessary, in some cases, to curtail off-task and/or aggressive actions.

For many children with ADHD the optimal treatment approach may be the combination of behavioral interventions with psycho-stimulant medication (e.g., methylphenidate). In school settings, stimulant medication can enhance the attention span, task completion and accuracy, and compliance with classroom rules of the majority of treated children. Given that the behavioral effects of stimulants are moderated by dose and individual responsivity, each child's treatment response *must* be assessed in an objective manner across a range of therapeutic doses. School-based professionals should play a major role in helping physicians to evaluate stimulant-induced changes in children's behavior across a variety of crucial functioning areas (e.g., educational performance, social relationships, and compliance with classroom rules). A subset of the same methods that were used in the initial evaluation of ADHD can be tapped on a continuous basis over several weeks to objectively determine whether an individual responds to pharmacotherapy and which dose optimizes the student's academic and social functioning.

Regardless of the well-established efficacy of stimulant medication and behavioral interventions, no single treatment approach will be sufficient in ameliorating ADHD-related difficulties. The chronic exhibition of problem behaviors across settings and with different caretakers likely will necessitate the implementation of a multimodal treatment approach over several years or longer. A number of intervention strategies can be used to supplement the use of classroom behavioral interventions and psychotropic medications. These may include both school-based (e.g., social skills training) and home-based (e.g., parent training) treatments. The focus must be on designing an effective comprehensive program to treat a variety of functional areas while acknowledging the necessity for long-term treatment. Concurrently, educators and parents, in particular, will need to set their sights on achieving short-term objectives throughout the school year to promote gradual improvements in the child's overall adjustment.

School-based professionals should carefully evaluate the documented efficacy of proposed treatments for ADHD, as there are a number of therapies that have been touted as "effective" in the treatment of this disorder (e.g., Feingold diet) that actually have limited or no empirical support. Given the allure of alternatives to medication or behavior modification among the general public, it is important that someone on the child's treatment team take a cautious, data-based stance toward newly proposed therapies that are purported to "cure" ADHD. Specifically, the quality and quantity of empirical support for the treatment should be evaluated closely. More often than not, it is necessary to point out the limitations of unsupported treatment modalities in an effort to maintain energy and resources focused on those interventions more likely to help the child.

Usually, a number of individuals are involved in the treatment of a child diagnosed with ADHD. Thus, the student and his or her parents often interact with both school-based (e.g., teachers, school psychologists, administrators, school nurse, and guidance counselors) and community-based (e.g., physician, clinical psychologist) professionals. This necessitates the adoption of a team approach to treatment wherein the provision of services is coordinated across professionals through ongoing communication. Unfortunately, the latter is more of an ideal than a commonplace circumstance in the real world. Nevertheless, it is assumed that the more teamwork is involved in treatment, the better the outcome for the child.

The team approach can be fostered by ensuring that all school professionals are aware of what ADHD is, how to identify students who may potentially require intervention, and how to treat problems related to the disorder. Educators aligned with both general and special education need to understand that ADHD-related behaviors are chronic and rarely fully eliminated, especially in the context of a single academic year. Thus, the focus of professional efforts should be on modifying the classroom and school environment to meet the needs of students with this disorder in order to promote attainment of short-term goals. As short-term improvements in attention, impulse control, and activity level are attained, gradual progress toward long-term amelioration of these problems is achieved. However, in our experience, to maintain the motivation of the student and treatment team members, it is necessary to promote concentration on making "small gains" rather than achieving a permanent "cure" within a short time period.

FUTURE DIRECTIONS FOR WORKING WITH STUDENTS WITH ADHD

Although there has been substantial progress over the past several decades in the school-based identification and treatment of students with ADHD, significant work remains to be done in a number of key areas. First, minimal attention has been paid to the difficulties and needs of middle, junior high, and senior high school students with ADHD. The latter typically exhibit myriad adjustment problems across academic, social, and behavioral areas of functioning. Given the greater emphasis on independence and individual responsibility for one's own behavior during the adolescent years, it is particularly crucial to determine the types of programming that will enhance scholastic success for these students. Second, the roles and responsibilities of school-based "case managers" must be delineated. Even during the elementary school years, students with ADHD work with a variety of professionals, thus implicating the need for someone to coordinate communication and services across home, school, and community environments. Third, instruction in how to meet the educational and behavioral needs of children with ADHD must occur at the preservice level of training (i.e., prior to receiving teacher certification) for both general educators and special education personnel. Currently, many teachers are not adequately prepared to work effectively with such children even after attending in-service workshops or reading relevant professional literature. Fourth, empirical investigations are sorely needed to determine practical, time-efficient ways to manage the behavior control difficulties associated with ADHD, while simultaneously enhancing the academic and social competencies of children and adolescents with this disorder.

Meeting the Needs of Adolescents with ADHD

As students with ADHD move from elementary school to middle school and beyond, they face a plethora of developmental "hurdles" that are substantially "higher" for them than for their peers. Furthermore, secondary settings are characteristically more demanding with respect to student organizational abilities, academic skills, and self-directedness. Specifically, secondary school students are expected to be able to study for tests and display adequate organizational skills (e.g., keep a neat notebook), as well as plan for their future beyond high school. It is presumed that if students with ADHD are able to meet the latter expectations then their chances for successful adjustment as adults are enhanced.

In most secondary schools, minimal instruction in study and organizational skills is provided. Students are assumed to develop these skills as they progress through the grade levels as a function of their burgeoning cognitive and emotional maturation. Although this assumption may be valid for many adolescents, it is clear that many students with ADHD do not acquire adequate study skills and that their academic performance is compromised accordingly (see Chapter 5 for additional discussion of study skills intervention). Thus, direct instruction in study and organizational strategies (for a review, see Gleason, Archer, & Colvin, 2002) must be provided to these students as early as possible in their schooling.

Despite the multiple and complex needs of adolescents with ADHD, minimal empirical work has been done with this age group. In fact, in their meta-analysis, DuPaul and Eckert (1997) found only a handful of research studies that have examined school interventions for secondary students with ADHD. Despite the dearth of research with adolescents, certain guidelines should be followed:

1. Initial instruction in how to study for tests and proper note taking should take place in the later elementary and early middle school years (i.e., fifth and sixth grades), when homework and long-term projects become more demanding. This instruction should be provided by either the general education classroom teacher or support personnel (e.g., guidance counselor, school psychologist) on an ongoing basis with ample opportunity for supervised practice.

2. Students with ADHD should be required to keep homework assignment books as soon as substantial amounts (i.e., more than 30 minutes per night) of such work are required. Both short- and long-term assignments should be recorded in this book. Initially, the teacher should check and initial the assignment book at the end of each school day to ensure that the proper assignments are recorded. Furthermore, parents should review the assignment book prior to each homework session to make sure that the student understands what is required. Home-based contingencies (e.g., preferred free-time activities) should be directly linked to compliance with assignment book responsibilities. The latter component is crucial because many youngsters with ADHD will not consistently write down their assignments unless there is a direct "payoff" for doing so. As the student demonstrates greater levels of individual responsibility in using the assignment book, the level of supervision by teachers and parents can be reduced. Nevertheless, students with ADHD should continue to be required to keep an assignment book throughout their schooling.

3. Compensations for the attentional and organizational deficits associated with ADHD should be made. First, these students should be allowed to tape-record lectures as a supplement to note taking. This is particularly helpful when the child is taught how to take notes by making transcriptions of the audiotaped lecture under the supervision of a teacher, older student, or peer. Second, an extra set of textbooks should be kept at home during the school year to prevent missed opportunities to complete homework assignments due to "forgetting" appropriate texts.

4. Continued direct instruction and monitoring of study, note-taking, and organizational skills may be necessary across several grade levels and should be considered an integral component of school-based programming for many adolescents with ADHD.

Although the above suggestions for educational practice are presumed to lead to improved student outcomes, there are still important questions in this domain that remain to be answered. At the most basic level, what are the specific deficits that students with ADHD demonstrate in the areas of study and organizational skills? Do these deficits endure over time, or are there some areas that improve or worsen as the child progresses through the grades? In terms of intervention, what are the best ways to teach study and organizational skills to this group of students? Should modes of instruction vary as a function of individual characteristics (e.g., presence of learning disabilities, grade level of the child)? Finally, what are the long-term effects of instruction in study skills? Do improvements in this area generalize across academic subjects and maintain over time? Is periodic monitoring and instruction in this functioning area necessary to ensure more durable improvements? Does study skill instruction make a difference in the eventual academic outcome of students with ADHD? Answers to these questions will certainly aid in promoting our ability to help these students in this crucial area of competence for independent learning.

In a related area of concern, as a function of their impulsivity, youngsters with ADHD frequently do not consider the long-term consequences of their actions, nor do they plan ahead with any consistency. Thus, students with this disorder often require greater guidance in planning for postsecondary school activities (i.e., entering the workforce or college). Although vocational and educational counseling are typically proffered to all secondary-level students at varying degrees of intensity, it is particularly crucial for individuals with ADHD to receive ongoing intensive advising in this area. The identification of interests and strengths at an earlier age than is common for other children may be necessary for students with this disorder. This should not be an effort to "pigeonhole" a child into one track (e.g., vocational education) versus another (e.g., college preparatory courses), but rather to encourage the student to develop a focus or interest area that will maintain his or her motivation for continuing schooling. One of the greatest risks facing this population is a loss of interest in education, resulting in leaving school prematurely. Thus, helping the child to look ahead and plan for the future may spur an interest in school, even if such interest is limited to selected subject areas. Beginning in middle school and continuing through each high school grade, students with ADHD should meet regularly with their guidance counselors or related personnel so that the latter can provide continuous assessment and programming related to vocational/collegiate aspirations.

As in the case of study skills, little empirical work has been conducted in the area of vocational programming for students with this disorder. We need information as to methods of career and academic counseling that are best suited to students with attention problems. How early in the child's educational program should interest assessment and vocational counseling take place? How frequent and specific must this counseling be to ensure greater success? What are the possible iatrogenic effects (e.g., premature determination of postsecondary plans) of career guidance and how can these be minimized? What methods can be used to encourage youngsters to take greater levels of responsibility for their own future? Even though most professionals working with these students would agree that this is a crucial area of investigation, it has received scant empirical attention to date.

The Use of a School-Based Case Manager

The successful treatment of ADHD frequently requires coordination of services among parents, student, teachers, other school professionals, physicians, and community-based service providers (e.g., clinical child psychologists). All too often, service providers associated with a given student's treatment program work independently of each other with little consistent communication occurring among them. This state of affairs increases the potential for redundancy of services or, worse still, the provision of conflicting treatment advice to parents and children. It seems reasonable to assume that effective communication among treatment team members and coordination of services could be enhanced by the efforts of one person serving in the role of a case manager. As children with ADHD spend much of their day in school settings, one cost-effective possibility is for a school-based professional (e.g., school psychologist) to take on case manager responsibilities (for additional discussion of the role of the case manager, see Power, Atkins, Osborne, & Blum, 1994).

An effective case manager would provide the following services to the child and treatment team:

1. Serve as the liaison between the school and the home by communicating on a regular basis with the student's teachers and parents. In addition, the case manager would have regular contact with all community-based professionals (e.g., physician) working with the student.

2. Coordinate school-based programming among teachers at the middle, junior high, or senior high school level. Either the case manager would meet with each teacher individually or would lead "team" meetings on a regular basis. This process would facilitate consistency in programming across classrooms while preventing potential miscommunication that could lead to ineffective treatment.

3. Coordinate home–school contingency management programming. When home-based contingencies are tied to a child's school performance, consistent communication between the student's parents and teachers is crucial. Also, it is important that all participants in the program are cognizant of their responsibilities and adhere to the tenets of the intervention. Intervention adherence can be facilitated by the case manager through maintaining contact with parents and teachers, as well as by periodically convening "team" meetings to assess progress and make changes in the format or content of the home–school program.

4. Communicate with physicians regarding medication effects on school behavior and academic performance. The importance of school-based data in determining a child's medication response as well as delineating an individual's optimal dose was discussed in Chapter 6. Having a designated person serve as the link between the physician and the school greatly enhances the probability of effective medication monitoring, and therefore improved outcomes. Thus, the case manager would collate and communicate information regarding changes in the child's school performance to the physician during the initial evaluation of medication response (see Appendices 8.4 and 8.5). In addition, he or she could apprise the physician and/or parents of any unusual changes in the child's behavior that may be occurring as a result of long-term medication administration. Also, the case manager could serve as a go-between when any changes in the child's medication or dosage need to be communicated by the parent or physician to members of the student's school-based team.

5. Serve as a child advocate to facilitate obtaining appropriate school- and community-based services. The case manager should develop an overview of the types of services that a student with ADHD may require versus those currently available. When gaps are found between existing and necessary services, the case manager should advocate for changes in the child's educational and community-based programming with appropriate members of the treatment team (e.g., school administrators, parents). In addition, advocacy for greater professional attention to student outcomes may be warranted.

The above list of case manager responsibilities is not intended to be exhaustive: there may well be other roles that the case manager could serve depending upon the child's needs. Furthermore, each of these responsibilities may not be pertinent in some cases. Nevertheless, there is a strong need for a single person to coordinate services on an ongoing basis. In many cases, this should be a school-based professional who can follow a child's education across grade levels (e.g., school psychologist or guidance counselor). School-based professionals have the advantage of daily contact with the child's teachers as well as the opportunity to make contacts with parents and community-based members of the child's treatment team. Ongoing coordination of services and communication among team members is assumed to enhance the overall efficacy of long-term treatment of this disorder.

Preservice Training in ADHD

One of the most frequent complaints voiced by parents of children with ADHD is that their children's teachers do not appear to have any background in working with students who have this disorder. Many teachers, particularly those in general education classrooms, readily acknowledge their limitations in working with these students. To address this problem, school systems have endeavored to provide in-service training to their staff in ways to identify, teach, and manage these children in both general and special education settings. Unfortunately, there are no empirical data to indicate that brief didactic training in how to work with children who have ADHD is effective in enhancing the knowledge and skills of educators. In fact, it appears that many teachers are not adequately prepared to work effectively with such children even after attending in-service workshops or reading the relevant professional literature.

Given this state of affairs, instruction in how to meet the educational and behavioral needs of children with ADHD should occur at the preservice level of training (i.e., prior to receiving teacher certification) for all teachers in training, as well as other school personnel. This training would afford the opportunity to provide not only didactic instruction in ADHD, but also supervised practice in effective teaching and behavior management strategies. The fact that every educator will typically work with *at least* one student who has ADHD per school year would warrant that this proposal receive serious consideration. Unfortunately, at the present time, intensive training in working with such children usually does not occur at the preservice level.

Although it seems reasonable to assume that preservice training in ADHD will enhance educators' skills in working with these children, there are currently no empirical data to support this claim. Thus, the efficacy of preservice training in ADHD should be examined in detail. Specifically, what training activities lead to greater levels of understanding of this disorder and an enhancement of teaching and management skills? Will the combination of didactic instruction, assigned readings, and supervised practice sufficiently prepare teachers to work effectively with this population? Are other training modalities (e.g., practicum placement in school for children with behavior disorders) necessary to teach adequate levels of skills in this area? These are important questions because adequate preservice training for teachers represents a proactive (i.e., preventative) model of service delivery for students with ADHD, and ultimately could reduce the need for more costly, more intensive programming at a later date.

School-Based Research on ADHD

Although various behavioral and cognitive-behavioral interventions for ADHD have been found effective in empirical studies (DuPaul & Eckert, 1997), there is still a great deal to be learned about how to enhance the school performance of students who have this disorder. Relative to the voluminous research literature examining stimulant medication treatment of this disorder, consideration of school-based, psychosocial, and instructional interventions is in its infancy. There are many directions that could be taken in this area; some of the more practice-relevant dimensions for future research are identified below.

Behavioral interventions that have been employed for ADHD are quite diverse in scope, content, and intensity. Little is known about the relative efficacies of intervention components (e.g., token reinforcement vs. response cost). What are the sufficient components of behavioral interventions for ADHD and how much should programming vary as a function of individual (e.g., age, gender, severity of the disorder) and environmental (e.g., general education vs. special education placement, level of teacher stress) factors? Practitioners need to know not only whether an intervention will work, but also which treatment will be most effective under a given set of circumstances.

Most of the intervention research has focused on manipulating consequences to change the behavior of students with ADHD. There is a dearth of information on what antecedent events (i.e., proactive procedures) can be used to reduce problematic behaviors and enhance academic performance. What are the most effective ways to present academic material to students with ADHD? Will the efficacy of various modes of instruction vary as a function of the behavioral and academic profile of the child? How can we improve children's attention to task directions? Are there ways that we can alter the stimulation level of academic material such that children with ADHD will be more likely to complete their work in a timely and accurate fashion? Greater knowledge of effective ways to manipulate antecedent events would presumably aid in preventing and/or reducing the severity of many of the behavioral control difficulties associated with this disorder, while enhancing academic skill achievement and performance.

Even though behavioral interventions have been found effective for

ADHD, these treatments often are not employed in classrooms. Despite their effectiveness, teachers frequently find such procedures unacceptable due to time constraints, lack of resources, or philosophical differences with the approach to intervening (Witt & Elliott, 1985). In other words, many interventions that work well in a research paradigm are not perceived to be very practical, particularly when implemented in general education classrooms. Thus, we need to know how to increase the acceptability of effective interventions. It is not enough to establish that a treatment works, we also must know if it is acceptable to the "consumers" (i.e., teachers, parents, and students) of these interventions. Are there modifications that can be made to currently available interventions that will increase their acceptability and hence their adoption into practice? How can the efficacy of interventions that have greater levels of acceptability, such as self-management strategies, be increased? The true test of whether research in this area contributes to practice will be the degree to which teachers and other school personnel actually implement empirically valid procedures on a consistent basis over lengthy time periods.

Researchers in the field of ADHD must develop and evaluate other methods for working with these children in school settings. This work should be aimed at directly enhancing educational outcomes rather than primarily controlling student problem behaviors. For example, procedures discussed in Chapter 5 included peer-mediated interventions and computer-assisted instruction. These technologies have great promise for students with ADHD, but they have not been studied in any great detail. Furthermore, it is unclear what process is optimal for deciding what academic interventions to employ in a given situation and whether ongoing modifications are needed to these strategies. For example, a data-based problem-solving model frequently is recommended for designing academic interventions (Elliott, Witt, Kratochwill, & Stoiber, 2002); however, there are no data regarding the cost-effectiveness of this model for making treatment decisions for students with ADHD. Does this more time-intensive model lead to greater improvements in academic performance relative to typical intervention design procedures that are more trial-and-error in nature?

Finally, with the current interpretation of federal regulations for special education, there is a great need to establish how and under what conditions children with ADHD might qualify for special services. Currently, the guidelines are quite vague as to how qualification decisions might be made. School systems are left to determine on their own how students with ADHD may be eligible for special education services. In an ideal world, there would be empirical guidelines available to facilitate eligibility decisions and to lead to effective programming. Under what conditions might students with ADHD benefit from special education? What assessment measures should be used to determine eligibility? What role do community-based professionals (e.g., physicians) play in making such decisions? What components should be included in a special education program for these students? Are these interventions different from what is currently available for students identified with learning disabilities and emotional disturbances? Certainly, these issues deserve further investigation.

CONCLUSIONS

It is quite humbling to realize that although our understanding of ADHD has been greatly advanced over the last several decades, children with this disorder continue to encounter significant difficulties succeeding in our schools. To correct this situation, gains must be made in two major areas. First, practitioners in the fields of psychology and education must increase their awareness and understanding of the limitations of students with this disorder. Those professionals possessing expertise in working with such children must educate their colleagues to be similarly proficient. Children with this disorder are encountered in every type of school setting. Therefore, all educators should possess, at the least, minimal competencies in identifying these children and designing effective educational programming to meet their needs and to help them to become successful, productive citizens. Second, the technology of assessing and treating children with ADHD must be improved. Assessment methodologies must be developed that go beyond the reports of significant others in order to enhance the ecological validity of the evaluation process. Third, treatment modalities that are effective on the one hand, while cost-efficient and acceptable to consumers, are sorely needed. Thus, the challenge is for research to lead to effective practice such that long-term improvements in school performance are attained for all children with ADHD. Until that goal is reached, however, the many suggestions contained herein can serve as starting points for guiding current practices to improve educational outcomes for these students.

References

♦

Abikoff, H. (1985). Efficacy of cognitive training intervention in hyperactive children: A critical review. *Clinical Psychology Review, 5,* 479–512.

Abikoff, H., & Gittelman, R. (1985). The normalizing effects of methylphenidate on the classroom behavior of ADDH children. *Journal of Abnormal Child Psychology, 13,* 33–44.

Abikoff, H., Gittelman-Klein, R., & Klein, D. (1977). Validation of a classroom observation code for hyperactive children. *Journal of Consulting and Clinical Psychology, 45,* 772–783.

Abramowitz, A. J., Eckstrand, D., O'Leary, S. G., & Dulcan, M. K. (1992). ADHD children's responses to stimulant medication and two intensities of a behavioral intervention. *Behavior Modification, 16,* 193–203.

Abramowitz, A. J., O'Leary, S. G., & Rosen, L. A. (1987). Reducing off-task behavior in the classroom: A comparison of encouragement and reprimands. *Journal of Abnormal Child Psychology, 15,* 153–163.

Achenbach, T. M. (1991a). *Manual for the Child Behavior Checklist and Revised Child Behavior Profile.* Burlington: University of Vermont, Department of Psychiatry.

Achenbach, T. M. (1991b). *Manual for the Teacher Report Form.* Burlington: University of Vermont, Department of Psychiatry.

Achenbach, T. M. (1991c). *Manual for the Youth Self-Report and 1991 Profile.* Burlington: University of Vermont, Department of Psychiatry.

Achenbach, T. M., & McConaughy, S. H. (1996). Relations between DSM-IV and empirically based assessment. *School Psychology Review, 25,* 329–341.

Achenbach, T. M., & Rescorla, L. A. (2000). *Manual for the ASEBA Preschool Forms and Profiles.* Burlington: University of Vermont, Department of Psychiatry.

Adams, M. J. (1990). *Beginning to read: Thinking and learning about print.* Cambridge, MA: MIT Press.

American Academy of Child and Adolescent Psychiatry. (2002). Practice parameter for the use of stimulant medications in the treatment of children, adolescents, and adults. *Journal of the American Academy of Child and Adolescent Psychiatry, 41*(2, Suppl.), 26S–49S.

American Academy of Pediatrics. (1999). *TIPP—The Injury Prevention Program.* Elk Grove Village, IL: Author.

American Academy of Pediatrics. (2000). Clinical practice guideline: Diagnosis and evaluation of the child with attention-deficit/hyperactivity disorder. *Pediatrics, 105,* 109–133.

American Academy of Pediatrics. (2001). Clinical practice guideline: Treatment of the child with attention-deficit/hyperactivity disorder. *Pediatrics, 105,* 1158–1170.

American Psychiatric Association. (1980). *Diagnostic and statistical manual of mental disorders* (3rd ed.). Washington, DC: Author.

American Psychiatric Association. (1987). *Diagnostic and statistical manual of mental disorders* (3rd ed., rev.). Washington, DC: Author.

American Psychiatric Association. (1994). *Diagnostic and statistical manual of mental disorders* (4th ed.). Washington, DC: Author.

American Psychiatric Association (2000). *Diagnostic and statistical manual of of mental disorders* (4th ed., rev.). Washington, DC: Author.

Anastopoulos, A. D., & Shelton, T. L. (2001). *Assessing attention-deficit/hyperactivity disorder.* New York: Kluwer Academic/Plenum Press.

Anastopoulos, A. D., Shelton, T. L., DuPaul, G. J., & Guevremont, D. C. (1993). Parent training for attention deficit hyperactivity disorder: Its impact on parent functioning. *Journal of Abnormal Child Psychology, 21,* 581–596.

Anastopoulos, A. D., Smith, J. M., & Wein, E. E. (1998). Counseling and training parents. In R. A. Barkley, *Attention-deficit hyperactivity disorder: A handbook for diagnosis and treatment* (2nd ed., pp. 373–393). New York: Guilford Press.

Anastopoulos, A. D., Spisto, M. A., & Maher, M. (1994). The WISC-III Freedom from Distractibility factor: Its utility in identifying children with attention deficit hyperactivity disorder. *Psychological Assessment, 6,* 368–371.

Anderson, R. C., Hiebert, E. H., Scott, J. A., & Wilkinson, I. A. G. (1985). *Becoming a nation of readers: The report of the commission on reading.* Washington, DC: National Institute of Education, U. S. Department of Education. (Available from the Center for the Study of Reading, University of Illinois, Champaign.)

Anesko, K. M., Schoiock, G., Ramirez, R., & Levine, F. M. (1987). The Homework Problem Checklist: Assessing children's homework difficulties. *Behavioral Assessment, 9,* 179–185.

Ang, R. P., & Hughes, J. N. (2002). Differential benefits of skills training with antisocial youth based on group composition: A meta-analytic investigation. *School Psychology Review, 31,* 164–185.

Archer, A., & Gleason, M. (1989). *Skills for school success (grades 3–6).* North Billerica, MA: Curriculum Associates.

Atkeson, B. M., & Forehand, R. (1979). Home-based reinforcement programs designed to modify classroom behavior: A review and methodological evaluation. *Psychological Bulletin, 86,* 1298–1308.

Atkins, M. S., Pelham, W. E., & Licht, M. H. (1985). A comparison of objective classroom measures and teacher ratings of attention deficit disorder. *Journal of Abnormal Child Psychology, 13,* 155–167.

August, G. J., & Garfinkel, G. D. (1989). Behavioral and cognitive subtypes of ADHD. *Journal of the American Academy of Child and Adolescent Psychiatry, 28,* 739–748.

August, G. J., & Garfinkel, G. D. (1990). Comorbidity of ADHD and reading disability among clinic-referred children. *Journal of Abnormal Child Psychology, 18,* 29–45.

August, G. J., & Holmes, C. S. (1984). Behavior and academic achievement in hyperactive subgroups and learning-disabled boys: A six-year follow-up. *American Journal of Diseases in Children, 138,* 1025–1029.

Ayllon, T., Layman, D., & Kandel, H. (1975). A behavioral–educational alternative to drug control of hyperactive children. *Journal of Applied Behavior Analysis, 8,* 137–146.

Baker, S., Gersten, R., & Grossen, B. (2002). Interventions for students with reading comprehension problems. In M. R. Shinn, H. M. Walker, & G. Stoner (Eds.), *Interventions for academic and behavior problems, II: Preventive and remedial approaches* (pp. 731–754). Bethesda, MD: National Association of School Psychologists.

Bambara, L. M., & Knoster, T. P. (1995). *Guidelines: Effective behavioral support.* Harrisburg: Pennsylvania Department of Education, Bureau of Special Education.

Bardon, J. I. (1988). Alternative educational delivery approaches: Implications for school psychology. In J. L. Graden, J. E. Zins, & M. J. Curtis (Eds.), *Alternative educational delivery systems: Enhancing instructional options for all students* (pp. 563–571). Washington, DC: National Association of School Psychologists.

Barkley, R. A. (1979). Using stimulant drugs in the classroom. *School Psychology Digest, 8,* 412–425.

Barkley, R. A. (1988). The effects of methylphenidate on the interactions of preschool ADHD children with their mothers. *Journal of the American Academy of Child and Adolescent Psychiatry, 27,* 336–341.

Barkley, R. A. (1989). Attention-deficit hyperactivity disorder. In E. J. Mash & R. A. Barkley (Eds.), *Treatment of childhood disorders* (pp. 39–72). New York: Guilford Press.

Barkley, R. A. (1990). *Attention-deficit hyperactivity disorder: A handbook for diagnosis and treatment.* New York: Guilford Press.

Barkley, R. A. (1991). The ecological validity of laboratory and analogue assessment methods of ADHD symptoms. *Journal of Abnormal Child Psychology, 19,* 149–178.

Barkley, R. A. (1997a). *ADHD and the nature of self-control.* New York: Guilford Press.

Barkley, R. A. (1997b). *Defiant children: A clinician's manual for assessment and parent training* (2nd ed.). New York: Guilford Press.

Barkley, R. A. (1998). *Attention-deficit hyperactivity disorder: A handbook for diagnosis and treatment* (2nd ed.). New York: Guilford Press.

Barkley, R. A. (2000). *Taking charge of ADHD: The complete, authoritative guide for parents* (rev. ed.). New York: Guilford Press.

Barkley, R. A. (2002). International consensus statement on ADHD. *Clinical Child and Family Psychology Review, 5,* 89–111.

Barkley, R. A., Anastopoulos, A. D., Guevremont, D. C., & Fletcher, K. E. (1991). Adolescents with attention deficit hyperactivity disorder: Patterns of behavioral adjustment, academic functioning, and treatment utilization. *Journal of the American Academy of Child and Adolescent Psychiatry, 30,* 752–861.

Barkley, R. A., & Biederman, J. (1997). Towards a broader definition of the age of onset criterion for attention deficit hyperactivity disorder. *Journal of the American Academy of Child and Adolescent Psychiatry, 36,* 1204–1210.

Barkley, R. A., Copeland, A., & Sivage, C. (1980). A self-control classroom for hyperactive children. *Journal of Autism and Developmental Disorders, 10,* 75–89.

Barkley, R. A., & Cunningham, C. E. (1978). Do stimulant drugs improve the academic performance of hyperkinetic children?: A review of outcome research. *Journal of Clinical Pediatrics, 17,* 85–92.

Barkley, R. A., DuPaul, G. J., & McMurray, M. B. (1990). A comprehensive evaluation of attention deficit disorder with and without hyperactivity as defined by research criteria. *Journal of Consulting and Clinical Psychology, 58,* 775–789.

Barkley, R. A., DuPaul, G. J., & McMurray, M. B. (1991). Attention deficit disorder with and without hyperactivity: Clinical response to three dose levels of methylphenidate. *Pediatrics, 87,* 519–531.

Barkley, R. A., Edwards, G., Laneri, M., Fletcher, K., & Metevia, L. (2001). The efficacy of problem-solving communication training alone, behavior management training alone, and their combination for parent–adolescent conflict in teenagers with ADHD and ODD. *Journal of Consulting and Clinical Psychology, 69,* 926–941.

Barkley, R. A., Fischer, M., Edelbrock, C. S., & Smallish, L. (1990). The adolescent outcome of hyperactive children diagnosed by research criteria: I. An 8-year prospective follow-up study. *Journal of the American Academy of Child and Adolescent Psychiatry, 29,* 546–557.

Barkley, R. A., Fischer, M., Newby, R., & Breen, M. (1988). Development of a multi-method clinical protocol for assessing stimulant drug responses in ADHD children. *Journal of Clinical Child Psychology, 17,* 14–24.

Barkley, R. A., Fischer, M., Smallish, L., & Fletcher, K. (2002). The persistence of attention-deficit/hyperactivity disorder into young adulthood as a function of reporting source and definition of disorder. *Journal of Abnormal Psychology, 111,* 279–289.

Barkley, R. A., Grodzinsky, G., & DuPaul, G. J. (1992). Frontal lobe functions in attention deficit disorder with and without hyperactivity: A review and research report. *Journal of Abnormal Child Psychology, 20,* 163–188.

Barkley, R. A., Guevremont, D. C., Anastopoulos, A. D., DuPaul, G. J., & Shelton, T. L. (1993). Driving-related risks and outcomes of attention deficit hyperactivity disorder in adolescents and young adults: A 3–5 year follow-up survey. *Pediatrics, 92,* 212–218.

Barkley, R. A., Guevremont, D. C., Anastopoulos, A. D., & Fletcher, K. E. (1992). A comparison of three family therapy programs for treating family conflicts in adolescents with attention-deficit hyperactivity disorder. *Journal of Consulting and Clinical Psychology, 60,* 450–462.

Barkley, R. A., Karlsson, J., Strzelecki, E., & Murphy, J. (1984). Effects of age and Ritalin dosage on the mother–child interactions of hyperactive children. *Journal of Consulting and Clinical Psychology, 52,* 750–758.

Barkley, R. A., McMurray, M. B., Edelbrock, C. S., & Robbins, K. (1989). The response of aggressive and non-aggressive ADHD children to two doses of methylphenidate. *Journal of the American Academy of Child and Adolescent Psychiatry, 28,* 873–881.

Barkley, R. A., McMurray, M. B., Edelbrock, C. S., & Robbins, K. (1990). The side effects of Ritalin in ADHD children: A systematic placebo-controlled evaluation of two doses. *Pediatrics, 86,* 184–192.

Barkley, R. A., & Murphy, K. R. (1998). *Attention-deficit hyperactivity disorder: A clinical workbook* (2nd ed.). New York: Guilford Press.

Barkley, R. A., Murphy, K., DuPaul, G. J., & Bush, T. (2002). Driving knowledge, performance, and adverse outcomes in teens and young adults with attention deficit hyperactivity disorder. *Journal of the International Neuropsychological Society, 8,* 655–672.

Barkley, R. A., Shelton, T. L., Crosswait, C., Moorehouse, M., Fletcher, K., Barrett, S., Jenkins, L., & Metevia, L. (2000). Multi-method psychoeducational intervention for preschool children with disruptive behavior: Preliminary results at post-treatment. *Journal of Child Psychology and Psychiatry, 41,* 319–332.

Barlow, D. H. (Ed.). (1981). *Behavioral assessment of adult disorders.* New York: Guilford Press.

Barnett, D. W., Hamlet, K., Conway-Hensley, L., Maples, K., Murdoch, A., Nelson, K., Sand-Niehaus, J., & Siemoens, S. (2002). Preparing school psychologists for early intervention settings. In M. R. Shinn, H. M. Walker, & G. Stoner (Eds.), *Interventions for academic and behavior problems, II: Preventive and remedial approaches* (pp. 1021–1045). Bethesda, MD: National Association of School Psychologists.

Barrios, B., & Hartmann, D. P. (1986). The contributions of traditional assessment: Concepts, issues, and methodologies. In R. O. Nelson & S. C. Hayes (Eds.), *Conceptual foundations of behavioral assessment* (pp. 81–110). New York: Guilford Press.

Beck, I. L., Perfetti, C. A., & McKeown, M. E. (1982). The effects of long-term vocabulary instruction on lexical access and reading comprehension. *Journal of Educational Psychology, 74,* 506–521.

Beitchman, J. H., Wekerle, C., & Hood, J. (1987). Diagnostic continuity from preschool to middle childhood. *Journal of the American Academy of Child and Adolescent Psychiatry, 26,* 694–699.

Bergan, J. R., & Kratochwill, T. R. (1990). *Behavioral consultation and therapy.* New York: Plenum Press.

Berliner, D. C. (1987). Simple views of effective teaching and a simple theory of classroom instruction. In D. C. Berliner & B. V. Rosenshine (Eds.), *Talks to teachers: A festschrift for N. L. Gage* (pp. 93–110). New York: Random House.

Berliner, D. C., & Rosenshine, B. V. (Eds.). (1987). *Talks to teachers: A festschrift for N. L. Gage.* New York: Random House.

Bersoff, D. N., & Hofer, P. T. (1990). The legal regulation of school psychology. In T. B. Gutkin & C. R. Reynolds (Eds.), *The handbook of school psychology* (2nd ed., pp. 939–961). New York: Wiley.

Biederman, J., Baldessarini, R. J., Wright, V., Knee, D., & Harmatz, J. S. (1989). A double-blind placebo-controlled study of desipramine in the treatment of ADHD: I. Efficacy. *Journal of the American Academy of Child and Adolescent Psychiatry, 28,* 777–784.

Biederman, J., Faraone, S. V., Milberger, S., Curtis, S., Chen, L., Marrs, A., Oullette, C., Moore, P., & Spencer, T. (1996). Predictors of persistence and remission of ADHD into adolescence: Results from a four-year prospective follow-up study. *Journal of the American Academy of Child and Adolescent Psychiatry, 35,* 343–351.

Biederman, J., Munir, K., Knee, D., Armentano, M., Autor, S., Waternaux, C., & Tsuang, M. (1987). High rate of affective disorders in probands with attention deficit disorders and in their relatives: A controlled family study. *American Journal of Psychiatry, 144,* 330–333.

Biederman, J., Wilens, T., Mick, E., Faraone, S. V., Weber, W., Curtis, S., Thornell, A., Pfister, K., Garcia Jetton, J., & Soriano, J. (1997). Is ADHD a risk factor for psychoactive substance use disorders?: Findings from a four-year prospective follow-up study. *Journal of the American Academy of Child and Adolescent Psychiatry, 36,* 21–29.

Biederman, J., Wilens, T., Mick, E., Spencer, T., & Faraone, S. V. (1999). Pharmacotherapy of attention-deficit/hyperactivity disorder reduces risk for substance use disorder. *Pediatrics, 104,* 20.

Bijur, P., Golding, J., Haslum, M., & Kurzon, M. (1988). Behavioral predictors of injury in school-age children. *American Journal of Diseases of Children, 142,* 1307–1312.

Blackman, J. A., Westervelt, V. D., Stevenson, R., & Welch, A. (1991). Management of preschool children with attention deficit-hyperactivity disorder. *Topics in Early Childhood Special Education, 11,* 91–104.

Boyajian, A. E., DuPaul, G. J., Wartel Handler, M., Eckert, T. L., & McGoey, K. E. (2001). The use of classroom-based brief functional analyses with preschoolers at-risk for attention deficit hyperactivity disorder. *School Psychology Review, 30,* 278–293.

Bremness, A. B., & Sverd, J. (1979). Methylphenidate-induced Tourette syndrome: Case report. *American Journal of Psychiatry, 136,* 1334– 1335.

Brestan, E. V., & Eyberg, S. M. (1998). Effective psychosocial treatments of conduct-disordered children and adolescents: 29 years, 82 studies, and 5,272 kids. *Journal of Clinical Child Psychology, 27,* 180–189.

Brown, R. T., & Borden, K. A. (1986). Hyperactivity at adolescence: Some misconceptions and new directions. *Journal of Clinical Child Psychology*, *15*, 194–209.

Brown, R. T., & Sammons, M. T. (2002). Pediatric psychopharmacology: A review of new developments and recent research. *Professional Psychology: Research and Practice*, *33*, 135–147.

Brown, R. T., & Sawyer, M. G. (1998). *Medications for school-age children: Effects on learning and behavior.* New York: Guilford Press.

Brown, R. T., & Sleator, E. K. (1979). Methylphenidate in hyperkinetic children: Differences in dose effects on impulsive behavior. *Pediatrics*, *64*, 408–411.

Budoff, M., Thormann, J., & Gras, A. (1984). *Microcomputers in special education.* Cambridge, MA: Brookline Books.

Buhrmester, D., Whalen, C. K., Henker, B., MacDonald, V., & Hinshaw, S. P. (1992). Prosocial behavior in hyperactive boys: Effects of stimulant medication and comparison with normal boys. *Journal of Abnormal Child Psychology*, *20*, 103–122.

Campbell, S. B. (2002). *Behavior problems in preschool children: Clinical and developmental issues* (2nd ed.). New York: Guilford Press.

Campbell, S. B., Endman, M. W., & Bernfield, G. (1977). A three year follow-up of hyperactive preschoolers into elementary school. *Journal of Child Psychology and Psychiatry*, *18*, 239–249.

Campbell, S. B., & Ewing, L. J. (1990). Follow-up of hard to manage preschoolers: Adjustment at age 9 and predictors of continuing symptoms. *Journal of Child Psychology and Psychiatry*, *31*, 871–889.

Campbell, S. B., Schleifer, M., & Weiss, G. (1978). Continuities in maternal reports and child behaviors over time in hyperactive and comparison groups. *Journal of Abnormal Child Psychology*, *6*, 33–45.

Cantwell, D. P. (1986). Attention deficit disorder in adolescents. *Clinical Psychology Review*, *6*, 237–247.

Cantwell, D. P., & Baker, L. (1991). Association between attention-deficit hyperactivity disorder and learning disorders. *Journal of Learning Disabilities*, *24*, 88–95.

Cantwell, D. P., & Satterfield, J. H. (1978). The prevalence of academic underachievement in hyperactive children. *Journal of Pediatric Psychology*, *3*, 168–171.

Carlson, C. L., & Mann, M. (2000). Attention-deficit/hyperactivity disorder predominantly inattentive subtype. *Child and Adolescent Psychiatric Clinics of North America*, *9*, 499–510.

Carnine, D., Kameenui, E., & Silbert, J. (1990). *Direct instruction reading.* Columbus, OH: Merrill.

Carnine, D., & Kinder, D. (1985). Teaching low performing students to apply generative and schema strategies to narrative and expository material. *Remedial and Special Education*, *6*, 20–30.

Carroll County Public Schools. (1997). *ADHD procedural guidelines.* Westminster, MD: Author.

Casat, C. D., Pleasants, D. Z., Schroeder, D. H., & Parler, D. W. (1989).

Bupropion in children with attention deficit disorder. *Psychopharmacology Bulletin, 25,* 198–201.

Castellanos, F. X., Giedd, J. N., Elia, J., Marsh, W. L., Ritcline, G. F., Hamburger, S. P., & Rapoport, J. L. (1997). Controlled stimulant treatment of ADHD and comorbid Tourette's syndrome: Effects of stimulant and dose. *Journal of the American Academy of Child and Adolescent Psychiatry, 36,* 589–596.

Chall, J. S. (1983). Literacy: Trends and explanations. *Educational Researcher, 12,* 3–8.

Chan, E., Zhan, C., & Homer, C. J. (2002). Health care use and costs for children with attention-deficit/hyperactivity disorder. *Archives of Pediatric and Adolescent Medicine, 156,* 504–511.

Chelune, G. J., Ferguson, W., Koon, R., & Dickey, T. O. (1986). Frontal lobe disinhibition in attention deficit disorder. *Child Psychiatry and Human Development, 16,* 221–234.

Christenson, S. L., Rounds, T., & Gorney, D. (1992). Family factors and student achievement: An avenue to increase students' success. *School Psychology Quarterly, 7,* 178–206.

Christenson, S. L., & Sheridan, S. M. (2001). *Schools and families: Creating essential connections for learning.* New York: Guilford Press.

Clay, M. M. (1979). *The early detection of reading difficulties* (3rd ed.). Auckland, New Zealand: Heinemann.

Columbia University DISC Development Group. (2000). *C-DISC 4 Young Child Version.* New York: Author.

Colvin, G. T., & Sugai, G. M. (1988). Proactive strategies for managing social behavior problems: An instructional approach. *Education and Treatment of Children, 11,* 341–348.

Comings, D. E., Gade-Andavolu, R., Gonzalez, N., Wu, S., Muhleman, D., Blake, H., Dietz, G., Saucier, G., & McMurray, J. P. (2000). Comparison of the role of dopamine, serotonin, and noradrenaline genes in ADHD, ODD and conduct disorder: Multivariate regression analysis of 20 genes. *Clinical Genetics, 57,* 178–196.

Cone, J. D. (1986). Idiographic, nomothetic, and related perspectives in behavioral assessment. In R. O. Nelson & S. C. Hayes (Eds.), *Conceptual foundations of behavioral assessment* (pp. 111–128). New York: Guilford Press.

Conners, C. K. (1995). *Conners' Continuous Performance Test.* Toronto: Multi-Health Systems.

Conners, C. K. (1997). *Conners' Rating Scales-Revised: Technical manual.* Toronto: Multi-Health Systems.

Conners, C. K., Epstein, J. N., March, J. S., Angold, A., Wells, K. C., Klaric, J., Swanson, J. M., Arnold, L. E., Abikoff, H. B., Elliott, G. R., Greenhill, L. L., Hechtman, L., Hinshaw, S. P., Hoza, B., Jensen, P. S., Kraemer, H. C., Newcorn, J. H., Pelham, W. E., Severe, J. B., Vitiello, B., & Wigal, T. (2001). Multimodal treatment of ADHD in the MTA: An alternative outcome analysis. *Journal of the American Academy of Child and Adolescent Psychiatry, 40,* 159–167.

Conners, C. K., Wells, K. C., Parker, J. D. A., Sitarenios, G., Diamond, J. M., &

Powell, J. W. (1997). A new self-report scale for assessment of adolescent psychopathology: Factor structure, reliability, validity, and diagnostic sensitivity. *Journal of Abnormal Child Psychology, 25,* 487–498.

Connor, D. F. (1998). Other medications in the treatment of child and adolescent ADHD. In R. A. Barkley, *Attention-deficit hyperactivity disorder: A handbook for diagnosis and treatment* (2nd ed., pp. 564–581). New York: Guilford Press.

Connor, D. F., Barkley, R. A., & Davis, H. T. (2000). A pilot study of methylphenidate, clonidine, or the combination in ADHD comorbid with aggressive oppositional defiant or conduct disorder. *Clinical Pediatrics, 39,* 15–25.

Connor, D. F., Fletcher, K. E., & Swanson, J. M. (1999). A meta-analysis of clonidine for symptoms of attention-deficit/hyperactivity disorder. *Journal of the American Academy of Child and Adolescent Psychiatry, 38,* 1551–1559.

Connor, D. F., Glatt, S. J., Lopez, I. D., Jackson, D., & Melloni, R. H. (2002). Psychopharmacology and aggression. I: A meta-analysis of stimulant effects on overt/covert aggression-related behaviors in ADHD. *Journal of the American Academy of Child and Adolescent Psychiatry, 41,* 253– 261.

Cooper, H., Lindsay, J. J., Nye, B., & Greathouse, S. (1998). Relationships among attitudes about homework, amount of homework assigned and completed, and student achievement. *Journal of Educational Psychology, 90,* 70–83.

Crenshaw, T. M., Kavale, K. A., Forness, S. R., & Reeve, R. E. (1999). Attention deficit hyperactivity disorder and the efficacy of stimulant medication: A meta-analysis. In T. Scruggs & M. Mastropieri (Eds.), *Advances in learning and behavioral disabilities* (Vol. 13, pp. 135–165). Stamford, CT: JAI Press.

Cunningham, C. E. (1998). A large-group community-based, family systems approach to parent training. In R. A. Barkley, *Attention-deficit hyperactivity disorder: A handbook for diagnosis and treatment* (2nd ed., pp. 394–412). New York: Guilford Press.

Cunningham, C. E., & Barkley, R. A. (1979). The interactions of hyperactive and normal children with their mothers during free play and structured task. *Child Development, 50,* 217–224.

Cunningham, C. E., Bremner, R., & Secord, M. (1998). *The Community Parent Education Program: A school-based family systems oriented workshop for parents of children with disruptive behavior disorders.* Hamilton, Ontario, Canada: Hamilton Health Sciences Corporation.

Cunningham, C. E., & Cunningham, L. J. (1998). Student-mediated conflict resolution programs. In R. A. Barkley, *Attention-deficit hyperactivity disorder: A handbook for diagnosis and treatment* (2nd ed., pp. 491–509). New York: Guilford Press.

Cunningham, C. E., Siegel, L. S., & Offord, D. R. (1985). A developmental dose response analysis of the effects of methylphenidate on the peer interactions of attention deficit disordered boys. *Journal of Child Psychology and Psychiatry, 26,* 955–971.

Daniel, S., Power, T. J., Karustis, J. L., & Leff, S. S. (1999, November). *Parent-mediated homework intervention for children with ADHD: Its impact on parent–child relationships and parenting stress.* Poster presented at the annual meeting of the Association for the Advancement of Behavior Therapy, Toronto, Ontario, Canada.

Davidson, L. L., Hughes, S. J., & O'Connor, P. A. (1988). Preschool behavior problems and subsequent risk of injury. *Pediatrics, 82,* 644–651.

Davila, R. R., Williams, M. L., & MacDonald, J. T. (1991, Sept. 16). *Clarification of policy to address the needs of children with attention deficit disorders within general and/or special education.* Unpublished letter to chief state school officers, U.S. Department of Education, Washington, DC.

Dawson, P., & Guare, R. (1998). *Coaching the ADHD student.* North Tonowanda, NY: Multi-Health Systems.

Demaray, M. K., & Elliott, S. N. (2001). Perceived social support by children with characteristics of attention-deficit/hyperactivity disorder. *School Psychology Quarterly, 16,* 68–90.

Denckla, M. B., & Rudel, R. G. (1978). Anomalies of motor development in hyperactive boys. *Annals of Neurology, 3,* 231–233.

Denckla, M. B., Rudel, R. G., Chapman, C., & Krieger, J. (1985). Motor proficiency in dyslexic children with and without attentional disorders. *Archives of Neurology, 42,* 228–231.

DeRisi, W. J., & Butz, G. (1975). *Writing behavioral contracts: A case simulation practice manual.* Champaign, IL: Research Press.

Deshler, D. D., & Schumaker, J. B. (1988). An instructional model for teaching students how to learn. In J. L. Graden, J. E. Zins, & M. J. Curtis (Eds.), *Alternative educational delivery systems: Enhancing instructional options for all students* (pp. 391–411). Washington, DC: National Association of School Psychologists.

DiPerna, J. C., & Elliott, S. N. (2000). *Academic Competence Evaluation Scale.* San Antonio, TX: Psychological Corporation.

DiScala, C., Lescohier, I., Barthel, M., & Li, G. (1998). Injuries to children with attention deficit hyperactivity disorder. *Pediatrics, 102,* 1415–1421.

Dishion, T. J., & Patterson, G. R. (1997). The timing and severity of antisocial behavior: Three hypotheses within an ecological framework. In D. M. Stoff, J. Breiling, & J. D. Maser (Eds.), *Handbook of antisocial behavior* (pp. 205–217). New York: Wiley.

Dishion, T. J., Patterson, G. R., & Kavanagh, K. A. (1992). An experimental test of the coercion model: Linking theory, measurement, and intervention. In J. McCord & R. E. Tremblay (Eds.), *Preventing antisocial behavior: Interventions from birth through adolescence* (pp. 253–282). New York: Guilford Press.

Donnelly, M., & Rapoport, J. L. (1985). Attention deficit disorders. In J. M. Wiener (Ed.), *Diagnosis and psychopharmacology of childhood and adolescent disorders* (pp. 179–197). New York: Wiley.

Dougherty, D. D., Bonab, A. A., Spencer, T. J., Rauch, S. L., Madras, B. K., & Fischmann, A. J. (1999). Dopamine transporter density in patients with attention deficit hyperactivity disorder. *Lancet, 354,* 2132–2133.

Douglas, V. I. (1980). Higher mental processes in hyperactive children: Implications for training. In R. Knights & D. Bakker (Eds.), *Treatment of hyperactive and learning disordered children* (pp. 65–92). Baltimore: University Park Press.

Douglas, V. A. (1984). The psychological processes implicated in ADD. In L. M. Bloomingdale (Ed.), *Attention deficit disorder: Diagnostic, cognitive, and therapeutic understanding* (pp. 147–162). New York: Spectrum.

Douglas, V. I., Barr, R. G., O'Neill, M. E., & Britton, B. G. (1986). Short term effects of methylphenidate on the cognitive, learning and academic performance of children with attention deficit disorder in the laboratory and the classroom. *Journal of Child Psychology and Psychiatry, 27,* 191–211.

Douglas, V. I., Barr, R. G., O'Neill, M. E., & Britton, B. G. (1988). Dosage effects and individual responsivity to methylphenidate in attention deficit disorder. *Journal of Child Psychology and Psychiatry, 29,* 453–475.

Dunlap, G., de Perczel, M., Clarke, S., Wilson, D., Wright, S., White, R., & Gomez, A. (1994). Choice making to promote adaptive behavior for students with emotional and behavioral challenges. *Journal of Applied Behavior Analysis, 27,* 505–518.

DuPaul, G. J. (1992). How to assess attention-deficit hyperactivity disorder within school settings. *School Psychology Quarterly, 7,* 60–74.

DuPaul, G. J., Anastopoulos, A. D., Kwasnik, D., Barkley, R. A., & McMurray, M. B. (1996). Methylphenidate effects on children with attention deficit hyperactivity disorder: Self-report of symptoms, side-effects, and self- esteem. *Journal of Attention Disorders, 1,* 3–15.

DuPaul, G. J., Anastopoulos, A. D., Shelton, T. L., Guevremont, D. C., & Metevia, L. (1992). Multimethod assessment of attention-deficit hyperactivity disorder: The diagnostic utility of clinic-based tests. *Journal of Clinical Child Psychology, 21,* 394–402.

DuPaul, G. J., & Barkley, R. A. (1992). Situational variability of attention problems: Psychometric properties of the revised home and school situations questionnaires. *Journal of Clinical Child Psychology, 21,* 178–188.

DuPaul, G. J., Barkley, R. A., & Connor, D. F. (1998). Stimulants. In R. A. Barkley, *Attention-deficit hyperactivity disorder: A handbook for diagnosis and treatment* (2nd ed., pp. 510–551). New York: Guilford Press.

DuPaul, G. J., Barkley, R. A., & McMurray, M. B. (1994). Response of children with ADHD to methylphenidate: Interaction with internalizing symptoms. *Journal of the American Academy of Child and Adolescent Psychiatry, 33,* 894–903.

DuPaul, G. J., & Eckert, T. L. (1994). The effects of social skills curricula: Now you see them, now you don't. *School Psychology Quarterly, 9,* 113–132.

DuPaul, G. J., & Eckert, T. L. (1997). School-based interventions for children with attention-deficit/hyperactivity disorder: A meta-analysis. *School Psychology Review, 26,* 5–27.

DuPaul, G. J., Eckert, T. K., & McGoey, K. E. (1997). Interventions for students with attention-deficit/hyperactivity disorder: One size does not fit all. *School Psychology Review, 26,* 369–381.

DuPaul, G. J., & Ervin, R. A. (1996). Functional assessment of behaviors related to attention-deficit/hyperactivity disorder: Linking assessment to intervention design. *Behavior Therapy, 27,* 601–622.

DuPaul, G. J., Ervin, R. A., Hook, C. L., & McGoey, K. E. (1998). Peer tutoring for children with attention deficit hyperactivity disorder: Effects on classroom behavior and academic performance. *Journal of Applied Behavior Analysis, 31,* 579–592.

DuPaul, G. J., Guevremont, D. C., & Barkley, R. A. (1991). Attention-deficit hyperactivity disorder in adolescence: Critical assessment parameters. *Clinical Psychology Review, 11,* 231–245.

DuPaul, G. J., Guevremont, D. C., & Barkley, R. A. (1992). Behavioral treatment of attention-deficit hyperactivity disorder in the classroom: The use of the Attention Training System. *Behavior Modification, 16,* 204–225.

DuPaul, G. J., & Henningson, P. N. (1993). Peer tutoring effects on the classroom performance of children with attention deficit hyperactivity disorder. *School Psychology Review, 22,* 134–143.

DuPaul, G. J., McGoey, K. E., Eckert, T. L., & VanBrakle, J. (2001). Preschool children with attention-deficit/hyperactivity disorder: Impairments in behavioral, social, and school functioning. *Journal of the American Academy of Child and Adolescent Psychiatry, 40,* 508–515.

DuPaul, G. J., & Power, T. J. (2000). Educational interventions for students with attention-deficit disorders. In T. E. Brown (Ed.), *Attention-deficit disorders and comorbidities in children, adolescents, and adults* (pp. 607–635). Washington, DC: American Psychiatric Press.

DuPaul, G. J., Power, T. J., Anastopoulos, A. D., & Reid, R. (1998). *ADHD Rating Scale–IV: Checklists, norms, and clinical interpretation.* New York: Guilford Press.

DuPaul, G. J., & Rapport, M. D. (1993). Does methylphenidate normalize the classroom performance of children with attention deficit disorder? *Journal of the American Academy of Child and Adolescent Psychiatry, 32,* 190–198.

DuPaul, G. J., Rapport, M. D., & Perriello, L. M. (1991). Teacher ratings of academic skills: The development of the Academic Performance Rating Scale. *School Psychology Review, 20,* 284–300.

DuPaul, G. J., & Stoner, G. (1999a). *Assessing ADHD in the schools* [Videotape]. New York: Guilford Press.

DuPaul, G. J., & Stoner, G. (1999b). *Classroom interventions for ADHD* [Videotape]. New York: Guilford Press.

DuPaul, G. J., & Stoner, G. (2002). Interventions for attention problems. In M. R. Shinn, H. M. Walker, & G. Stoner (Eds.), *Interventions for academic and behavior problems, II: Preventive and remedial approaches* (4th ed., pp. 913–938). Washington, DC: National Association of School Psychologists.

DuPaul, G. J., Stoner, G., & O'Reilly, M. J. (2002). Best practices in classroom interventions for attention problems. In A. Thomas & J. Grimes (Eds.), *Best practices in school psychology IV* (2nd ed., pp. 1115–1128). Washington, DC: National Association of School Psychologists.

Dyer, K., Dunlap, G., & Winterling, V. (1990). Effects of choice making on the serious problem behaviors of students with severe handicaps. *Journal of Applied Behavior Analysis, 23,* 515–524.

Dykman, R. A., & Ackerman, P. T. (1991). Attention deficit disorder and specific learning disability: Separate but often overlapping disorders. *Journal of Learning Disabilities, 24,* 96–103.

Eckert, T. L., DuPaul, G. J., McGoey, K. E., & Volpe, R. J. (2002). *Young children at-risk for attention-deficit/hyperactivity disorder: A needs assessment of parents, community service providers, and experts.* Manuscript submitted for publication.

Eddy, J. M., Reid, J. B., & Curry, V. (2002). The etiology of youth antisocial behavior, delinquency, and violence and a public health approach to prevention. In M. R. Shinn, H. M. Walker, & G. Stoner (Eds.), *Interventions for academic and behavior problems, II: Preventive and remedial approaches* (pp. 27–51). Bethesda, MD: National Association of School Psychologists.

Edwards, G., Barkley, R. A., Laneri, M., Fletcher, K., & Metevia, L. (2001). Parent–adolescent conflict in teenagers with ADHD and ODD. *Journal of Abnormal Child Psychology, 29,* 557–572.

Elia, J., & Rapoport, J. L. (1991). Ritalin versus dextroamphetamine in ADHD: Both should be tried. In L. L. Greenhill & B. B. Osman (Eds.), *Ritalin: Theory and patient management* (pp. 69–74). New York: Mary Ann Liebert.

Elliott, S. L., Witt, J. C., Kratochwill, T. R., & Stoiber, K. C. (2002). Selecting and evaluating classroom interventions. In M. R. Shinn, H. M. Walker, & G. Stoner (Eds.), *Interventions for achievement and behavior problems, II: Remedial and preventive approaches* (2nd ed., pp. 243–294). Washington, DC: National Association of School Psychologists.

Ellis, E. S., Deshler, D. D., & Schumaker, J. B. (1989). Teaching adolescents with learning disabilities to generate and use task specific strategies. *Journal of Learning Disabilities, 22,* 108–119, 130.

Epstein, J. L. (1986). Parents' reactions to teacher practices of parent involvement. *Elementary School Journal, 86,* 277–294.

Ervin, R., DuPaul, G. J., Kern, L., & Friman, P. (1996). *A functional assessment of the variables affecting classroom compliance for students with ADHD and ODD: Toward a proactive approach to classroom management.* Unpublished manuscript, Lehigh University, Bethlehem, PA.

Ervin, R. A., DuPaul, G. J., Kern, L., & Friman, P. C. (1998). Classroom-based functional and adjunctive assessments: Proactive approaches to intervention selection for adolescents with attention deficit hyperactivity disorder. *Journal of Applied Behavior Analysis, 31,* 65–78.

Ervin, R. A., Ehrhardt, K. E., & Poling, A. (2001). Functional assessment: Old wine in new bottles. *School Psychology Review, 30,* 173–179.

Evans, I. M., & Meyer, L. H. (1985). *An educative approach to behavior problems.* Baltimore: Paul H. Brookes.

Evans, R. W., Gualtieri, C. T., & Amara, I. (1986). Methylphenidate and memory: Dissociated effects in hyperactive children. *Psychopharmacology, 90,* 211–216.

Evans, S. W., & Pelham, W. E. (1991). Psychostimulant effects on academic and behavioral measures for ADHD junior high school students in a lecture format classroom. *Journal of Abnormal Child Psychology, 19,* 537–552.

Evans, S. W., Pelham, W., & Grudberg, M. V. (1995). The efficacy of notetaking to improve behavior and comprehension of adolescents with attention deficit hyperactivity disorder. *Exceptionality, 5,* 1–17.

Evans, S. W., Pelham, W. E., Smith, B. H., Bukstein, O., Gnagy, E. M., Greiner, A. R., Altenderfer, L., & Baron-Myak, C. (2001). Dose–response effects of methylphenidate on ecologically valid measures of academic performance and classroom behavior in adolescents with ADHD. *Experimental and Clinical Psychopharmacology, 9,* 163–175.

Fabiano, G. A., Pelham, W. E., Gnagy, E. M., Kipp, H., Lahey, B. B., Burrows-MacLean, L., Chronis, A. M., Onyango, A. N., & Morrisey, S. (1999, November). *The reliability and validity of the Children's Impairment Rating Scale: A practical measure of impairment in children with ADHD.* Poster presented at the annual meeting of the Association for the Advancement of Behavior Therapy, Toronto, Ontario, Canada.

Faraone, S. V. (2000). Genetics of childhood disorders: XX. ADHD, Part 4: Is ADHD genetically heterogeneous? *Journal of the American Academy of Child and Adolescent Psychiatry, 39,* 1455–1457.

Faraone, S. V., Biederman, J., Krifcher, B., Lehmann, B., Keenan, K., Norman, D., Seidman, L. J., Kolodny, R., Kraus, I., Perrin, J., & Chen, W. J. (1993). Evidence for the independent familial transmission of attention deficit hyperactivity disorder and learning disabilities: Results from a family genetic study. *American Journal of Psychiatry, 150,* 891–895.

Faraone, S. V., Biederman, J., Weber, W., & Russell, R. L. (1998). Psychiatric, neuropsychological, and psychosocial features of DSM-IV subtypes of attention-deficit/hyperactivity disorder: Results from a clinically-referred sample. *Journal of the American Academy of Child and Adolescent Psychiatry, 37,* 185–193.

Feil, E. G., Walker, H. M., & Severson, H. H. (1995). Young children with behavior problems: Research and development of the Early Screening Project. *Journal of Emotional and Behavioral Disorders, 3,* 194–202.

Feingold, B. (1975). *Why your child is hyperactive.* New York: Random House.

Felton, R. H., Wood, F. B., Brown, I. S., Campbell, S. K., & Harter, M. R. (1987). Separate verbal memory and naming deficits in attention deficit disorder and reading disability. *Brain and Language, 31,* 171–184.

Fergusson, D. M., & Horwood, L. J. (1992). Attention deficit and reading achievement. *Journal of Child Psychology and Psychiatry, 33,* 375–385.

Fergusson, D. M., & Horwood, L. J. (1995). Early disruptive behavior, IQ, and later school achievement and delinquent behavior. *Journal of Abnormal Child Psychology, 23,* 183–199.

Fergusson, D. M., Horwood, L. J., & Lynskey, M. T. (1993). The effects of conduct disorder and attention deficit in middle childhood on offending and scholastic ability at age 13. *Journal of Child Psychology and Psychiatry, 34,* 899–916.

Fergusson, D. M., Lynskey, M. T., & Horwood, L. J. (1997). Attentional difficulties in middle childhood and psychosocial outcomes in young adulthood. *Journal of Child Psychology and Psychiatry, 38*, 633–644.

Fielding, L. T., Murphy, R. J., Reagan, M. W., & Peterson, T. L. (1980). An assessment program to reduce drug use with the mentally retarded. *Hospital and Community Psychiatry, 31*, 771–773.

Finn, C. A., & Sladeczek, I. E. (2001). Assessing the social validity of behavioral interventions: A review of treatment acceptability measures. *School Psychology Quarterly, 16*, 176–206.

Fischer, M. (1990). Parenting stress and the child with attention deficit hyperactivity disorder. *Journal of Clinical Child Psychology, 19*, 337–346.

Flicek, M. (1992). Social status of boys with both academic problems and attention-deficit hyperactivity disorder. *Journal of Abnormal Child Psychology, 20*, 353–366.

Forehand, R. L., & McMahon, R. J. (1981). *Helping the noncompliant child: A clinician's guide to parent training.* New York: Guilford Press.

Forness, S. R., & Kavale, K. A. (2001). ADHD and a return to the medical model of special education. *Education and Treatment of Children, 24*, 224–247.

Forness, S. R., Kavale, K. A., Sweeney, D. P., & Crenshaw, T. M. (1999). The future of research and practice in behavioral disorders: Psychopharmacology and its school treatment implications. *Behavioral Disorders, 24*, 305–318.

Fowler, M. (1992). *C.H.A.D.D. educators manual: An in-depth look at attention deficit disorders from an educational perspective.* Plantation, FL: C.H.A.D.D.

Frick, P. J., Kamphaus, R. W., Lahey, B. B., Loeber, R., Christ, M. A. G., Hart, E. L., & Tannenbaum, L. E. (1991). Academic underachievement and the disruptive behavior disorders. *Journal of Consulting and Clinical Psychology, 59*, 289–294.

Frick, P. J., & Lahey, B. B. (1991). Nature and characteristics of attention-deficit hyperactivity disorder. *School Psychology Review, 20*, 163–173.

Fuchs, L. S., Fuchs, D., Phillips, N., Hamlett, C. L., & Karns, K. (1995). Acquisition and transfer effects of class wide peer-assisted learning strategies in mathematics for students with varying learning histories. *School Psychology Review, 24*, 604–620.

Fuerst, D. R., Fisk, J. L., & Rourke, B. P. (1989). Psychosocial functioning of learning-disabled children: Replicability of statistically derived subtypes. *Journal of Consulting and Clinical Psychology, 57*, 275–280.

Gadow, K. D. (1986). *Children on medication, Vol. 1: Hyperactivity, learning disabilities, and mental retardation.* Boston: Little, Brown.

Gadow, K. D. (1993). A school-based medication evaluation program. In J. L. Matson (Ed.), *Handbook of hyperactivity in children* (pp. 186–219). Boston: Allyn & Bacon.

Gadow, K. D., Nolan, E. E., Paolicelli, L. M., & Sprafkin, J. (1991). A procedure for assessing the effects of methylphenidate on hyperactive children in public school settings. *Journal of Clinical Child Psychology, 20*, 268–276.

Gadow, K. D., Nolan, E. E., Sverd, J., Sprafkin, J., & Paolicelli, L. (1990). Methylphenidate in aggressive-hyperactive boys: I. Effects on peer aggression in public school settings. *Journal of the American Academy of Child and Adolescent Psychiatry, 29,* 710–718.

Gadow, K. D., & Sprafkin, J. (1997). *Early Childhood Inventory-4: Norms manual.* Stony Brook, NY: Checkmate Plus.

Gadow, K. D., Sprafkin, J., Carlson, C. A., Schneider, J., Nolan, E. E., Mattison, R. E., & Rundberg-Rivera, V. (2002). A DSM-IV-referenced, adolescent self-report rating scale. *Journal of the American Academy of Child and Adolescent Psychiatry, 41,* 671–679.

Gadow, K. D., Sprafkin, J., & Nolan, E. E. (1996). *ADHD School Observation Code.* Stony Brook, NY: Checkmate Plus.

Gadow, K. D., Sverd, J., Sprafkin, J., Nolan, E. E., & Ezor, S. (1995). Efficacy of methylphenidate for attention-deficit hyperactivity disorder in children with tic disorder. *Archives of General Psychiatry, 52,* 444–455.

Garmezy, N. (1978). DSM-III. Never mind the psychologists: Is it good for the children? *The Clinical Psychologist, 31,* 1–6.

Gaub, M., & Carlson, C. L. (1997). Gender differences in ADHD: A meta-analysis and critical review. *Journal of the American Academy of Child and Adolescent Psychiatry, 36,* 1036–1045.

Gersten, R., & Chard, D. (1999). Number sense: Rethinking arithmetic instruction for students with mathematical disabilities. *Journal of Special Education, 33,* 18–28.

Gittelman, R., Mannuzza, S., Shenker, R., & Bonagura, N. (1985). Hyperactive boys almost grown up. *Archives of General Psychiatry, 42,* 937–947.

Gleason, M. M., Archer, A. L., & Colvin, G. (2002). Interventions for improving study skills. In M. R. Shinn, H. M. Walker, & G. Stoner (Eds.), *Interventions for achievement and behavior problems, II: Preventive and remedial approaches* (2nd ed., pp. 651–680). Washington, DC: National Association of School Psychologists.

Goldstein, S., & Goldstein, M. (1998). *Managing attention deficit hyperactivity disorder in children: A guide for practitioners* (2nd ed.). New York: Wiley.

Good, R. H., Gruba, J., & Kaminski, R. A. (2002). Best practices in using dynamic indicators of basic early literacy skills (DIBELS) in an outcomes-driven model. In A. Thomas & J. Grimes (Eds.), *Best practices in school psychology IV* (4th ed., pp. 699–720). Washington, DC: National Association of School Psychologists.

Gordon, M. (1983). *The Gordon diagnostic system.* DeWitt, NY: Gordon Systems.

Gordon, M. (1986). How is a computerized attention test used in the diagnosis of attention deficit disorder? *Journal of Children in Contemporary Society, 19,* 53–64.

Graham, S., & Harris, K. R. (2002). Prevention and intervention for struggling writers. In M. R. Shinn, H. M. Walker, & G. Stoner (Eds.), *Interventions for academic and behavior problems, II: Preventive and remedial approaches* (pp. 589–610). Bethesda, MD: National Association of School Psychologists.

Greene, R. W., Beszterczey, S. K., Katzenstein, T., Park, K., & Goring, J. (2002).

Are students with ADHD more stressful to teach?: Patterns of teacher stress in an elementary school sample. *Journal of Emotional and Behavioral Disorders, 10,* 79–89.

Greene, R. W., Biederman, J., Faraone, S. V., Ouellette, C. A., Penn, C., & Griffin, S. (1996). Toward a new psychometric definition of social disability in children with attention-deficit hyperactivity disorder. *Journal of the American Academy of Child and Adolescent Psychiatry, 35,* 571–578.

Greenhill, L. L. (1984). Stimulant related growth inhibition in children: A review. In L. Greenhill & B. Shopsin (Eds.), *The psychobiology of childhood* (pp. 135–157). New York: Spectrum.

Greenhill, L. L. (2000). *The preschool attention treatment study (PATS).* New York: Department of Psychiatry, Columbia-Presbyterian Medical Center.

Greenwood, C. R., Delquadri, J., & Carta, J. J. (1988). *Classwide peer tutoring.* Seattle: Educational Achievement Systems.

Greenwood, C. R., Maheady, L., & Delquadri, J. (2002). Classwide peer tutoring programs. In M. R. Shinn, H. M. Walker, & G. Stoner (Eds.), *Interventions for academic and behavior problems, II: Preventive and remedial approaches* (pp. 611–649). Bethesda, MD: National Association of School Psychologists.

Gregory, R. J. (1996). *Psychological testing: History, principles, and applications* (2nd ed). Boston: Allyn & Bacon.

Gresham, F. M. (1989). Assessment of treatment integrity in school consultation and prereferral intervention. *School Psychology Review, 18,* 37–50.

Gresham, F. M. (1991). Conceptualizing behavior disorders in terms of resistance to intervention. *School Psychology Review, 20,* 23–36.

Gresham, F. M. (2002). Teaching social skills to high-risk children and youth: Preventive and remedial strategies. In M. R. Shinn, H. M. Walker, & G. Stoner (Eds.), *Interventions for academic and behavior problems, II: Preventive and remedial approaches* (2nd ed., pp. 403–432). Washington, DC: National Association of School Psychologists.

Gresham, F. M., & Elliott, S. N. (1990). *Social skills rating system.* Circle Pines, MN: American Guidance Service.

Gresham, F. M., & Gansle, K. A. (1992a). Misguided assumptions of DSM-III-R: Implications for school psychological practice. *School Psychology Quarterly, 7,* 79–95.

Gresham, F. M., & Gansle, K. A. (1992b). Misological or misconstrued: Rejoinder to Reynolds and Hynd. *School Psychology Quarterly, 7,* 108–111.

Gresham, F. M., Watson, T. S., & Skinner, C. H. (2001). Functional behavioral assessment: Principles, procedures, and future directions. *School Psychology Review, 30,* 156–172.

Griffin, S. A., Case, R., & Siegler, R. S. (1994). Rightstart: Providing the central conceptual prerequisites for first formal learning of arithmetic to students at risk for school failure. In K. McGilly (Ed.), *Classroom lessons: Integrating cognitive theory and classroom practice* (pp. 25–49). Cambridge, MA: MIT Press.

Grossen, B., & Carnine, D. (1991). Strategies for maximizing reading success in the regular classroom. In G. Stoner, M. R. Shinn, & H. M. Walker (Eds.),

Interventions for achievement and behavior problems (pp. 333–355). Silver Spring, MD: National Association of School Psychologists.

Gureasko-Moore, S., DuPaul, G. J., & White, G. P. (in press). The effects of self-management in general education classrooms on the organizational skills of adolescents with AD/HD. *Behavior Modification.*

Guevara, J., Lozano, P., Wickizer, T., Mell, L., & Gephart, H. (2001). Utilization and cost of health care services for children with attention-deficit/hyperactivity disorder. *Pediatrics, 108,* 71–78.

Guevremont, D. C. (1990). Social skills and peer relationship training. In R. A. Barkley, *Attention-deficit hyperactivity disorder: A handbook for diagnosis and treatment* (pp. 540–572). New York: Guilford Press.

Hakola, S. (1992). Legal rights of students with attention deficit disorder. *School Psychology Quarterly, 7,* 285–297.

Halperin, J. M., Gittelman, R., Klein, D. F., & Rudel, R. G. (1984). Reading-disabled hyperactive children: A distinct subgroup of attention deficit disorder with hyperactivity? *Journal of Abnormal Child Psychology, 12,* 1–14.

Halperin, J. M., Sharma, V., Greenblatt, E., & Schwartz, S. T. (1991). Assessment of the continuous performance test: Reliability and validity in a nonreferred sample. *Psychological Assessment: A Journal of Consulting and Clinical Psychology, 3,* 603–608.

Hamlett, K. W., Pellegrini, D. S., & Conners, C. K. (1987). An investigation of executive processes in the problem-solving of attention deficit disorder-hyperactive children. *Journal of Pediatric Psychology, 12,* 227–240.

Hammer, E. F. (1975). *The clinical application of projective drawings.* Springfield, IL: Charles C Thomas.

Handler, M. W., & DuPaul, G. J. (2002). Diagnosis of childhood ADHD: Differences across psychology specialty areas. *ADHD Report, 10*(3), 7–9.

Hansen, C., Weiss, D., & Last, C. G. (1999). ADHD boys in young adulthood: Psychosocial adjustment. *Journal of the American Academy of Child and Adolescent Psychiatry, 38,* 165–171.

Hart, B., & Risley, T. R. (1995). *Meaningful differences in the everyday experience of young American children.* Baltimore: Paul H. Brookes.

Hartsough, C. S., & Lambert, N. M. (1985). Medical factors in hyperactive and normal children: Prenatal, developmental, and health history findings. *American Journal of Orthopsychiatry, 55,* 190–210.

Hayes, S. C., Barlow, D. H., & Nelson-Gray, R. O. (1999). *The scientist-practitioner: Research and accountability in the age of managed care* (2nd ed.). Boston: Allyn & Bacon.

Haynes, S. N. (1986). The design of intervention programs. In R. O. Nelson & S. C. Hayes (Eds.), *Conceptual foundations of behavioral assessment* (pp. 386–429). New York: Guilford Press.

Hersen, M., & Barlow, D. H. (1982). *Single case experimental designs: Strategies for studying behavior change.* Elmsford, NY: Pergamon Press.

Hinshaw, S. P. (1991). Stimulant medication and the treatment of aggression in children with attentional deficits. *Journal of Clinical Child Psychology, 20,* 301–312.

Hinshaw, S. P. (1992a). Academic underachievement, attention deficits, and aggression: Comorbidity and implications for intervention. *Journal of Consulting and Clinical Psychology, 60,* 893–903.

Hinshaw, S. P. (1992b). Externalizing behavior problems and academic underachievement in childhood and adolescence: Causal relationships and underlying mechanisms. *Psychological Bulletin, 111,* 127–155.

Hinshaw, S. P., Henker, B., & Whalen, C. K. (1984). Self-control in hyperactive boys in anger-inducing situations: Effects of cognitive-behavioral training and of methylphenidate. *Journal of Abnormal Child Psychology, 12,* 55–77.

Hinshaw, S. P., Henker, B., Whalen, C. K., Erhardt, D., & Dunnington, R. E., Jr. (1989). Aggressive, prosocial, and nonsocial behavior in hyperactive boys: Dose effects of methylphenidate in naturalistic settings. *Journal of Consulting and Clinical Psychology, 57,* 636–643.

Hinshaw, S. P., & Melnick, S. (1992). Self-management therapies and attention-deficit hyperactivity disorder: Reinforced self-evaluation and anger control interventions. *Behavior Modification, 16,* 253–273.

Hinshaw, S. P., Zupan, B. A., Simmel, C., Nigg, J. T., & Melnick, S. (1997). Peer status in boys with and without attention-deficit hyperactivity disorder: Predictions from overt and covert antisocial behavior, social isolation, and authoritative parenting beliefs. *Child Development, 68,* 880–896.

Hodgens, J. B., Cole, J., & Boldizar, J. (2000). Peer-based differences among boys with ADHD. *Journal of Clinical Child Psychology, 29,* 443–452.

Hoff, K., & DuPaul, G. J. (1998). Reducing disruptive behavior in general education classrooms: The use of self-management strategies. *School Psychology Review, 27,* 290–303.

Hoff, K. E., & Robinson, S. L. (2002). Best practices in peer-mediated interventions. In A. Thomas & J. Grimes (Eds.), *Best practices in school psychology IV* (pp. 1555–1567). Bethesda, MD: National Association of School Psychologists.

Holborow, P. L., & Berry, P. S. (1986). Hyperactivity and learning difficulties. *Journal of Learning Disabilities, 19,* 426–431.

Hook, C. L., & DuPaul, G. J. (1999). Parent tutoring for students with attention deficit hyperactivity disorder: Effects on reading at home and school. *School Psychology Review, 28,* 60–75.

Horn, W. F., Ialongo, N., Popovich, S., & Peradotto, D. (1987). Behavioral parent training and cognitive-behavioral self-control therapy with ADD-H children: Comparative and combined effect. *Journal of Clinical Child Psychology, 16,* 57–68.

Horner, R. H., Albin, R. W., & O'Neill, R. E. (1991). Supporting students with severe intellectual disabilities and severe challenging behaviors. In G. Stoner, M. R. Shinn, & H. M. Walker (Eds.), *Interventions for achievement and behavior problems* (pp. 269–287). Silver Spring, MD: National Association of School Psychologists.

Horner, R. H., Dunlap, G., & Koegel, R. L. (1988). *Generalization and maintenance: Lifestyle changes in applied settings.* Baltimore: Paul H. Brookes.

Hoza, B., Pelham, W. E., Sams, S. E., & Carlson, C. (1992). An examination of the "dosage" effects of both behavior therapy and methylphenidate on the

classroom performance of two ADHD children. *Behavior Modification, 16,*
164–192.

Hunt, R. D., Lau, S., & Ryu, J. (1991). Altenative therapies for ADHD. In L. L.
Greenhill & B. B. Osman (Eds.), *Ritalin: Theory and patient management*
(pp. 75–95). New York: Mary Ann Liebert.

Hunt, R. D., Mindera, R. B., & Cohen, D. J. (1985). Clonidine benefits children
with attention deficit disorder and hyperactivity: Report of a double-blind
placebo-crossover therapeutic trial. *Journal of the American Academy of
Child and Adolescent Psychiatry, 24,* 617–629.

Hynd, G. W. (1992). Misrepresentation or simply misinformed? Comment on
Gresham and Gansle's vitriolic diatribe regarding the DSM. *School Psychology Quarterly, 7,* 100–103.

Ingersoll, B., & Goldstein, S. (1993). *Attention deficit disorder and learning disabilities: Realities, myths, and controversial treatments.* New York: Doubleday.

Jacob, R. G., O'Leary, K. D., & Rosenblad, C. (1978). Formal and informal
classroom settings: Effects on hyperactivity. *Journal of Abnormal Child
Psychology, 6,* 47–59.

Jacobsen, N. S., & Truax, P. (1991). Clinical significance: A statistical approach
to defining meaningful change in psychotherapy research. *Journal of Consulting and Clinical Psychology, 59,* 12–19.

James, R. S., Sharp, W. S., Bastain, T. M., Lee, P. P., Walter, J. M., Czarnolewski,
M., & Castellano, F. X. (2001). Double-blind, placebo-controlled study of
single-dose amphetamine formulations in ADHD. *Journal of the American
Academy of Child and Adolescent Psychiatry, 40,* 1268–1276.

Jensen, P. S., Martin, D., & Cantwell, D. P. (1997). Comorbidity in ADHD: Implications for research, practice, and DSM-V. *Journal of the American
Academy of Child and Adolescent Psychiatry, 36,* 1065–1079.

Jenson, W. R., Clark, E., Walker, H. M., & Kehle, T. (1991). Behavior disorders:
Training needs for school psychologists. In G. Stoner, M. R. Shinn, & H.
M. Walker (Eds.), *Interventions for achievement and behavior problems*
(pp. 763–787). Silver Spring, MD: National Association of School Psychologists.

Johnson, R. A., Kenney, J. B., & Davis, J. B. (1976, November). Developing
school policy for use of stimulant drugs for hyperactive children. *School
Review,* pp. 78–96.

Johnson, R. C., & Rosén, L. A. (2000). Sports behavior of ADHD children.
Journal of Attention Disorders, 4, 150–160.

Johnson, T. C., Stoner, G., & Green, S. K. (1996). Demonstrating the experi-
menting society model with classwide behavior management interventions.
School Psychology Review, 25, 198–213.

Johnston, C., & Mash, E. J. (2001). Families of children with attention-deficit/
hyperactivity disorder: Review and recommendations for future research.
Clinical Child and Family Psychology Review, 4, 183–207.

Johnston, C., Pelham, W. E., Hoza, J., & Sturges, J. (1987). Psychostimulant rebound in attention deficit disordered boys. *Journal of the American Academy of Child and Adolescent Psychiatry, 27,* 806–810.

Kameenui, E. J. (1993). Diverse learners and the tyranny of time: Don't fix blame, fix the leaky roof. *Reading Teacher, 46,* 376–383.

Kameenui, E. J., & Simmons, D. C. (1990). *Designing instructional strategies: The prevention of academic learning problems.* Columbus, OH: Merrill.

Kaminski, R. A., & Good, R. H. (1996). Toward a technology for assessing basic early literacy skills. *School Psychology Review, 25,* 215–227.

Kaplan, B. J., Crawford, S. G., Dewey, D. M., & Fisher, G. C. (2000). The IQs of children with ADHD are normally distributed. *Journal of Learning Disabilities, 33,* 435–432.

Karustis, J. L., Power, T. J., Rescorla, L. A., Eiraldi, R. B., & Gallagher, P. R. (1998). *The contribution of internalizing symptoms to functional impairment in children with attention-deficit/hyperactivity disorder.* Manuscript submitted for publication.

Karustis, J. L., Power, T. J., Rescorla, L. A., Eiraldi, R. B., & Gallagher, P. R. (2000). Anxiety and depression in children with ADHD: Unique associations with academic and social functioning. *Journal of Attention Disorders, 4,* 133–149.

Kavale, K. A., & Mattson, P. D. (1983). One jumped off the balance beam: Meta-analysis of perceptual-motor training. *Journal of Learning Disabilities, 16,* 165–173.

Kazdin, A. E. (1992). *Research design in clinical psychology* (2nd ed.). Boston: Allyn & Bacon.

Kazdin, A. E. (2000). *Psychotherapy for children and adolescents: Directions for research and practice.* London: Oxford University Press.

Keenan, K., Shaw, D. S., Walsh, B., Deliquadri, E., & Giovanelli, J. (1997). DSM-III-R disorders in preschool children from low-income families. *Journal of the American Academy of Child and Adolescent Psychiatry, 36,* 620–627.

Kelley, M. L. (1990). *School–home notes: Promoting children's classroom success.* New York: Guilford Press.

Kelly, K. (2001). *An assessment of the peer relationships of elementary school children diagnosed with attention deficit hyperactivity disorder.* Unpublished doctoral dissertation, Lehigh University, Bethlehem, PA.

Kendall, P. C., & Braswell, L. (1985). *Cognitive-behavioral therapy for impulsive children.* New York: Guilford Press.

Keogh, B. A. (1971). Hyperactivity and learning disorders: Review and speculation. *Exceptional Children, 38,* 101–109.

Kern, L., Childs, K. E., Dunlap, G., Clarke, S., & Falk, G. D. (1994). Using assessment-based curricular intervention to improve the classroom behavior of a student with emotional and behavioral challenges. *Journal of Applied Behavior Analysis, 27,* 7–19.

Klein, S. D. (1993). The challenge of communicating with parents. *Journal of Developmental and Behavioral Pediatrics, 14,* 184–191.

Klorman, R., Brumaghim, J. T., Salzman, L. F., Strauss, J., Borgsted, A. D., McBride, M. C., & Loeb, S. (1988). Effects of methylphenidate on attention-deficit hyperactivity disorder with and without aggressive/noncompliant features. *Journal of Abnormal Psychology, 97,* 413–422.

Koegel, R. L., Dyer, K., & Bell, L. K. (1987). The influence of child-preferred activities on autistic children's social behavior. *Journal of Applied Behavior Analysis, 20*, 243–252.

Kohler, F. W., Schwartz, I., Cross, J., & Fowler, S. A. (1989). The effects of two alternating intervention roles on independent work skills. *Education and Treatment of Children, 12*, 205–218.

Kohler, F. W., & Strain, P. S. (1990). Peer-assisted interventions: Early promises, notable achievements, and future aspirations. *Clinical Psychology Review, 10*, 441–452.

Kratochwill, T. R., & Bergan, J. (1990). *Behavioral consultation in applied settings: An individual guide.* New York: Plenum Press.

La Greca, A. M. (1990). *Through the eyes of the child.* Boston: Allyn & Bacon.

Lahey, B. B. (2000, October). *Assessment issues in doing research with preschoolers.* Paper presented at the annual convention of the American Academy of Child and Adolescent Psychiatry (Research Forum), New York.

Lahey, B. B., Applegate, B., McBurnett, K., Biederman, J., Greenhill, L., Hynd, G. W., Barkley, R. A., Newcorn, J., Jensen, P., Richters, J., Garfinkel, B., Kerdyk, L., Frick, P. J., Ollendick, T., Perez, D., Hart, E. L., Waldman, I., & Shaffer, D. (1994). DSM-IV field trials for attention deficit hyperactivity disorder in children and adolescents. *American Journal of Psychiatry, 151*, 1673–1685.

Lahey, B. B., & Carlson, C. (1992). Validity of the diagnostic category of attention deficit disorder without hyperactivity: A review of the literature. In S. E. Shaywitz & B. A. Shaywitz (Eds.), *Attention deficit disorder comes of age: Toward the twenty-first century* (pp. 119–144). Austin, TX: Pro-Ed.

Lahey, B. B., Pelham, W. E., Stein, M. A., Loney, J., Trapani, C., Nugent, K., Kipp, H., Schmidt, E., Lee, S., Cale, M., Gold, E., Hartung, C. M., Willcutt, E., & Baumann, B. (1998). Validity of DSM-IV attention-deficit/hyperactivity disorder for younger children. *Journal of the American Academy of Child and Adolescent Psychiatry, 37*, 695–702.

Lahey, B. B., Piacentini, J. C., McBurnett, K., Stone, P., Hartdagen, S., & Hynd, G. (1988). Psychopathology in the parents of children with conduct disorder and hyperactivity. *Journal of the American Academy of Child and Adolescent Psychiatry, 27*, 163–170.

Lam, A. L., Cole, C. L., Shapiro, E. S., & Bambara, L. M. (1994). Relative effects of self-monitoring on-task behavior, academic accuracy, and disruptive behavior in students with behavior disorders. *School Psychology Review, 23*, 44–58.

Lambert, N. M., & Sandoval, J. (1980). The prevalence of learning disabilities in a sample of children considered hyperactive. *Journal of Abnormal Child Psychology, 8*, 33–50.

Landau, S., Milich, R., & Widiger, T. A. (1991). Conditional probability of child interview symptoms in the diagnosis of attention deficit disorder. *Journal of Child Psychology and Psychiatry, 32*, 501–513.

Lavigne, J. V., Gibbons, R. D., Christoffel, K. K., Arend, R., Rosenbaum, D., Binns, H., Dawson, N., Sobel, H., & Isaacs, C. (1996). Prevalence rates and correlates of psychiatric disorders among preschool children. *Journal of the American Academy of Child and Adolescent Psychiatry, 35*, 204–214.

Levin, H., Glass, G., & Meister, G. (1984). *Cost-effectiveness of four educational interventions* (Report No. 84–A11). Stanford, CA: Stanford University Institute for Research in Educational Finance and Governance.

Levine, M. D., Busch, B., & Aufseeser. C. (1982). The dimension of inattention among children with school problems. *Pediatrics, 70*, 387–395.

Levy, F., Hay, D. A., McStephen, M., Wood, C., & Waldman, I. (1997). Attention-deficit hyperactivity disorder: A category or a continuum? Genetic analysis of a large-scale twin study. *Journal of the American Academy of Child and Adolescent Psychiatry, 36*, 737–744.

Lillie, D. L., Hannun, W. H., & Stuck, G. B. (1989). *Computers and effective instruction.* New York: Longman.

Lindsley, O. R. (1991). From technical jargon to plain English for application. *Journal of Applied Behavior Analysis, 24*, 449–458.

Livingston, R. (1990). Psychiatric comorbidity with reading disability: A clinical study. *Advances in Learning and Behavioral Disabilities, 6*, 143–155.

Lochman, J. E., & Curry, J. F. (1986). Effects of social problem-solving and self-instruction training with aggressive boys. *Journal of Clinical Child Psychology, 15*, 159–164.

Loney, J., & Milich, R. (1982). Hyperactivity, inattention, and aggression in clinical practice. In D. Routh & M. Wolraich (Eds.), *Advances in developmental and behavioral pediatrics* (Vol. 3, pp. 113–147). Greenwich, CT: JAI Press.

Loney, J., Weissenburger, F. E., Woolson, R. F., & Lichty, E. C. (1979). Comparing psychological and pharmacological treatments for hyperkinetic boys and their classmates. *Journal of Abnormal Child Psychology, 7*, 133–143.

Lord, C., Rutter, M., & Le Couteur, A. (1994). Autism Diagnostic Interview—Revised: A revised version of a diagnostic interview for caregivers of individuals with possible pervasive developmental disorders. *Journal of Autism and Developmental Disabilities, 24*, 659–685.

Lovejoy, M. C., & Rasmussen, N. H. (1990). The validity of vigilance tasks in differential diagnosis of children referred for attention and learning problems. *Journal of Abnormal Child Psychology, 18*, 671–681.

Madsen, C. H., Becker, W. C., & Thomas, D. R. (1968). Rules, praise, and ignoring: Elements of elementary classroom control. *Journal of Applied Behavior Analysis, 1*, 139–150.

Mannuzza, S., Gittelman-Klein, R., Bessler, A., Malloy, P., & LaPadula, M. (1993). Adult outcome of hyperactive boys: Educational achievement, occupational rank, and psychiatric status. *Archives of General Psychiatry, 50*, 565–576.

Mariani, M., & Barkley, R. A. (1997). Neuropsychological and academic functioning in preschool children with attention deficit hyperactivity disorder. *Developmental Neuropsychology, 13*, 111–129.

Marston, D. B. (1989). A curriculum-based measurement approach to assessing academic performance: What it is and why do it. In M. R. Shinn (Ed.), *Curriculum-based measurement: Assessing special children* (pp. 18–78). New York: Guilford Press.

Martens, B. K. (1992). The difference between a good theory and a good treatment is a matter of degree. *School Psychology Quarterly, 7,* 104–107.

Martens, B. K., & Kelly, S. Q. (1993). A behavioral analysis of effective teaching. *School Psychology Quarterly, 8,* 10–26.

McBurnett, K., Pfiffner, L. J., & Frick, P. (2001). Symptom properties as a function of ADHD type: An argument for continued study of sluggish cognitive tempo. *Journal of Abnormal Child Psychology, 29,* 207–213.

McConaughy, S. H., Achenbach, T. M., & Gent, C. L. (1988). Multiaxial empirically based assessment: Parent, teacher, observational, cognitive, and personality correlates of child behavior profile types for 6- to 11-year-old boys. *Journal of Abnormal Child Psychology, 16,* 485–509.

McConaughy, S. H., Mattison, R. E., & Peterson, R. L. (1994). Behavioral/emotional problems of children with serious emotional disturbance and learning disabilities. *School Psychology Review, 23,* 81–98.

McConnell, S. R., & Hecht, M. (1991). Instructional problems and interventions: Training needs for school psychologists. In G. Stoner, M. R. Shinn, & H. M. Walker (Eds.), *Interventions for achievement and behavior problems* (pp. 741–761). Silver Spring, MD: National Association of School Psychologists.

McDermott, P. A., Leigh, N. M., & Perry, M. A. (2002). Development and validation of the Preschool Learning Behaviors Scale. *Psychology in the Schools, 39,* 353–365.

McGee, R., & Share, D. L. (1988). Attention deficit disorder-hyperactivity and academic failure: Which comes first and what should be treated? *Journal of the American Academy of Child and Adolescent Psychiatry, 27,* 318–325.

McGee, R. A., Clark, S. E., & Symons, D. K. (2000). Does the Conners' Continuous Performance Test aid in ADHD diagnosis? *Journal of Abnormal Child Psychology, 28,* 415–424.

McGee, R., Williams, S., & Silva, P. A. (1984). Behavioral and developmental characteristics of aggressive, hyperactive, and aggressive-hyperactive boys. *Journal of the American Academy of Child and Adolescent Psychiatry, 23,* 270–279.

McGoey, K. E., Bradley-Klug, K., Crone, D., Shelton, T. L., & Radcliffe, J. (2000, April). *Normative data of the ADHD-Rating Scale-IV—Preschool version.* Paper presented at the annual convention of the National Association of School Psychologists, New Orleans, LA.

McGoey, K. E., & DuPaul, G. J. (2000). Token reinforcement and response cost procedures: Reducing the disruptive behavior of preschool children with ADHD. *School Psychology Quarterly, 15,* 330–343.

McGoey, K. E., DuPaul, G. J., Eckert, T. L., VanBrakle, J., & Volpe, R. J. (2002). *Early intervention for young children at-risk for ADHD: Home and school outcomes.* Manuscript submitted for publication.

McGoey, K. E., Eckert, T. L., & DuPaul, G. J. (2002). Early intervention for preschool-age children with ADHD: A literature review. *Journal of Emotional and Behavioral Disorders, 10*, 14–28.

Meichenbaum, D., & Goodman, J. (1971). Training impulsive children to talk to themselves: A means of developing self-control. *Journal of Abnormal Psychology, 77*, 115–126.

Merrell, K. (1994). *Preschool and Kindergarten Behavior Scales.* Longmont, CO: Sopris-West.

Merrrell, K. (1999). *Behavioral, social, and emotional assessment of children and adolescents.* Mahwah, NJ: Erlbaum.

Meyer, L. H., & Evans, I. M. (1989). *Nonaversive interventions for behavior problems: A manual for home and community.* Baltimore: Paul H. Brookes.

Michelson, D., Allen, A. J., Busner, J., Casat, C., Dunn, D., Kratochvil, C., Newcorn, J., Sallee, F. R., Sangal, R. B., Saylor, K., West, S., Kelsey, D., Wernicke, J., Trapp, N. J., & Harder, D. (2002). Once-daily atomoxetine treatment for children and adolescents with attention deficit hyperactivity disorder: A randomized, placebo-controlled study. *American Journal of Psychiatry, 159*, 1896–1901.

Mick, E., Biederman, J., Faraone, S. V., Sayer, J., & Kleinman, S. (2002). Case–control study of attention-deficit hyperactivity disorder and maternal smoking, alcohol use, and drug use during pregnancy. *Journal of the American Academy of Child and Adolescent Psychiatry, 41*, 378–385.

Mick, E., Biederman, J., Prince, J., Fischer, M. J., & Faraone, S. V. (2002). Impact of low birth weight on attention-deficit hyperactivity disorder. *Journal of Developmental and Behavioral Pediatrics, 23*, 16–22.

Milberger, S., Biederman, J., Faraone, S. V., Chen, L., & Jones, J. (1996). Is maternal smoking during pregnancy a risk factor for attention deficit hyperactivity disorder in children? *American Journal of Psychiatry, 153*, 1138–1142.

Milich, R., Balentine, A. C., & Lynam, D. R. (2001). ADHD combined type and ADHD predominately inattentive type are distinct and unrelated disorders. *Clinical Psychology: Science and Practice, 8*, 463–488.

Milich, R., Carlson, C. L., Pelham, W. E., Jr., & Licht, B. G. (1991). Effects of methylphenidate on the persistence of ADHD boys following failure experiences. *Journal of Abnormal Child Psychology, 19*, 519–536.

Milich, R., Landau, S., Kilby, G., & Whitten, P. (1982). Preschool peer perceptions of the behavior of hyperactive and aggressive children. *Journal of Abnormal Child Psychology, 10*, 497–510.

Minuchin, S. (1974). *Families and family therapy.* Cambridge, MA: Harvard University Press.

Morgan, D. L., & Morgan, R. K. (2001). Single-participant research design: Bringing science to managed care. *American Psychologist, 56*, 119–127.

MTA Cooperative Group. (1999). A 14–month randomized clinical trial of treatment strategies for attention-deficit/hyperactivity disorder. *Archives of General Psychiatry, 56*, 1073–1086.

Murray, H. A. (1943). *Thematic apperception test.* Cambridge, MA: Harvard University Press.

Murray, L. K., & Kollins, S. H. (2000). Effects of methylphenidate on sensitivity to reinforcement in children diagnosed with attention deficit hyperactivity disorder: An application of the matching law. *Journal of Applied Behavior Analysis, 33,* 573–591.

Naglieri, J. A., LeBuffe, P. A., & Pfeiffer, S. I. (1994). *The Devereux Scales of Mental Disorders.* San Antonio, TX: Psychological Corporation.

National Association of School Psychologists. (1998). *Position statement on students with attention problems.* Washington, DC: Author.

National Association of School Psychologists. (2000). *Professional conduct manual: Principles for professional ethics. Standards for the provision of school psychological services.* Bethesda, MD: Author.

National Institutes of Health. (1998). Diagnosis and treatment of attention-deficit/hyperactivity disorder. *NIH Consensus Statement, 16(2),* 1–37.

National Reading Panel. (2000). *Teaching children to read: An evidence-based assessment of the scientific research literature on reading and its implications for reading instruction* [Online]. Available: www.nichd.nih.gov/publications/nrp/smallbook.htm

National Research Council. (1998). *Preventing reading difficulties in young children.* Washington, DC: National Academy Press.

Nebrig, M., & DuPaul, G. J. (2001). *The effects of bupropion hydrochloride on the classroom performance of students with attention-deficit/hyperactivity disorder.* Manuscript submitted for publication.

Nelson, J. R., Roberts, M. L., & Smith, D. L. (1998). *Conducting functional behavioral assessments.* Longmont, CO: Sopris-West.

Ninio, A., & Bruner, J. (1978). The achievement and antecedents of labeling. *Journal of Child Language, 7,* 565–573.

Nixon, R. D. (2002). Treatment of behavior problems in preschoolers: A review of parent training programs. *Clinical Psychology Review, 22,* 525–546.

Northup, J., Fusilier, I., Swanson, V., Huete, J., Bruce, T., Freeland, J., Gulley, V., & Edwards, S. (1999). Further analysis of the separate and interactive effects of methylphenidate and common classroom contingencies. *Journal of Applied Behavior Analysis, 32,* 35–50.

Northup, J., & Gulley, V. (2001). Some contributions of functional analysis to the assessment of behaviors associated with attention deficit hyperactivity disorder and the effects of stimulant medication. *School Psychology Review, 30,* 227–238.

Northup, J., Jones, K., Broussard, C., DiGiovanni, G., Herring, M., Fusilier, I., & Hanchey, A. (1997). A preliminary analysis of interactive effects between common classroom contingencies and methylphenidate. *Journal of Applied Behavior Analysis, 30,* 121–125.

Northup, J., Wacker, D., Sasso, G., Steege, M., Cigrand, K., Cook, J., & DeRaad, A. (1991). A brief functional analysis of aggressive and alternative behavior in an outclinic setting. *Journal of Applied Behavior Analysis, 24,* 509–522.

Notari-Syverson, A., O'Connor, R. E., & Vadasy, P. F. (1998). *Ladders to literacy: A preschool activity book.* Baltimore: Paul H. Brookes.

Nussbaum, N. L., Grant, M. L., Roman, M. J., Poole, J. H., & Bigler, E. (1990).

Attention deficit disorder and the mediating effect of age on academic and behavioral variables. *Developmental Behavioral Pediatrics, 11,* 22–26.

Office of Technology Assessment. (1988). *Power on!: New tools for teaching and learning* (OTA-SET-379). Washington, DC: U.S. Government Printing Office.

O'Leary, K. D. (1980). Pills or skills for hyperactive children. *Journal of Applied Behavior Analysis, 13,* 191–204.

O'Leary, K. D., Pelham, W. E., Rosenbaum, A., & Price, G. H. (1976). Behavioral treatment of hyperkinetic children: An experimental evaluation of its usefulness. *Clinical Pediatrics, 15,* 510–515.

Olfson, M., Marcus, S. C., Weissman, M. M., & Jensen, P. S. (2002). National trends in the use of psychotropic medications by children. *Journal of the American Academy of Child and Adolescent Psychiatry, 41,* 514–521.

Olympia, D. E., Jenson, W. R., & Hepworth-Neville, M. (1996). *Sanity savers for parents: Tips for tackling homework.* Longmont, CO: Sopris-West.

O'Neill, R. E., Horner, R. H., Albin, R. W., Storey, K., & Sprague, J. R. (1997). *Functional analysis of problem behavior: A practical assessment guide* (2nd ed.). Pacific Grove, CA: Brookes/Cole.

O'Reilly, M. J. (2002). *Early literacy skill development of kindergartners and first-graders at-risk for externalizing behavior disorders.* Manuscript submitted for publication.

O'Shea, L. J., Sindelar, P. T., & O'Shea, D. J. (1987) The effects of repeated readings and attentional cues on the reading fluency and comprehension of learning disabled readers. *Learning Disabilities Research, 2,* 103–109.

Ota, K. R., & DuPaul, G. J. (2002). Task engagement and mathematics performance in children with attention deficit hyperactivity disorder: Effects of supplemental computer instruction. *School Psychology Quarterly, 17,* 242–257.

Pagani, L., Tremblay, R. E., Vitaro, F., Boulerice, B., & McDuff, P. (2001). Effects of grade retention on academic performance and behavioral development. *Development and Psychopathology, 13,* 297–315.

Paine, S., & Paine, C. K. (2002). Promoting safety and success in school by developing students' strengths. In M. R. Shinn, H. M. Walker, & G. Stoner (Eds.), *Interventions for academic and behavior problems II: Preventive and remedial approaches* (pp. 89–111). Bethesda, MD: National Association of School Psychologists.

Paine, S. C., Radicchi, J., Rosellini, L. C., Deutchman, L., & Darch, C. B. (1983). *Structuring your classroom for academic success.* Champaign, IL: Research Press.

Paniagua, F. A. (1992). Verbal–nonverbal correspondence training with ADHD children. *Behavior Modification, 16,* 226–252.

Pany, D., Jenkins, J. R., & Schreck, J. (1982). Vocabulary instruction: Effects on word knowledge and reading comprehension. *Learning Disability Quarterly, 5,* 202–214.

Parker, H. C. (1992). *The ADD hyperactivity handbook for schools: Effective strategies for identifying and teaching students with attention deficit disorders in elementary and secondary schools.* Plantation, FL: Impact.

Parker, J. G., & Asher, S. R. (1987). Peer relations and later personal adjustment: Are low-accepted children at risk? *Psychological Bulletin, 102,* 357–389.

Pastor, P. N., & Reuben, C. A. (2002). Attention deficit disorder and learning disability: United States, 1997–98. In *National Center for Health Statistics: Vital Health Statistics* (DHHS Publication No. PHS 2002–1534). Hyattsville, MD: Department of Health and Human Services.

Patterson, G. R., & Chamberlain, P. (1994). A functional analysis of resistance during parent-training therapy. *Clinical Psychology: Science and Practice, 1,* 53–70.

Patterson, G. R., Reid, J. B., & Dishion, T. J. (1992). *Antisocial boys.* Eugene, OR: Castalia.

Pelham, W. E. (1989). Behavior therapy, behavioral assessment, and psychostimulant medication in treatment of attention deficit disorders: An interactive approach. In J. Swanson & L. Bloomingdale (Eds.), *Attention deficit disorders, IV: Current concepts and emerging trends in attentional and behavior disorders of childhood* (pp. 169–195). London: Pergamon Press.

Pelham, W. E., Bender, M. E., Caddell, J., Booth, S., & Moorer, S. H. (1985). Methylphenidate and children with attention deficit disorder. *Archives of General Psychiatry, 42,* 948–952.

Pelham, W. E., Carlson, C., Sams, S. E., Vallano, G., Dixon, M. J., & Hoza, B. (1993). Separate and combined effects of methylphenidate and behavior modification on boys with attention deficit-hyperactivity disorder in classroom. *Journal of Consulting and Clinical Psychology, 61,* 506–515.

Pelham, W. E., & Hoza, J. (1987). Behavioral assessment of psychostimulant effects on ADD children in a summer day treatment program. In R. Prinz (Ed.), *Advances in behavioral assessment of children and families* (Vol. 3, pp. 3–33). Greenwich, CT: JAI Press.

Pelham, W. E., McBurnett, K., Harper, G. W., Milich, R., Murphy, D. A., Clinton, J., & Thiel, C. (1990). Methylphenidate and baseball playing in ADHD children: Who's on first? *Journal of Consulting and Clinical Psychology, 58,* 130–133.

Pelham, W. E., & Milich, R. (1991). Individual differences in response to Ritalin in classwork and social behavior. In L. L. Greenhill & B. B. Osman (Eds.), *Ritalin: Theory and patient management* (pp. 203–221). New York: Mary Ann Liebert.

Pelham, W. E., & Murphy, H. A. (1986). Attention deficit and conduct disorders. In M. Hersen (Ed.), *Pharmacological and behavioral treatment: An integrative approach* (pp. 108–148). New York: Wiley.

Pelham, W. E., Vodde-Hamilton, M., Murphy, D. A., Greenstein, J. L., & Vallano, G. (1991). The effects of methylphenidate on ADHD adolescents in recreational, peer group, and classroom settings. *Journal of Clinical Child Psychology, 20,* 293–300.

Pelham, W. E., Wheeler, T., & Chronis, A. (1998). Empirically-supported psychosocial treatments for ADHD. *Journal of Clinical Child Psychology, 27,* 190–205.

Peterson, L., Homer, A. L., & Wonderlich, S. A. (1982). The integrity of independent variables in behavior analysis. *Journal of Applied Behavior Analysis, 15,* 477–492.

Pfiffner, L. J., & Barkley, R. A. (1998). Treatment of ADHD in school settings. In R. A. Barkley, *Attention-deficit hyperactivity disorder: A handbook for diagnosis and treatment* (2nd ed., pp. 458–490). New York: Guilford Press.

Pffifner, L. J., & O'Leary, S. G. (1987). The efficacy of all-positive management as a function of the prior use of negative consequences. *Journal of Applied Behavior Analysis, 20,* 265–271.

Pfiffner, L. J., & O'Leary, S. G. (1993). School-based psychological treatments. In J. L. Matson (Ed.), *Handbook of hyperactivity in children* (pp. 234–255). Boston: Allyn & Bacon.

Pfiffner, L. J., O'Leary, S. G., Rosen, L. A., & Sanderson, W. C., Jr. (1985). A comparison of the effects of continuous and intermittent response cost and reprimands in the classroom. *Journal of Clinical Child Psychology, 14,* 348–352.

Phelps, L., Brown, R. T., & Power, T. J. (2001). *Pediatric psychopharmacology: Combining medical and psychosocial intervention.* Washington, DC: American Psychological Association.

Pierce, E. W., Ewing, L. J., & Campbell, S. B. (1999). Diagnostic status and symptomatic behavior of hard-to-manage preschool children in middle childhood and early adolescence. *Journal of Clinical Child Psychology, 28,* 44–57.

Platzman, K. A., Stoy, M. R., Brown, R. T., Coles, C. D., Smith, I. E., & Falek, A. (1992). Review of observational methods in attention deficit hyperactivity disorder (ADHD): Implications for diagnosis. *School Psychology Quarterly, 7,* 155–177.

Pliszka, S. R., Carlson, C. L., & Swanson, J. M. (1999). *ADHD with comorbid disorders: Clinical assessment and management.* New York: Guilford Press.

Power, T. J. (2002). Preparing school psychologists as interventionists and preventionists. In M. R. Shinn, H. M. Walker, & G. Stoner (Eds.), *Interventions for academic and behavior problems, II: Preventive and remedial approaches* (pp. 1047–1065). Bethesda, MD: National Association of School Psychologists.

Power, T. J., Atkins, M., Osborne, M., & Blum, N. (1994). The school psychologist as manager of programming for ADHD. *School Psychology Review, 23,* 279–291.

Power, T. J., DuPaul, G. J., Shapiro, E. S., & Kazak, A. (2003). *Promoting children's health: Integrating school, family, and community.* New York: Guilford Press.

Power, T. J., Karustis, J. L., & Habboushe, D. F. (2001). *Homework success for children with ADHD: A family–school intervention program.* New York: Guilford Press.

Rapoport, J. L. (1986). Antidepressants in childhood attention deficit disorder and obsessive–compulsive disorder. *Psychosomatics, 27,* 30–36.

Rapoport, J., Buchsbaum, M., Weingartner, H., Zahn, T., Ludlow, C., Bartko, J.,

Mikkelson, E., Langer, D., & Bunney, W. (1980). Dextroamphetamine: Cognitive and behavioral effects in normal and hyperactive boys and normal adult males. *Archives of General Psychiatry, 37,* 933–946.

Rapport, M. D. (1987a). Attention deficit disorder with hyperactivity. In M. Hersen & V. B. Van Hasselt (Eds.), *Behavior therapy with children and adolescents* (pp. 325–361). New York: Wiley.

Rapport, M. D. (1987b). *The attention training system: User's manual.* DeWitt, NY: Gordon Systems, Inc.

Rapport, M. D., Carlson, G. A., Kelly, K. L., & Pataki, C. (1993). Methylphenidate and desipramine in hospitalized children: I. Separate and combined effects on cognitive function. *Journal of the American Academy of Child and Adolescent Psychiatry, 32,* 333–342.

Rapport, M. D., Chung, K. M., Shore, G., Denney, C. B., & Isaacs, P. (2000). Upgrading the science and technology of assessment and diagnosis: Laboratory and clinic-based assessment of children with ADHD. *Journal of Clinical Child Psychology, 29,* 555–568.

Rapport, M. D., & Denney, C. B. (1997). Titrating methylphenidate in children with attention-deficit/hyperactivity disorder: Is body mass predictive of clinical response? *Journal of the American Academy of Child and Adolescent Psychiatry, 36,* 523–530.

Rapport, M. D., & Denney, C. B. (2000). Attention deficit hyperactivity disorder and methylphenidate: Assessment and prediction of clinical response. In L. L. Greenhill & B. B. Osman (Eds.), *Ritalin: Theory and practice* (2nd ed., pp. 45–70). Larchmont, NY: Mary Ann Liebert.

Rapport, M. D., Denney, C. B., DuPaul, G. J., & Gardner, M. J. (1994). Attention deficit disorder and methylphenidate: Normalization rates, clinical effectiveness, and response prediction in 76 children. *Journal of the American Academy of Child and Adolesecent Psychiatry, 33,* 882–893.

Rapport, M. D., DuPaul, G. J., & Kelly, K. L. (1989). Attention-deficit hyperactivity disorder and methylphenidate: The relationship between gross body weight and drug response in children. *Psychopharmacology Bulletin, 25,* 285–290.

Rapport, M. D., DuPaul, G. J., & Smith, N. F. (1985). Rate-dependency and hyperactivity: Methylphenidate effects upon operant performance. *Pharmacology, Biochemistry, and Behavior, 23,* 77–83.

Rapport, M. D., DuPaul, G. J., Stoner, G., & Jones, J. T. (1986). Comparing classroom and clinic measures of attention deficit disorder: Differential, idiosyncratic, and dose–response effects of methylphenidate. *Journal of Consulting and Clinical Psychology, 54,* 334–341.

Rapport, M. D., Jones, J. T., DuPaul, G. J., Kelly, K. L., Gardner, M. J., Tucker, S. B., & Shea, M. S. (1987). Attention deficit disorder and methylphenidate: Group and single-subject analyses of dose effects on attention in clinic and classroom settings. *Journal of Clinical Child Psychology, 16,* 329–338.

Rapport, M. D., & Kelly, K. L. (1991). Psychostimulant effects on learning and cognitive function: Findings and implications for children with attention-deficit hyperactivity disorder. *Clinical Psychology Review, 11,* 61–92.

Rapport, M. D., & Moffitt, C. (2002). Attention deficit/hyperactivity disorder and methylphenidate: A review of height/weight, cardiovascular, and somatic complaint side effects. *Clinical Psychology Review, 22,* 1107–1131.

Rapport, M. D., Murphy, A., & Bailey, J. S. (1980). The effects of a response cost treatment tactic on hyperactive children. *Journal of School Psychology, 18,* 98–111.

Rapport, M. D., Murphy, A., & Bailey, J. S. (1982). Ritalin vs. response cost in the control of hyperactive children: A within subject comparison. *Journal of Applied Behavior Analysis, 15,* 205–216.

Rapport, M. D., Scanlan, S. W., & Denney, C. B. (1999). Attention-deficit/hyperactivity disorder and scholastic achievement: A model of dual developmental pathways. *Journal of Child Psychology and Psychiatry, 40,* 1169–1183.

Rapport, M. D., Stoner, G., DuPaul, G. J., Birmingham, B. K., & Tucker, S. (1985). Methylphenidate in hyperactive children: Differential effects of dose on academic, learning, and social behavior. *Journal of Abnormal Child Psychology, 13,* 227–244.

Rapport, M. D., Stoner, G., DuPaul, G. J., Kelly, K. L., Tucker, S. B., & Schoeler, T. (1988). Attention deficit disorder and methylphenidate: A multilevel analysis of dose–response effects on children's impulsivity across settings. *Journal of the American Academy of Child and Adolescent Psychiatry, 27,* 60–69.

Rapport, M. D., Tucker, S. B., DuPaul, G. J., Merlo, M., & Stoner, G. (1986). Hyperactivity and frustration: The influence of size and control over rewards in delaying gratification. *Journal of Abnormal Child Psychology, 14,* 191–204.

Reeve, E., & Garfinkel, B. (1991). Neuroendocrine and growth regulation: The role of sympathomimetic medication. In L. L. Greenhill & B. B. Osman (Eds.), *Ritalin: Theory and patient management* (pp. 289–300). New York: Mary Ann Liebert.

Reich, W. (2000). *Diagnostic Interview for Children and Adolescents: Preschool version.* St. Louis, MO: Washington University.

Reid, J. B., & Eddy, J. M. (1997). The prevention of antisocial behavior: Some considerations in the search for effective interventions. In D. M. Stoff, J. Breiling, & J. D. Maser (Eds.), *Handbook of antisocial behavior* (pp. 343–356). New York: Wiley.

Reid, R., DuPaul, G. J., Power, T. J., Anastopoulos, A. D., & Riccio, C. (1998). Assessing culturally different students for attention deficit hyperactivity disorder using behavior rating scales. *Journal of Abnormal Child Psychology, 26,* 187–198.

Reith, H., Bahr, C., Polsgrove, L, Okolo, C., & Eckert, R. (1987). The effects of microcomputers on the secondary special education classroom ecology. *Journal of Special Education Technology, 8,* 36–45.

Reschly, D. J. (1988). Special education reform: School psychology revolution. *School Psychology Review, 17,* 459–475.

Reschly, D. J. (2000). Assessment and eligibility determination in the Individuals with Disabilities Education Act of 1997. In C. F. Telzrow & M. Tankersley (Eds.), *IDEA amendments of 1997: Practice guidelines for school-based teams* (pp. 65–104). Bethesda, MD: National Association of School Psychologists.

Reschly, D. J., Tilly, W. D. III, & Grimes, J. P. (1999). *Special education in transition: Functional assessment and noncategorical programming.* Longmont, CO: Sopris-West.

Reynolds, C. R. (1992). Misguided epistemological shifting, misdirected misology, and dogma in diagnosis. *School Psychology Quarterly, 7,* 96–99.

Reynolds, C. R., & Kamphaus, R. W. (1992). *BASC: Behavior Assessment System for Children manual.* Circle Pines, MN: American Guidance.

Reynolds, M. C. (1988). Alternative educational approaches: Implications for school psychology. In J. L. Graden, J. E. Zins, & M. J. Curtis (Eds.), *Alternative educational delivery systems: Enhancing instructional options for all students* (pp. 555–562). Washington, DC: National Association of School Psychologists.

Reynolds, W. M. (1987). *Reynolds Adolescent Depression Scale: Professional manual.* Odessa, FL: Psychological Assessment Resources.

Rhode, G., Morgan, D. P., & Young, K. R. (1983). Generalization and maintenance of treatment gains of behaviorally handicapped students from resource rooms to regular classrooms using self-evaluation procedures. *Journal of Applied Behavior Analysis, 16,* 171–188.

Riggs, P. D., Leon, S. L., Mikulich, S. K., & Pottle, L. C. (1998). An open trial of bupropion for ADHD in adolescents with substance use disorders and conduct disorder. *Journal of the American Academy of Child and Adolescent Psychiatry, 37,* 1271–1278.

Risley, T. R., & Hart, B. (1968). Developing correspondence between the nonverbal and verbal behavior of preschool children. *Journal of Applied Behavior Analysis, 1,* 267–281.

Roberts, M. L., & Landau, S. (1995). Using curriculum-based data for assessing children with attention deficits. *Journal of Psychoeducational Assessment, ADHD Special Edition,* 75–88.

Robin, A. L. (1998). *ADHD in adolescents: Diagnosis and treatment.* New York: Guilford Press.

Robin, A. L., & Foster, S. L. (1989). *Negotiating parent–adolescent conflict: A behavioral-family systems approach.* New York: Guilford Press.

Robinson, P. W., Newby, T. J., & Ganzell, S. L. (1981). A token system for a class of underachieving hyperactive children. *Journal of Applied Behavior Analysis, 14,* 307–315.

Rose, T. L., & Sherry, L. (1984). Relative effects of two previewing procedures on LD adolescents' oral reading performance. *Learning Disability Quarterly, 7,* 39–44.

Rosen, L. A., O'Leary, S. G., Joyce, S. A., Conway, G., & Pfiffner, L. J. (1984). The importance of prudent negative consequences for maintaining the appropriate behavior of hyperactive students. *Journal of Abnormal Child Psychology, 12,* 581–604.

Rosenshine, B. V. (1987). Explicit teaching. In D. C. Berliner & B. V. Rosenshine (Eds.), *Talks to teachers: A festschrift for N. L. Gage* (pp. 75– 92). New York: Random House.

Rosvold, H. E., Mirsky, A. F., Sarason, I., Bransome, E. D., & Beck, L. H. (1956). A continuous performance test of brain damage. *Journal of Consulting Psychology, 20,* 343–350.

Rourke, B. P. (1988). Socioemotional disturbances of learning disabled children. *Journal of Consulting and Clinical Psychology, 56,* 801–810.

Rowe, K. J., & Rowe, K. S. (1992). The relationship between inattentiveness in the classroom and reading achievement, Part B: An explanatory study. *Journal of the American Academy of Child and Adolescent Psychiatry, 31,* 357–368.

Safer, D. J., & Zito, J. M. (2000). Pharmacoepidemiology of methylphenidate and other stimulants for the treatment of attention deficit hyperactivity disorder. In L. L. Greenhill & B. B. Osman (Eds.), *Ritalin: Theory and practice* (2nd ed., pp. 7–26). Larchmont, NY: Mary Ann Liebert.

Salvia, J., & Ysseldyke, J. (1998). *Assessment in special and remedial education* (7th ed.). Boston: Houghton Mifflin.

Samuels, S. J. (1979). The method of repeated readings. *Reading Teacher, 32,* 403–408.

Saudargas, R. A., & Creed, V. (1980). *State-event classroom observation system.* Knoxville: University of Tennessee, Department of Psychology.

Schacar, R., Rutter, M., & Smith, A. (1981). The characteristics of situationally and pervasively hyperactive children: Implications for syndrome definition. *Journal of Child Psychology and Psychiatry, 22,* 375–392.

Schacht, T., & Nathan, P. E. (1977). But is it good for the psychologists?: Appraisal and status of DSM-III. *American Psychologist, 32,* 1017–1025.

Schopler, E., Reichler, R. J., & Renner, B. R. (1988). *The Childhood Autism Rating Scale (CARS).* Los Angeles, CA: Western Psychological Services.

Schrag, P., & Divoky, D. (1975). *The myth of the hyperactive child.* New York: Pantheon.

Schumaker, J. B., Deschler, D. D., & McKnight, P. (2002). Ensuring success in the secondary general education curriculum through the use of teaching routines. In M. R. Shinn, H. M. Walker, & G. Stoner (Eds.), *Interventions for academic and behavior problems, II: Preventive and remedial approaches* (pp. 791–823). Bethesda, MD: National Association of School Psychologists.

Schwartz, I. S., & Baer, D. M. (1991). Social validity assessments: Is current practice state of the art? *Journal of Applied Behavior Analysis, 24,* 189–204.

Semrud-Clikeman, M., Biederman, J., Sprich-Buckminster, S., Lehman, B. K., Faraone, S. V., & Norman, D. (1992). Comorbidity between ADDH and learning disability: A review and report in a clinically referred sample. *Journal of the American Academy of Child and Adolescent Psychiatry, 31,* 439–448.

Shapiro, E. S. (Ed.). (1992). Response/dialogue: The social maladjustment exclusion clause [Special issue]. *School Psychology Review, 21,* 11–44.

Shapiro, E. S. (1996). *Academic skills problems: Direct assessment and Intervention* (2nd ed.). New York: Guilford Press.

Shapiro, E. S., & Cole, C. L. (1994). *Behavior change in the classroom: Self-management interventions.* New York: Guilford Press.

Shapiro, E. S., DuPaul, G. J., & Bradley, K. L. (1998). Self-management as a strategy to improve the classroom behavior of adolescents with ADHD. *Journal of Learning Disablities, 31,* 545–555.

Shapiro, E. S., DuPaul, G. J., Bradley, K. L., & Bailey, L. T. (1996). A school-based consultation program for service delivery to middle school students with attention-deficit/hyperactivity disorder. *Journal of Emotional and Behavioral Disorders, 4,* 73–81.

Shapiro, E. S., & Kratochwill, T. R. (Eds.). (2000). *Behavioral assessment in schools: Theory, research, and clinical foundations* (2nd ed.). New York: Guilford Press.

Shaywitz, B. A., Fletcher, J. M., & Shaywitz, S. E. (1995). Defining and classifying learning disabilities and attention-deficit/hyperactivity disorder. *Journal of Child Neurology, 10,* 50–57.

Shaywitz, B. A., & Shaywitz, S. E. (1991). Comorbidity: A critical issue in attention deficit disorder. *Journal of Child Neurology, 6,* 13–22.

Shelton, T. L., Barkley, R. A., Crosswait, C., Moorehouse, M., Fletcher, K., Barrett, S., Jenkins, L., & Metevia, L. (1998). Psychiatric and psychological morbidity as a function of adaptive disability in preschool children with aggressive and hyperactive–impulsive–inattentive behavior. *Journal of Abnormal Child Psychology, 26,* 475–494.

Shelton, T. L., Barkley, R. A., Crosswait, C., Moorehouse, M., Fletcher, K., Barrett, S., Jenkins, L., & Metevia, L. (2000). Multimethod psychoeducational intervention for preschool children with disruptive behavior: Two-year post-treatment follow-up. *Journal of Abnormal Child Psychology, 28,* 253–266.

Shelton, T. L., Woods, J. E., Williford, A. P., Dobbins, T. R., & Neal, J. M. (2002). *Project Mastery: Early intervention with Head Start preschoolers at risk for AD/HD.* Manuscript submitted for publication.

Sheridan, S. M. (1995). *The tough kid social skills book.* Longmont, CO: Sopris-West.

Sheridan, S. M., Dee, C. C., Morgan, J. C., McCormick, M. E., & Walker, D. (1996). A multimethod intervention for social skills deficits in children with ADHD and their parents. *School Psychology Review, 25,* 57–76.

Sheridan, S. M., Kratochwill, T. R., & Bergan, J. (1996). *Conjoint behavioral consultation: A procedural manual.* New York: Plenum Press.

Shinn, M. R. (Ed.). (1989). *Curriculum-based measurement: Assessing special children.* New York: Guilford Press.

Shinn, M. R. (Ed.). (1998). *Advanced applications of curriculum-based measurement.* New York: Guilford Press.

Shinn, M. R., Walker, H. M., & Stoner, G. (Eds.). (2002). *Interventions for academic and behavior problems, II: Preventive and remedial approaches.* Bethesda, MD: National Association of School Psychologists.

Silver, L. B. (1981). The relationship between learning disabilities, hyperactivity, distractibility, and behavioral problems. *Journal of the American Academy of Child and Adolescent Psychiatry, 20,* 385–397.

Silver, L. B. (1990). Attention deficit-hyperactivity disorder: Is it a learning disability or a related disorder? *Journal of Learning Disabilities, 23,* 394–397.

Simeon, J. G., Ferguson, H. B., & Van Wyck Fleet, J. (1986). Bupropion effects in attention deficit and conduct disorders. *Canadian Journal of Psychiatry, 31*, 581–585.

Simmons, D. C., Kame'enui, E. J., Good, R. H. III, Harn, B. A., Cole, C., & Braun. D. (2002). Building, implementing, and sustaining a beginning reading improvement model: Lessons learned school by school. In M. R. Shinn, H. M. Walker, & G. Stoner (Eds.), *Interventions for academic and behavior problems, II: Preventive and remedial approaches* (pp. 537–569). Bethesda, MD: National Association of School Psychologists.

Sindelar, P. T., Lane, H. B., Pullen, P. C., & Hudson, R. F. (2002). Remedial interventions for students with reading decoding problems. In M. R. Shinn, H. M. Walker, & G. Stoner (Eds.), *Interventions for academic and behavior problems, II: Preventive and remedial approaches* (pp. 703–729). Bethesda, MD: National Association of School Psychologists.

Sindelar, P. T., & Stoddard, K. (1991). Teaching reading to mildly disabled students in regular classes. In G. Stoner, M. R. Shinn, & H. M. Walker (Eds.), *Interventions for achievement and behavior problems* (pp. 357–378). Silver Spring, MD: National Association of School Psychologists.

Skinner, C. H., Johnson, C. W., Larkin, M. J., Lessley, D. J., & Glowacki, M. L. (1995). The influence of rate of presentation during taped-words interventions on reading performance. *Journal of Emotional and Behavior Disorders, 4*, 214–223.

Smith, B. H., Pelham, W. E., Jr., Evans, S., Gnagy, E., Molina, B., Bukstein, O., Greiner, A., Myak, C., Presnell, M., & Willouhby, M. (1998). Dosage effects of methylphenidate on the social behavior of adolescents diagnosed with attention-deficit hyperactivity disorder. *Experimental and Clinical Psychopharmacology, 6*, 187–204.

Smith, B. H., Pelham, W. E., Jr., Gnagy, E., Molina, B., & Evans, S. (2000). The reliability, validity, and unique contributions of self-report by adolescents receiving treatment for attention-deficit/hyperactivity disorder. *Journal of Consulting and Clinical Psychology, 68*, 489–499.

Smith, D. J., Young, K. R., Nelson, J. R., & West, R. P. (1992). The effect of a self- management procedure on the classroom academic behavior of students with mild handicaps. *School Psychology Review, 21*, 59–72.

Snow, C. E., & Goldfield, B. A. (1983). Turn the page please: Relationships during the preschool years. *Harvard Educational Review, 53*, 1165–1189.

Sokil, N. G. (2002). *Early Numeracy Screening Assessment.* Unpublished manuscript, Department of Education and Human Services, Lehigh University, Bethlehem, PA.

Solanto, M. V. (1984). Neuropharmacological basis of stimulant drug action in attention deficit disorder with hyperactivity: A review and synthesis. *Psychological Bulletin, 95*, 387–409.

Solanto, M. V. (2000). Dose–response effects of Ritalin on cognitive self-regulation, learning and memory, and academic performance. In L. L. Greenhill & B. B. Osman (Eds.), *Ritalin: Theory and practice* (2nd ed., pp. 219–236). Larchmont, NY: Mary Ann Liebert.

Solanto, M. V., & Wender, E. H. (1989). Does methylphenidate constrict cognitive functioning? *Journal of the American Academy of Child and Adolescent Psychiatry, 28,* 897–902.

Speer, D. C. (1992). Clinically significant change: Jacobson and Truax (1991) revisited. *Journal of Consulting and Clinical Psychology, 60,* 402–408.

Spencer, T. J., Biederman, J., & Wilens, T. (1998). Pharmacotherapy of ADHD with antidepressants. In R. A. Barkley, *Attention-deficit hyperactivity disorder: A handbook for diagnosis and treatment* (2nd ed., pp. 552–563). New York: Guilford Press.

Spencer, T. J., Biederman, J., Wilens, T., Harding, M., O'Donnell, D., & Griffin, S. (1996). Pharmacotherapy of attention-deficit hyperactivity disorder across the life cycle. *Journal of the American Academy of Child and Adolescent Psychiatry, 35,* 409–432.

Spencer, T. J., Biederman, J., Wilens, T., Steingard, R., & Geist, D. (1993). Nortriptyline in the treatment of children with attention deficit hyperactivity disorder and tic disorder or Tourette's syndrome. *Journal of the American Academy of Child and Adolescent Psychiatry, 32,* 205– 210.

Spencer, T., Biederman, J., Wright, V., & Danon, M. (1992). Growth deficits in children treated with desipramine: A controlled study. *Journal of the American Academy of Child and Adolescent Psychiatry, 31,* 235–243.

Spires, H. A., & Stone, D. P. (1989). The directed notetaking activity: A self-questioning approach. *Journal of Reading, 33,* 36–39.

Spivack, G., & Shure, M. B. (1974). *Social adjustment of young children: A cognitive approach to solving real-life problems.* San Francisco: Jossey-Bass.

Sprafkin, J., Grayson, P., Gadow, K. D., Nolan, E. E., & Paolicelli, L. M. (1986). *Code for Observing Social Activity (COSA).* Stony Brook: State University of New York, Department of Psychiatry and Behavioral Science.

Sprague, R. K., & Sleator, E. K. (1977). Methylphenidate in hyperkinetic children: Differences in dose effects on learning and social behavior. *Science, 198,* 1274–1276.

Sprick, R. S., Borgmeier, C., & Nolet, V. (2002). Prevention and management of behavior problems in secondary schools. In M. R. Shinn, H. M. Walker, & G. Stoner (Eds.), *Interventions for academic and behavior problems, II: Preventive and remedial approaches* (pp. 373–401). Bethesda, MD: National Association of School Psychologists.

Stein, M. A., & Pao, M. (2000). Attention deficit hyperactivity disorder and Ritalin side effects: Is sleep delayed, disrupted, or disturbed? In L. L. Greenhill & B. B. Osman (Eds.), *Ritalin: Theory and practice* (2nd ed., pp. 287–300). Larchmont, NY: Mary Ann Liebert.

Stokes, T. F., & Baer, D. M. (1977). An implicit technology of generalization. *Journal of Applied Behavior Analysis, 10,* 349–367.

Stokes, T. F., & Osnes, P. G. (1989). An operant pursuit of generalization. *Behavior Therapy, 20,* 337–355.

Stoner, G., & Carey, S. P. (1992). Serving students with ADD: Avoiding deficits in professional attention. *School Psychology Quarterly, 7,* 302–307.

Stoner, G., Carey, S. P., Ikeda, M. J., & Shinn, M. R. (1994). The utility of curriculum-based measurement for evaluating the effects of methylphenidate on academic performance. *Journal of Applied Behavior Analysis, 27,* 101–114.

Stoner, G., & Green, S. K. (1992a). *A pilot study of instruction in and understanding of classroom rules in the primary grades.* Unpublished manuscript, College of Education, University of Oregon, Eugene.

Stoner, G., & Green, S. K. (1992b). Reconsidering the scientist-practitioner model for school psychology practice. *School Psychology Review, 21,* 154–165.

Stormont, M. (2001). Social outcomes of children with AD/HD: Contributing factors and implications for practice. *Psychology in the Schools, 38,* 521–531.

Stormont, M., & Stebbins, M. S. (2001). Teachers' comfort and importance ratings for interventions for preschoolers with AD/HD. *Psychology in the Schools, 38,* 259–267.

Strayhorn, J. M., & Weidman, C. S. (1989). Reduction of attention deficit and internalizing symptoms through parent–child interaction training. *Journal of the American Academy of Child and Adolescent Psychiatry, 28,* 888–896.

Strayhorn, J. M., & Weidman, C. S. (1991). Follow-up one year after parent–child interaction training: Effects on behavior of preschool children. *Journal of the American Academy of Child and Adolescent Psychiatry, 30,* 138–143.

Sugai, G., Horner, R. H., & Gresham, F. M. (2002). Behaviorally effective school environments. In M. R. Shinn, H. M. Walker, & G. Stoner (Eds.), *Interventions for academic and behavior problems, II: Preventive and remedial approaches* (pp. 315–350). Bethesda, MD: National Association of School Psychologists.

Sulzer-Azaroff, B., & Mayer, G. R. (1991). *Behavior analysis for lasting change.* Fort Worth, TX: Holt, Rinehart & Winston.

Swanson, J., & Kinsbourne, M. (1975). Stimulant-related state-dependent learning in hyperactive children. *Science, 192,* 1354–1357.

Swanson, J. M., Kraemer, H. C., Hinshaw, S. P., Arnold, L. E., Conners, C. K., Abikoff, H. B., Clevenger, W., Davies, M., Elliott, G. R., Greenhill, L. L., Hechtman, L., Hoza, B., Jensen, P. S., March, J. S., Newcorn, J. H., Owens, E. B., Pelham, W. E., Schiller, E., Severe, J. B., Simpson, S., Vitiello, B., Wells, K., Wigal, T., & Wu, M. (2001). Clinical relevance of the preliminary findings of the MTA: Success rates based on severity of ADHD and ODD symptoms at the end of treatment. *Journal of the American Academy of Child and Adolescent Psychiatry, 40,* 168–179.

Swanson, J. M., Sunohora, G. A., Kennedy, J. L., Regino, R., Fineberg, E., Wigal, T., Lerner, M., Williams, L., LaHoste, G. J., & Wigal, S. (1998). Association of the dopamine receptor D4 (DRD4) gene with a refined phenotype of attention deficit hyperactivity disorder (ADHD): A family-based approach. *Molecular Psychiatry, 3,* 38–41.

Szatmari, P., Offord, D. R., & Boyle, M. H. (1989). Ontario Child Health Study: Prevalence of attention deficit disorder with hyperactivity. *Journal of Child Psychology and Psychiatry, 30,* 219–230.

Tannock, R. (1998). Attention deficit hyperactivity disorder: Advances in cognitive, neurobiological, and genetic research. *Journal of Child Psychology and Psychiatry, 39,* 65–99.

Tant, J. L., & Douglas, V. I. (1982). Problem solving in hyperactive, normal, and reading-disabled boys. *Journal of Abnormal Child Psychology, 10,* 285–306.

Teeter, P. A. (1998). *Interventions for ADHD: Treatment in developmental context.* New York: Guilford Press.

Telzrow, C. F., & Tankersley, M. (2000). *IDEA amendments of 1997: Practice guidelines for school-based teams.* Bethesda, MD: National Association of School Psychologists.

Todd, R. D., Sitdhirakso, N., Reich, W., Ji, T. H., Joyner, C. A., Heath, A. C., & Neuman, R. J. (2002). Discrimination of DSM-IV and latent class attention-deficit/hyperactivity disorder subtypes by educational and cognitive performance in a population-base sample of child and adolescent twins. *Journal of the American Academy of Child and Adolescent Psychiatry, 41,* 820–828.

Torgesen, J. K., & Young, K. A. (1983). Priorities for the use of microcomputers with learning disabled children. *Journal of Learning Disabilities, 16,* 234–237

Touchette, P. E., MacDonald, R. F., & Langer, S. N. (1985). A scatter plot for identifying stimulus control of problem behavior. *Journal of Applied Behavior Analysis, 18,* 343–351.

Tremblay, R. E., Vitaro, F., Bertrand, L., LeBlanc, M., Beauchesne, H., Boileau, H., & David, L. (1992). Parent and child training to prevent early onset of delinquency: The Montréal Longitudinal–Experimental Study. In J. McCord & R. E. Tremblay (Eds.), *Preventing antisocial behavior: Interventions from birth through adolescence* (pp. 117–138). New York: Guilford Press.

Turnbull, A. P., & Turnbull, H. R. (1986). *Families, professionals, and exceptionality: A special partnership.* Columbus, OH: Merrill.

Ullman, D. G., Barkley, R. A., & Brown, H. W. (1978). The behavioral symptoms of hyperkinetic children who successfully responded to stimulant drug treatment. *American Journal of Orthopsychiatry, 48,* 425–437.

Ullmann, R. K., Sleator, E. K., & Sprague, R. L. (1985). Introduction to the use of the ACTeRS. *Psychopharmacology Bulletin, 21,* 915–920.

U.S. Department of Education. (1999). *20th Annual Report to Congress, on the implementation of the Individuals with Disabilities Education Act.* Washington, DC: Author.

Van der Oord, E. J. C. G., Boomsa, D. I., & Verhulst, F. C. (1994). A study of problem behaviors in 10- to 15–year old biologically related and unrelated international adoptees. *Behavior Genetics, 24,* 193–205.

Vatz, B. C. (1990, April). *Behavioral subtypes of learning disabled children.* Paper presented at the annual convention of the National Association of School Psychologists, San Francisco.

Voelker, S. L., Carter, R. A., Sprague, D. J., Gdowski, C. L., & Lachar, D. (1989). Developmental trends in memory and metamemory in children with attention deficit disorder. *Journal of Pediatric Psychology, 14,* 75–88.

Volpe, R. J., & Lorah, K. S. (2000). *The Systematic Hybrid Observation Code* for Kids (SHOCK). Bethlehem, PA: Department of Education and Human Services, Lehigh University.

Vyse, S. A., & Rapport, M. D. (1989). The effects of methylphenidate on learning in children with ADDH: The stimulus equivalence paradigm. *Journal of Consulting and Clinical Psychology, 57,* 425–435.

Walker, H. M., Block-Pedego, A., Todis, B., & Severson, H. (1998). *School archival records search (SARS): User's guide and technical manual.* Longmont, CO: Sopris-West.

Walker, H. M., & McConnell, S. R. (1988). *Walker–McConnell Scale of Social Competence and School Adjustment.* Austin, TX: Pro-Ed.

Walker, H. M., & Severson, H. (1988). *Systematic screening for behavior disorders assessment system.* Longmont, CO: Sopris-West.

Wallander, J. L., Schroeder, S. R., Michelli, J. A., & Gualtieri, C. T. (1987). Classroom social interactions of attention deficit disorder with hyperactivity children as a function of stimulant medication. *Journal of Pediatric Psychology, 12,* 61–76.

Webster-Stratton, C. (1994). Advancing videotape parent training: A comparison study. *Journal of Consulting and Clinical Psychology, 62,* 585–593.

Webster-Stratton, C. (1996). *The parents and children series: A comprehensive course divided into four programs.* Seattle, WA: Author.

Webster-Stratton, C. (1998). Preventing conduct problems in Head Start children: Strengthening parenting competencies. *Journal of Consulting and Clinical Psychology, 66,* 715–730.

Webster-Stratton, C., Hollinsworth, T., & Kolpacoff, M. (1989). The long-term effectiveness and clinical significance of three cost-effective training programs for families with conduct-problem children. *Journal of Consulting and Clinical Psychology, 57,* 550–553.

Weiss, G., & Hechtman, L. T. (1993). *Hyperactive children grown up: ADHD in children, adolescents, and adults* (2nd ed.). New York: Guilford Press.

Weiss, G., Kruger, E., Danielson, U., & Elman, M. (1975). Effects of long-term treatment of hyperactive children with methylphenidate. *Canadian Medical Association Journal, 112,* 159–165.

Wells, K. C., Pelham, W. E., Jr., Kotkin, R. A., Hoza, B., Abikoff, H. B., Abaramowitz, A., Arnold, L. E., Cantwell, D. P., Conners, C. K., Del Carmen, R., Elliott, G., Greenhill, L. L., Hechtman, L., Hibbs, E., Hinshaw, S. P., Jensen, P. S., March, J. S., Swanson, J. M., & Schiller, E. (2000). Psychosocial treatment strategies in the MTA Study: Rationale, methods, and critical issues in design and implementation. *Journal of Abnormal Child Psychology, 28,* 483–506.

Werry, J. S., & Aman, M. (Eds.). (1999). *Practitioner's guide to psychoactive drugs for children and adolescents* (2nd ed.). New York: Plenum Press.

Werry, J. S., Elkind, G. S., & Reeves, J. C. (1987). Attention deficit, conduct, oppositional, and anxiety disorders in children: III. Laboratory differences. *Journal of Abnormal Child Psychology, 15,* 409–428.

Werry, J. S., Sprague, R. L., & Cohen, M. N. (1975). Conners' Teacher Rating Scale for use in drug studies with children: An empirical study. *Journal of Abnormal Child Psychology, 3,* 217–229.

Whalen, C. K., Collins, B. E., Henker, B., Alkus, S. R., Adams, D., & Stapp, J. (1978). Behavior observations of hyperactive children and methylphenidate (Ritalin) effects in systematically structured classroom environments: Now you see them, now you don't. *Journal of Pediatric Psychology, 3*, 177–187.

Whalen, C. K., Henker, B., Buhrmester, D., Hinshaw, S. P., Huber, A., & Laski, K. (1989). Does stimulant medication improve the peer status of hyperactive children? *Journal of Consulting and Clinical Psychology, 57*, 545–549.

Whalen, C. K., Henker, B., Collins, B. E., Finck, D., & Dotemoto, S. (1979). A social ecology of hyperactive boys: Medication effects in structured classroom environments. *Journal of Applied Behavior Analysis, 12*, 65–81.

Whalen, C. K., Henker, B., & Dotemoto, S. (1981). Teacher response to methylphenidate (Ritalin) versus placebo status of hyperactive boys in the classroom. *Child Development, 52*, 1005–1014.

White, M. A. (1975). Natural rates of teacher approval and disapproval in the classroom. *Journal of Applied Behavior Analysis, 8*, 367–372.

Wierson, M., & Forehand, R. (1994). Parental behavioral training for child noncompliance: Rationale, concepts, and effectiveness. *Current Directions in Psychological Science, 3*, 146–150.

Willcutt, E. G., Chhabildas, N., & Pennington, B. F. (2001). Validity of the DSM-IV subtypes of ADHD. *ADHD Report, 9*(1), 2–5.

Willcutt, E. G., Pennington, B. F., Chhabildas, N. A., Friedman, M. C., & Alexander, J. (1999). Psychiatric comorbidity associated with DSM-IV ADHD in a nonreferred sample of twins. *Journal of the American Academy of Child and Adolescent Psychiatry, 38*, 1355–1362.

Wilson, L. J., & Jennings, J. N. (1996). Parents' acceptability of alternative treatments for attention-deficit hyperactivity disorder. *Journal of Attention Disorders, 1*, 114–121.

Wirt, R. D., Lachar, D., Klinedinst, J. K., & Seat, P. D. (1977). *Multidimensional description of child personality: A manual for the Personality Inventory for Children*. Los Angeles, CA: Western Psychological Services.

Witt, J. C., Daly, E. M., & Noell, G. (2000). *Functional assessments: A step-by-step guide to solving academic and behavior problems*. Longmont, CO: Sopris-West.

Witt, J. C., & Elliott, S. N. (1985). Acceptability of classroom management strategies. In T. R. Kratochwill (Ed.), *Advances in school psychology* (Vol. 4, pp. 251–288). Hillsdale, N. J. : Erlbaum.

Wixon, K. K. (1986). Vocabulary instruction and children's comprehension of basal stories. *Reading Research Quarterly, 21*, 317–329.

Wolraich, M. L., Hannah, J. N., Pinnock, T. Y., Baumgaertel, A., & Brown, J. (1996). Comparison of diagnostic criteria for attention-deficit/hyperactivity disorder in a county-wide sample. *Journal of the American Academy of Child and Adolescent Psychiatry, 35*, 319–324.

Woodward, J., Carnine, D., & Collins, M. T. (1986). *Closing the performance gap in secondary education*. Unpublished manuscript, College of Education, University of Oregon, Eugene.

Ysseldyke, J. E., & Christenson, S. L. (1987). *The Instructional Environment Scale*. Austin, TX: Pro-Ed.

Ysseldyke, J. E., & Christenson, S. L. (1988). Linking assessment to intervention. In J. L. Graden, J. E. Zins, & M. J. Curtis (Eds.), *Alternative educational delivery systems: Enhancing instructional options for all students* (pp. 91–110). Washington, DC: National Association of School Psychologists.

Zametkin, A., Rapoport, J. L., Murphy, D. L., Linnoila, M., & Ismond, D. (1985). Treatment of hyperactive children with monoamine oxidase inhibitors: I. Clinical efficacy. *Archives of General Psychiatry, 42,* 962–966.

Zentall, S. S. (1988). Production deficiencies in elicited language but not in the spontaneous verbalizations of hyperactive children. *Journal of Abnormal Child Psychology, 16,* 657–673.

Zentall, S. S. (1989). Attentional cuing in spelling tasks for hyperactive and comparison regular classroom children. *Journal of Special Education, 23,* 83–93.

Zentall, S. S., & Leib, S. L. (1985). Structured tasks: Effects on activity and performance of hyperactive and comparison children. *Journal of Educational Research, 79,* 91–95.

Zentall, S. S., & Meyer, M. J. (1987). Self-regulation of stimulation for ADD-H children during reading and vigilance task performance. *Journal of Abnormal Child Psychology, 15,* 519–536.

Zito, J. M., Safer, D. J., dos Reis, S., Gardner, J. F., Boles, M., & Lynch, F. (2000). Trends in the prescribing of psychotropic medications to preschoolers. *Journal of the American Medical Association, 283,* 1025–1030.

Zirkel, P. A. (1992). A checklist for determining legal eligibility of ADD/ADHD students. *Special Educator, 8*(7), 93–97.

Zirkel, P. A., & Aleman, S. R. (2000). *Section 504, the ADA and the schools* (2nd ed.). Horsham, PA: LRP Publications.

Index

◆